Also by Elizabeth Somer

*The Origin Diet*

*Age-Proof Your Body*

*Food & Mood*

*Nutrition for a Healthy Pregnancy*

*The Essential Guide to Vitamins and Minerals*

*The Nutrition Desk Reference*

# *Nutrition for Women*

# ELIZABETH SOMER, M.A., R.D.

# Nutrition for Women

*How Eating Right Can Help You*

*Look and Feel Your Best*

· SECOND EDITION ·

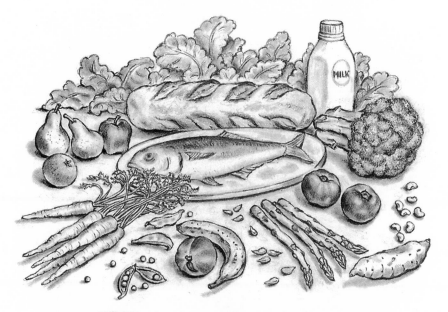

AN OWL BOOK

*Henry Holt and Company · New York*

Henry Holt and Company, LLC
*Publishers since 1866*
115 West 18th Street
New York, New York 10011

Henry Holt® is a registered trademark of
Henry Holt and Company, LLC.

Library of Congress Cataloging-in-Publication Data

Somer, Elizabeth.
    Nutrition for women : how eating right can help you look and
feel your best / Elizabeth Somer.—2nd ed.
        p.   cm.
    "An Owl book."
    Includes bibliographical references and index.
    ISBN 0-8050-7081-8
    1. Women—Nutrition.  2. Women—Health and hygiene.  I. Title.
    RA778 .S644 2003
    613.2'082—dc21                                        2002068804

First published in hardcover in 1993 by Henry Holt and Company

First Owl Books Edition 1995
Second Owl Books Edition 2003

*Illustration on pages v, 1, 159, and 235 by Kathryn Parise*

Printed in the United States of America
1   3   5   7   9   10   8   6   4   2

Every woman needs remarkable women in her life.
I have been surrounded by many, including my mother, Miriam,
my sisters, Gayle and Lovey, and my dear friends
Sandra, Karen, Francesca, and Julie.

A woman is lucky to find one good man. I have had two:
my father, Rolly, and my husband, Patrick.

This book is dedicated to them.

The nutritional and health advice presented in this book is based on an in-depth review of the current scientific literature. It is intended only as an informative resource guide to help you make informed decisions; it is not meant to replace the advice of a physician or to serve as a guide to self-treatment. Always seek competent medical help for any health condition or if there is any question about the appropriateness of a procedure or health recommendation.

# Contents

# *Foreword*

Having been *Shape* magazine's editor in chief for the past fifteen years and observing American women's food and fitness habits closely, I can honestly say that today, it is harder than ever to eat healthfully—or easier than ever—depending on the nutrition knowledge you apply. Calorically dense, high-fat, and sugar-laden foods are everywhere. Clever marketing and an eat-on-the-go lifestyle make it easy to eat without thinking, taking in too many calories and overeating the wrong foods. Compounding today's environment is misinformation (i.e., carbs are bad), fad diets (high-protein is "in"!), and magic bullets (ginseng for energy). It's more essential now than ever to be conscious about our food choices and properly informed about nutrition science. Having smart, practical eating strategies is a must. The right information is there if you can find it.

We can be thankful that there are nutritionists like Elizabeth Somer who patiently and persistently decipher the details and synthesize hundreds of studies, year upon year, swept up in a love affair with their topic. Going ever deeper to know more, the veil separating them from their subject eventually dissolves. Such teachers, including Elizabeth, are a wellspring of intimate knowledge.

The information in this new edition of *Nutrition for Women* will unlock food mysteries and guide you to negotiate your particular nutrition challenges. Whether you want to revamp and start a completely new path or simply refine and build upon your already healthy eating habits, this book will help.

I always learn something new when I read Elizabeth's work. This time around I learned yet another helpful nutrition idea. Her strategy for stress is to create a plan of small, nutrient-rich meals eaten at regular intervals, limiting or bypassing the alcohol, sugar, or caffeine. Our ability to limit these foods is compromised when we're stressed so she recommends to either steer clear or only eat them with a meal. Smart advice!

Enjoy the excellent science and hundreds of strategies contained herein. When it comes to making your nutrition changes, think evolution, not revolution. You have your whole lifetime to eat better and smarter and to get more pleasure from your food—all of which are also very good for your body, mind, and soul and will serve you well in this very adventurous time in which we're living.

Barbara Harris
Editor in Chief, *Shape* magazine

# *Acknowledgments*

A huge thank-you to all the people that helped make this book possible, including my friends and agent David Smith, editor Deborah Brody, assistant Martha Kaufman, and researcher Victoria Dolby-Toews. Thank-you to my family—Patrick, Lauren, and William—for putting up with the long hours away from the dinner table making sure this book met the deadline.

I can write books and articles only because of the dedicated researchers who supply me with the thousands of scientific studies necessary to bring accurate information to my readers. Those researchers who took time out of their busy schedules to explain their research deserve a special thank-you and include Jeffrey Blumberg, Ph.D., at Tufts University; Fergus Clydesdale, Ph.D., at the University of Massachusetts; Winston Craig, Ph.D., R.D., at Andrews University; Adam Drewnowski, Ph.D., at the University of Washington; Anne Fletcher, M.S., R.D.; John Foreyt, Ph.D., at Baylor College of Medicine; JoAnn Hattner, R.D., M.P.H., at Stanford University; Mary Lou Klem, Ph.D., at the University of Pittsburgh; Susan Krebs-Smith, Ph.D., at the National Cancer Institute; David Levitsky, Ph.D., at Cornell University; Lauren Mellin, M.A., R.D.; Mark Messina, Ph.D.; Vince Nistico, M.S., ACE; Judith Putnam, at the U.S. Department of Agriculture; Barbara Rolls, Ph.D., at Pennsylvania State University; David Schardt, at the Center for Science in the Public Interest; Amy Subar, Ph.D., R.D., at the National Cancer Institute; Cyndi Thomson, Ph.D., R.D., with the American Dietetic Association; Evelyn Tribole, M.S., R.D.; Varro Tyler, Ph.D., Sc.D., formerly at Purdue University; Zoe Warwick, Ph.D., at the University of Maryland; Debra Waterhouse, M.P.H.; Ronald Watson, Ph.D., at Arizona Health Sciences Center; Walter Willett, M.D., Dr.P.H., at the Harvard School of Public Health; and John Wolf, M.D., at Baylor College of Medicine.

# *Preface*

I'm told that coffee causes heart disease, then I hear that coffee is OK. Which one should I believe?"

"First pasta was touted as the perfect food, then it's fattening. Butter was bad for your heart, then margarine is the culprit. Iron is essential for boosting 'tired blood,' then we're told that mineral causes heart disease. I don't know about you, but this nutritional Ping-Pong game is giving me a headache!"

"One source tells me the only way to make sure I get enough vitamins is to supplement my diet; someone else says supplements are useless and possibly harmful. How can I make sense out of such different opinions?"

For more than twenty years, I have listened to the frustration in women's voices. Women want to know what to believe, how to cut through the nutrition hype to reach the facts, and where to get accurate nutrition information. They are willing to make changes in their diets to improve health and the quality of their lives, but are often confused, and sometimes overwhelmed, at the conflicting news. That is why I wrote this book.

*Nutrition for Women* is an easy-to-read reference guide about and for women. It is the only book of its kind to provide a bottom-line summary of the scientific nutrition research, from thousands of the most recent studies, on the issues pertinent to women's health. *Nutrition for Women* distills scientific jargon into simple, understandable terms. It dispels the myths, presents the facts, and provides practical, easy advice on how to eat to feel and look your best, reduce your risk for disease, and live vitally.

# *What's New?*

Since the first edition of this book was published in 1993, much has changed regarding women's diets and health issues. This second edition didn't just get a face-lift, it is completely revised with more practical and accurate information on the latest findings. You'll find answers to questions, such as:

- What is your biggest health threat? (Hint: If you said breast cancer, you're wrong.)
- How much sugar are you eating every day? Ten to twenty teaspoons? Twenty to forty teaspoons? Forty to sixty teaspoons?
- What foods reduce wrinkling and aging of the skin?
- What is the number one source of saturated fat—the fat that causes heart disease and cancer—in your diet? (If you said red meat, guess again.)
- What nutrients do you need most during times of stress?
- Are sugar substitutes, such as aspartame, Splenda, and saccharin, safe?
- Should you take extra supplements or sports supplements like creatine if you exercise?
- Can diet lessen hot flashes and other symptoms of menopause?
- How much should you spend a month for all your supplements?
- Are the medications you take, even aspirin or birth control pills, affecting your nutritional status?
- Is it possible that what you eat during pregnancy could affect the future risk of your baby for heart disease, cancer, diabetes, high blood pressure, and even obesity?
- Is organic food worth the extra cost?

You'll also learn that it doesn't cost more, take more time, or require sacrificing taste in order to eat well. If you have the time to pull up to a drive-through window to order a hamburger, you have time to fuel your body with the best foods possible to keep you young, healthy, and energetic.

This second edition also includes:

- A total revision of the Healthy Woman's Diet based on the latest research on how phytochemicals in fruits and vegetables, omega-3 fats in fish, phytoestrogens in soy, and fiber in whole grains lower your risk for disease.

- New information on how to shop for and prepare foods, based on the wealth of new fat-free and healthful fast foods at the grocery store.
- How to eat well when traveling—including healthy foods in airports, hotels, in the air, on the road, and brown-bag lunches—since so many of us are on the road as much as we are in our kitchens.
- Expanded chapters on shopping, quick-fix cooking, and how to dine out without sacrificing your health or your waistline.
- New research on what really works for long-term weight loss.
- Antiaging guidelines based on new evidence that aging is not inevitable, but rather results from years of neglecting our health.
- A complete update of the diseases and health conditions most important to women, including a review of the research on disorders from cancer and heart disease to fibromyalgia and mood swings.
- How to eat to boost energy, and which foods protect your memory.

## A Quick-Reference Guide for Women

You probably don't have a private secretary, gardener, nanny, maid, and wife to accomplish everything that you need to get done in a day. Trying to squeeze in time to read a book on women's nutrition might seem close to impossible. That's why *Nutrition for Women* is written in a quick-reference style. Don't feel you have to read this book from cover to cover. Rather, jump in and check out the topics that are important to you. If you want to know what to eat, turn to the Healthy Woman's Diet in chapter 2. Shopping tips are in chapter 3, quick-fix cooking ideas are in chapter 4, eating out is outlined in chapter 5, and the answers to all your questions about how to supplement are found in chapter 6. The second section of this book covers the nutritional needs of women at the different stages of our lives, and the third section addresses, in a quick-reference format, the health conditions and diseases most pertinent to women.

## Simple Answers to Complex Issues

Nutrition is a new and evolving science. While everyone wants absolute answers, often only limited information is available for making dietary recommendations.

It is this battlefield between incomplete supply and high demand that is fertile ground for misinformation.

One of my pet peeves is when people report or make recommendations based on one study. There are no black-and-white answers in nutrition. Every topic has pros and cons. One study is never reason to make a conclusion. What you must do is review all the evidence and make decisions based on where the weight of the evidence lies. That is what I have done in this book. Every recommendation, every tip, every word of wisdom, is based on a thorough review of the scientific literature. If only one study or a handful of studies is available, I'll mention that so you know we need more evidence before conclusions can be drawn.

Researching and writing this book on and for women has been a joy. I hope it serves you well.

# Nutrition for Women

# PART I

# *How to Eat*

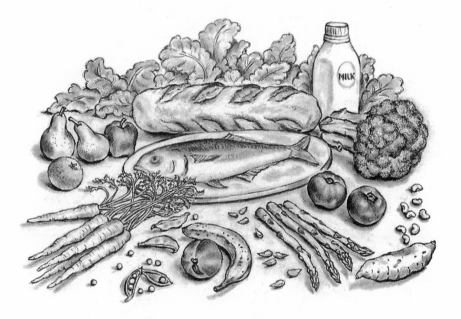

# Introduction

## It's Not "All in Your Head"

As women, it's refreshing to know that never before has our health been taken more seriously. In the past, women's health complaints were dismissed as "all in their heads." Insecurity, depression, or irritability the week before menstruation signaled a woman was too emotional; a craving for sweets showed lack of willpower. Reporting these symptoms to a physician, husband, or friend was met with a smile and a not-so-soothing suggestion to take it easy. The symptoms, such as lethargy, mood swings, headaches, or even fluid retention, were vague and poorly understood by the medical community.

Times have changed. Many emotional and physical symptoms that at one time went undiagnosed are now known to stem from body processes often affected by diet. The mood swings, food cravings, and anxiety many of us experience before our periods now have a name—premenstrual syndrome (PMS)—and can be partially alleviated by changes in what you eat and how much you exercise. Poor concentration, memory problems, and fatigue could be a result of something as simple as iron deficiency. Other mood and emotional problems have been linked to sugar, vitamin deficiencies, and even caffeine consumption. Even the symptoms of chronic fatigue and fibromyalgia might improve with changes in what we eat and how much we move.

We're also fighting back when it comes to aging. Until recently, growing old was considered inevitable. The frail, stooped old lady with the protruding abdomen and confused mind was our destiny. Well, forget all of that. While we can't avoid getting older, we don't have to age. A wealth of research is showing us that it's not age, but years of abuse that wear down our bodies. Just about every aspect of aging—from sun spots, wrinkles, and such age-related diseases as heart disease, diabetes, hypertension, and osteoporosis to memory loss, middle-age spread, and even the frailty, feebleness, and loss of independence that so many of us fear—can be slowed, halted, and even in some cases reversed by making a few simple changes in *what we eat* and *how much we move.* There is every reason to expect we can live robustly, passionately, vitally into our nineties and beyond! With so much at stake when it comes to what we eat, why are so many of us eating so poorly?

## Women's Diets: State of the Union

A good friend of mine always complained about how she ate so well, munching mostly on veggies, yet was still thirty pounds overweight.

I always suspected that something about my friend's diet was amiss. No one gains weight on small servings of vegetables. So I followed her throughout a typical day, writing down everything she ate. She was correct about her serving sizes being small, at least those that made it to the plate. However, she more than made up for lost calories by finishing her sons' leftover eggs and buttered toast in the morning, putting cream in her coffee, and finishing off a bag of cookies. She consumed almost 400 calories by repeatedly tasting while making dinner, then sitting down for the meal. And, oops, it completely slipped her mind about the potato chips. (But the calories don't count if you eat them standing up and straight out of the bag, right?)

My friend's misconceptions about her diet are not unusual. In fact, according to a Gallup poll conducted by Weight Watchers and the American Dietetic Association, 90 percent of women think their diets are pretty healthy. Most of them are delusional.

### The Hourglass Diet

The latest national nutrition survey of Americans' eating habits found that only 1 percent of us meet even minimum standards of a balanced diet. According to a U.S.D.A. study, of women who rated their diets as excellent, only 18 percent actually ate reasonably well; women under the age of thirty-nine were the ones most likely to eat poorly.

"Our eating styles are more like an hourglass than a pyramid," says Judith

Putnam, an economist at the U.S. Department of Agriculture. We gobble lots of sugar and fat from the top of the Food Pyramid and platters of refined grains from the bottom tier, but we are sorely lacking in the vegetables, fruits, low-fat milk products, and other nutritious foods in the middle of the Pyramid. "Fat, sugar, and refined grains are found together in the same processed foods, and people don't want to admit they eat much of these," says Putnam.

It's not that we don't know better. Nine out of ten women know it's important to limit sugary and fatty foods, yet we're gobbling these foods in record amounts. Only a third of us meet the recommendations to keep fat at no more than 30 percent of calories, many of us unknowingly eat too much cholesterol, and we're whole-grain phobic. "Most Americans are missing out on whole grains, often consuming less than one serving a day, yet are eating record amounts of refined grains," says Putnam.

Of course there are also a few of us who are too hard on ourselves. "Many women think they are doing worse than they are," says Debra Waterhouse, M.P.H., a registered dietitian and author of *Outsmarting Female Fatigue* (Hyperion, 2001). They think they are eating too much fat, sugar, and calories, when in fact they are doing just fine. "That's why I encourage women to 'eat write,' that is write down everything they eat so they have a clear picture of how they really are eating. Many find they are eating too much, but a surprising number of women find they are eating too little," says Waterhouse.

## Lie, Cheat, 'n' Steal

One reason why our beliefs don't match our reality is that few women tell the truth about what they eat. In one study, more than 80 percent of the people underestimated their daily food intake by about 700 calories! The more overweight we are or the more we diet, the more we fudge the numbers. "Some people underreport everything, even healthy food and how many vegetables they eat, but they really fudge on servings when it comes to desserts, snack items, and other foods high in fat and sugar," says Amy Subar, Ph.D., R.D., research nutritionist at the National Cancer Institute in Bethesda, Maryland. (By the way, this is a peculiarity of American women, since women in other cultures accurately report their eating habits.)

The more we graze from the Pyramid's top tier, the more we fall from nutritional grace. According to a report from U.S.D.A., half of women think their diets are adequate in calcium, yet only 20 percent met the daily recommendations of

## Then and Now

The more nutrition conscious we've become, the more we are making not-so-healthy food choices. Based on the latest diet statistics from the U.S. Department of Agriculture, here's a comparison of what we were eating in the 1970s and what we're eating today.

- Although we're eating more grain products, almost all of them are refined grains such as pasta, white bread, white rice, etc. Our consumption of grains has jumped 45 percent since the 1970s, from 138 pounds of grains per person per year to 200 pounds! Only 2 percent of the wheat flour is consumed as whole wheat.
- We're eating more fruits and vegetables, but that's because the U.S.D.A. includes French fries and potato chips as a vegetable. Potato products account for almost a third of our "produce" choices. Our next favorite selection is iceberg lettuce (the nutritional equivalent of crunchy water), accounting for 16 percent of all vegetable choices.
- We're drinking 23 percent less whole milk, but we've more than doubled our cheese intake. Cheese now outranks meat as the number one source of saturated fat in our diets.
- We've cut back on red meat, but have more than made up for the loss by increasing our intake of chicken (much of it dark meat and/or fried), so that we're eating 13 pounds more meat today than we did back in the 1970s.
- We're guzzling three times more carbonated soft drinks than milk, compared to the 1970s when we drank twice as much milk as soda.
- We're pouring twice as much vegetable oil on our food and salads and even though we're using 25 percent less butter on our toast, our total added fat intake has increased 32 percent.
- "Americans' weight gain over the last twenty years is no mystery," says Judith Putnam, an economist at the U.S. Department of Agriculture. We consume roughly 150 to 300 calories more every day than people did thirty years ago and we sit at computers or in front of TV instead of riding our bikes or working in the yard. "People are surprised to learn that we are consuming more calories in today's sedentary society than did our vigorously active ancestors in the early 1900s," adds Putnam.

1,000 to 1,200 mg. More than half of women think they get enough iron, but only 62 percent of these actually do. Our diets also are low in vitamins A, D, C, E, and $B_6$, as well as folic acid, magnesium, and zinc.

Yet some of us eat better than we think. In these cases, we fool ourselves into thinking we're not doing enough. "Society's pressure to be thin and fit has caused women to be overly judgmental about their eating habits," says Waterhouse. "We mistakenly label some foods, such as junk food or sugary foods, as bad and so the logic follows that our diets must be bad if we include even a few of these," she adds.

## Nutrition in a Nutshell

OK, so some of us are in serious diet denial. The good news is it takes only a few minor changes in what we're eating to produce big-time results. "If women focused on increasing their vegetables, fruits, and whole grains, and minimizing added fats, especially when eating out, they would be well on their way to eating better," says Dr. Subar. Here's a quick look at what we're doing, versus what we should be doing, based on the Healthy Woman's Diet (see chapter 2).

**Vegetables and Fruits** (Goal: Eight or more servings a day)

*What We're Eating:* Our fruit and vegetable intakes have increased in the past twenty-five years, but only by 1/5 of a serving. We say that eating fruits and vegetables is a top priority, but most women average only about 3.1 servings a day and more than half of all women don't eat fruit at all on any given day. Many women choose nutritional duds, including French fries, iceberg lettuce, apple juice, and other potatoes. Less than a 0.2 serving of dark green leafy vegetables makes it to the plate each day and nine out of ten women don't choose even one serving of deep yellow vegetables on any four days.

*The Improvement Plan:* Include two fruits and/or vegetables at every meal and snack. Select mostly deep-colored produce, such as carrots, sweet potatoes, spinach, blueberries, dried plums, and green peas. Choose only 100 percent juice, such as orange, grapefruit, or pineapple juice.

**Grains** (Goal: Six or more servings a day)

*What We're Eating:* According to U.S.D.A.'s Healthy Eating Index—which ranks Americans' eating habits from 1 to 10 in ten categories for a perfect score of 100—we get a D score for grains, averaging only 6.1 out of 10 points. Eighty-five percent of our grains are refined, which contributes to a huge fiber shortfall, not to mention the phytochemicals, vitamins, and minerals that are lost from processed grains. Many highly processed grains, such as cakes, cookies, doughnuts, and muffins, are so high in fat that they rank fourth as a source of saturated fat.

*The Improvement Plan:* Focus on whole grains. Choose whole-wheat bread, brown rice, and plain oatmeal instead of white bread, white rice, and granola bars. Skip the pastry case and the snack aisle in favor of air-popped popcorn, baked corn chips, and whole-wheat crackers. Sprinkle wheat germ into batters for pancakes, waffles, muffins, and breads. Use whole-wheat flour when possible.

**Nonfat milk** (Goal: Three servings a day, 1,000 to 1,200 mg calcium)

*What We're Eating:* Only one out of every five women consumes enough calcium from milk, with most women averaging about 1½ servings a day and a little over 600 mg of calcium. Cheese is now the number one source of saturated fat in our diets.

*The Improvement Plan:* Include at least 3 fat-free, calcium-rich foods in the daily menu, such as nonfat milk or yogurt, fortified soy milk or orange juice, or canned salmon. Otherwise, take a 500-mg calcium supplement to fill in the gaps.

**Legumes, Fish, Poultry Breast** (Goal: Two to three servings a day)

*What We're Eating:* While we eat record amounts of meat and chicken, we fall far short of optimal for legumes. We average less than ¾ cup of cooked legumes a week.

*The Improvement Plan:* Limit red meat, select poultry breast, and add one to two servings of beans per week, such as kidney beans in salads, fat-free refried beans in burritos, and hummus spread for sandwiches. Include two fish dishes in the weekly plan, such as baked salmon, tuna salad, or grilled fish taco.

**Oils and Fats** (Limit intake)

*What We're Eating:* We've cut back a little on butter and margarine, but are eating record amounts of vegetable oils. In fact, salad dressing is the number one source of fat in women's diets. "What is startling is that our intake of added fats [margarine, salad oils, butter, fats used to process foods, etc.] totals almost all the fat a woman should consume in order to fall within the limits of a 30 percent fat diet," says Putnam. Add onto that the fats in meat and dairy and . . . oops, we've blown our low-fat diets. Besides the unnecessary calories, the more fat a woman eats the less likely she is to get enough vegetables, fruit, whole grains, fish, nonfat milk, and vitamins C and A, folic acid, and fiber.

*The Improvement Plan:* The more unprocessed a food, the lower its fat content. So choose a baked potato instead of French fries or chips, whole-wheat bread instead of a scone or croissant, and grilled instead of fried foods. Use fat-free salad dressing and mayonnaise, moderate amounts of olive oil, and limit cookies, pastries, processed snack items, and most fast foods to once a week. Read labels and select only those processed foods that contain no more than 3 grams of fat per 100 calories.

**Sugar** (Goal: Limit added sugars to about 7 percent of calories—6 teaspoons for a 1,600 calorie diet, 12 teaspoons for a 2,200 calorie diet)

*What We're Eating:* Sugar intake has never been so high. Today the average woman consumes 20 to 32 teaspoons a day of added sugars. Much of that comes from the 54 gallons of soft drinks we each drink annually. Three-quarters of our sugar is hidden in processed foods, from fruited yogurts to flavored oatmeal. The number one source of sugar is soda pop.

*The Improvement Plan:* Limit soda pop to one or two 12-ounce cans a week. Limit pastries and desserts. Read labels: Avoid foods that list sugar as one of the first three ingredients or that contain several types of sugar, such as sucrose, high-fructose corn syrup, or glucose. (Hint: There are four grams in every teaspoon of sugar, so a product that lists sugar content as 26 grams means it contains 6½ teaspoons of sugar.)

## *It Pays to Eat Well*

OK, so some of us have a long way to go before our diets are pristine. Don't despair. You'll find that eating well takes no more time than it does to pull up to a drive-through window or to order takeout. Eating well also costs less than junk food. And, most importantly, good food tastes great!

Switching from a diet of hamburgers, fries, and a cola to a diet based on real food will take a change in priorities and a little planning up front. But, I guarantee the small amount of effort will be worth it. Women who have adopted the dietary guidelines outlined in this book continually tell me "I never knew I could feel this good!" They have more energy, sleep better, lose weight, look ten years younger, lower their risk for all age-related diseases from heart disease to cancer, and often with the consent of their physicians are able to reduce or completely eliminate medications.

Before you tackle your diet and your health, take a moment to assess just what needs changing. Take the following quiz, "Are You Eating as Well as You Think?" Then read on.

## Are You Eating as Well as You Think?

Be honest. Do you skip breakfast sometimes? Snack at the vending machine at work? Occasionally live on takeout? Sneak bags of chips or cookies? Now is the time to really take a look at what you're eating. No need to show this assessment to anyone. Answer the questions (honestly!) then score your points to see how you rate and what needs a little nutritional housecleaning.

Rank your answers 0 to 2 (0 = never, 1 = sometimes, 2 = always).

1. I include at least 8 servings of fruits and/or vegetables, not counting French fries or other fried potatoes, in my daily menu.    _____
2. I choose only dark-colored produce, such as Romaine lettuce, spinach, blueberries, carrots, cantaloupe, sweet potatoes, and broccoli.    _____
3. I eat primarily whole grains, including whole-grain breads, cereals, pastas, and crackers.    _____
4. I average three servings daily of nonfat milk, milk products, and/or calcium-fortified soy milk/cheese or orange juice.    _____
5. I limit my protein-rich foods to two to three every day and my choices are poultry breast, fish, and/or legumes.    _____
6. I limit fats. What fats I do eat come from nuts, seeds, olive or canola oil, avocados, fish, olives, and/or nut butters.    _____
7. I use fat-free salad dressings and mayonnaise.    _____
8. I avoid processed foods that contain added fats, such as fried foods, snack items, and convenience foods.    _____
9. I select only foods with little or no added sugars.    _____

**10.** I eat minimeals and snacks throughout the day so that no more
than four hours go by between meals.                                    _____

**11.** I drink at least eight glasses of water every day.                 _____

**12.** I bake, steam, broil, poach, or grill food, rather than fry, sauté,
or use sauces and gravies that contain fat.                            _____

**13.** At restaurants, I order low-fat, healthy foods and watch portions. _____

**14.** I drink alcohol in moderation or not at all (one drink or less/day). _____

**15.** I take a moderate-dose multiple vitamin and mineral supplement.   _____


## Score:

20 to 30:    *Outstanding.* You can stick with your current eating plan, or aim for turning one or two lower scores into a 2.

15 to 19:    *Average.* You fit right in with most women, which means there are some changes to be made. Identify three or four 0 and 1 scores that you want to boost into the 1 to 2 range. When you've successfully accomplished this, tackle two or three more.

0 to 14:     *Needs improvement.* Time to start taking your health more seriously. Set a goal to gradually improve your score by 3 points every month until your score is above 19.

# CHAPTER 1

# *Nutrition Basics*

It is a relief to know that many of the health problems women face are not "all in our heads." There is something we can do to stay well or return to wellness when we've been sick. On the other hand, knowing that health is within our grasp means we are responsible for taking charge of our nutritional status.

The first step in being your own nutrition advocate is to stay informed. You need accurate information and an understanding of nutrition basics in order to design an individualized diet and supplement plan. For those of you who don't want or have the time to spend hours in the local medical library or the desire to take a college nutrition class, here is a crash course in basic nutrition.

## *Nutrition 101*

Given the right mix of foods, your body has an amazing ability to mend itself. It can manufacture most of the chemicals and compounds you need for health, in many cases, making one nutrient from other nutrients. For example, vitamin D can be manufactured from a cholesterol-like compound when skin is exposed to sunlight, or one amino acid (the building blocks for protein) can be made from another amino acid supplied in the diet.

More than forty-five nutrients and several thousand health-enhancing compounds cannot be manufactured either in sufficient quantities or at all, so they must be obtained from the diet. These nutrients are grouped into seven categories:

- Protein
- Carbohydrates, including fiber

- Fat
- Vitamins
- Minerals
- Phytochemicals
- Water

All the nutrients in these categories are obtained from a variety of "real" foods (that is, minimally processed, nutrient-packed foods) in a wide variety of combinations and calorie intakes.

## Nutrients Work in Teams

The essential nutrients in these seven categories work in teams, with each of the millions of metabolic processes in the body requiring two or more nutrients for normal function. For example, most women know they need iron to build red blood cells. However, red blood cells also need calories, protein, vitamin E, vitamin C, most of the B vitamins, copper, zinc, and other minerals to function properly. Poor dietary intake of one or more of these nutrients, even if iron intake is adequate, will reduce the formation or activity of red blood cells and compromise energy and health. With the exception of sugar and fat, which are exclusively carbohydrate and fat, respectively, all foods are a combination of nutrients.

## Why Five Food Groups?

Foods are categorized into five basic food groups. A food is placed into one of these groups based on its nutrient content.

- Grains: Breads, cereals, rice, noodles, and other grains tend to be high in carbohydrates, B vitamins, and iron. If they are whole grains, they also supply fiber, other trace minerals and vitamins, and some phytochemicals. (All of these terms are described in detail below.)
- Vegetables/Fruits: From apples to zucchini, these foods supply vitamins A and C, folic acid, trace minerals, and fiber. Colorful produce typically also is an excellent source of antioxidant phytochemicals, calcium, and iron.
- Milk: Milk and fortified soy milk are the diet's best sources of calcium. Milk or fortified soy milk also supplies ample amounts of protein,

vitamin D, vitamin B$_2$, and vitamin B$_{12}$. Your best choices here are nonfat or 1 percent low-fat selections, since whole milk and cheeses contain too much saturated fat.

- Meat and legumes: Meat, poultry, fish, and cooked dried beans, peas, and lentils are some of the diet's best sources of protein, iron, zinc, and B vitamins. Extra-lean cuts supply all the nutrients without the saturated fat.
- Extras: The last group—sugary or fatty foods—is high in calories and low in nutrients.

The rationale behind grouping foods into these categories is to make it easy to eyeball your diet and see how you're doing. Diets based on at least six servings of whole grains, eight to ten servings of vegetables and fruit, two to three servings of calcium-rich foods, and two servings of meat or beans guarantee a wide array of nutrient-packed foods and stack the deck in favor of getting all the nutrients you need. Cut back or eliminate one or more groups, and you make it difficult to reach your optimal nutrient intake. For example, the milk group supplies about 40 percent of most people's calcium needs. You are hard-pressed to ensure strong bones if you fail to meet your quota in this group. Women who cut back on meat are likely to be low in iron, while people who skimp on vegetables typically consume inadequate amounts of antioxidants, placing themselves at high risk for numerous diseases, from heart disease and diabetes to cancer and cataracts. Of course, anyone who focuses on highly processed foods in the sugar and fat category will fall short of optimal for a variety of vitamins, minerals, fiber, and phytochemicals, not to mention increasing the risk for weight problems.

## The Myth of Variety

All diet experts worth their weight in nutrition credentials always emphasize the importance of variety in your menu. Rightfully so. For hundreds of thousands of years, our ancient ancestors thrived on hundreds of different plants and animals. Their flexible food choices are one reason why our species survived while others didn't during times of famine or climatic changes. In short, variety is so basic to our nutritional needs that it is embedded in our genetic upbringing.

The reason why nutrition experts push for variety is that the wider a person's food choices, the more likely all the nutrients will be supplied and the less likely there will be toxicities from overconsumption of any one food. It makes sense, but does it apply in today's food supply?

Not really. With the thousands of highly processed foods available on grocery stores shelves, you could easily eat a variety of junk and come out a nutritional dud. Especially since Americans are much more likely to choose pizza, doughnuts, and soda pop rather than split-pea soup, whole-wheat bread, and soy milk.

Variety is still a very good idea, but within limits. Eat a wide variety of real foods. That means unprocessed vegetables, fruits, juices, whole grains, nonfat milk products, extra-lean meats, fish and shellfish, nuts, seeds, and legumes. A varied diet is not five different cookies, six different chips, several different frozen potato products, and a variety of deep-fat-fried meats.

## The Calorie-Containing Nutrients

The nutrients that supply calories are protein, carbohydrate, and fat. Alcohol also supplies calories but is not considered a nutrient since it is not necessary for life and is harmful to health when consumed in excess. Consume too much of any calorie-containing food and you gain weight.

Foods that supply a large amount of calories for relatively few nutrients are called "calorie-dense." These foods are usually high in sugar and/or fat, such as butter and oils, cheese and sour cream, fatty cuts of meat, fatty or sugary desserts, and many highly processed foods. In contrast, foods that supply large amounts of nutrients for few calories are called "nutrient-dense." Examples of nutrient-dense foods include selections you usually consider "healthy," such as fresh vegetables and fruits, cooked dried beans and peas, nonfat milk, whole-grain breads and cereals, fish, extra-lean meat, and poultry breast without the skin.

Most foods contain a mixture of protein, carbohydrates, and/or fats, although the combination varies greatly from one food to another. For example,

- Nuts are primarily fat, but also contain protein.
- Meat is considered a protein-rich food, but also supplies fat.
- Cooked dried beans and peas are excellent sources of both protein and carbohydrate, with a little fat.
- Whole grains supply mostly complex carbohydrates, but also some protein and fat.

- Milk contains protein, carbohydrate (as lactose or milk sugar), and varying amounts of fat depending on whether it is nonfat, low-fat, or whole milk.

One guideline for balancing these nutrients is to consume approximately 12 to 15 percent of calories from protein, 20 percent but no more than 30 percent from fat, and the rest from high-quality carbohydrates (55 percent or more).

## Protein

Protein is comprised of large strings of amino acids. Eight to ten amino acids cannot be manufactured in the body and are called the "essential" amino acids, not because they are more important than other amino acids, but because it is *essential* that they be supplied regularly from food. Most foods contain at least some protein, with the exception of fruit and all sugars, oils, and fats. The best sources of protein include extra-lean meat, chicken, fish, low-fat milk products, soy products, and cooked dried beans and peas combined with whole-grain breads and cereals.

*Why Do We Need Protein?* Protein is essential for tissue repair, maintenance, and growth. Many essential body compounds are comprised of protein, including hemoglobin in red blood cells, many hormones, all enzymes (the body's catalysts for all metabolic reactions), and antibodies in the immune system. Protein also maintains the fluid balance in the body and buffers against changes in the acid-base balance. When you don't consume enough calories, the body uses protein for energy, which prevents protein from being used to repair and maintain tissues.

*Too Much Protein:* While too little protein can damage many body processes, more typically American women eat too much. The overemphasis on protein in current fad diets and the American tradition of planning menus around meat has led to an excess of protein, with most people consuming two to four times as much protein as they need. For example,

- A breakfast of eggs, bacon, toast, and milk provides almost the entire day's requirement for protein.
- A bowl of oatmeal, toast, and milk provides more than a third of the day's protein allotment.
- An athlete's typical diet contains more protein than she needs to build muscle. Seldom, if ever, does someone need protein powders.

Women who follow high-protein diets in an effort to lose weight increase the chances of consuming too much protein. Excess protein flushes calcium out of the body increasing the risk for osteoporosis, raises blood fat levels (high-protein foods tend to be high-fat foods), and elevates your risk for developing kidney stones. (See chapter 9 for more information on protein and bodybuilding.) That's why it's important to get enough, but not too much protein.

## Carbohydrates: Sugar, Starches, and Fiber

When it comes to carbohydrates, do you feel like a Ping-Pong ball? First, grains are good for you. Then you hear they're bad. Let's set the record straight once and for all. Grains *are* good for you. The trick is choosing the right ones, in the right amounts.

*Sugar versus Starch:* Carbohydrates are the simple sugars in fruits, honey, and refined sugar and the complex carbohydrates or starches in grains, beans, and starchy vegetables. Processed foods high in sugars are calorie-dense, nutrient-poor selections, even if they are fortified with a handful of nutrients. In contrast, the simple sugars in fruit come packaged with fiber, vitamins, minerals, phytochemicals, and water and are nutrient-packed foods. The starch in processed white breads, rice, noodles, and other grains are long strings of sugar units that break down slowly to enter the bloodstream. These carbohydrates supply some vitamins and minerals, but are nutritional duds compared to minimally processed complex carbohydrates in whole grains, legumes, and vegetables, since they have lost much of their original nutrients in processing. Whole grains and other unprocessed starchy foods supply hefty amounts of vitamins, minerals, fiber, and phytochemicals, and moderate amounts of protein.

*Why Do We Need Carbohydrates?* Carbohydrate-rich foods supply our bodies with the primary source of fuel—glucose. Glucose is blood sugar, while packages of glucose stored in the liver and muscles for future use are called glycogen. Glucose is the main fuel for the nervous system, including the brain, and the primary quick fuel for muscles and organs. Glucose from carbohydrates also is essential for the efficient burning of body fat and for sparing protein so it can be used to build muscles and other protein-rich tissues.

Granted, the current claim in many fad diet books that carbohydrates make you fat is partly right. In the past few decades, our appetites have dramatically increased for thousands of highly refined, calorie-dense grain-based foods, from doughnuts, cookies, white pasta, and sweetened cereals to white bread and bagels, sports bars, and snack foods. Along with our increasingly sedentary lives, these carbs have packed on the weight, especially with the super-sized portions that we're so used to. Along with the pounds has come an escalating risk for disease.

The main paradox in the controversy over carbohydrates is that refined grains *cause* the same diseases that whole grains help to *prevent*. Fiber-rich whole grains lower our risks for everything from heart disease and cancer to diabetes, and they fill us up without filling us out, so they help keep us lean and fit. Unlike processed refined grains, whole grains are low-fat, high-fiber, nutrient-packed foods loaded with vitamins, minerals, fiber, and antioxidant phytochemicals. In short, making sure at least half the grains you eat every day are whole grains, along with loading the plate with tons of vegetables and fruit, is the smartest thing a woman can do for her health and waistline.

*What Is Fiber?* Fiber is an umbrella term for a family of compounds that are indigestible. Dietary fiber adds bulk to the stool and helps move waste through the intestine, but is not absorbed. Insoluble fibers, such as cellulose, are found in wheat bran, celery, and other vegetables and reduce a woman's risk for intestinal cancers and digestive tract disorders, such as constipation and diverticulosis.

---

**TABLE 1.1    Whole Grains**

The following grains are the mainstay of any healthful diet. Most can be found at your local supermarket or health-food store.

| GRAIN | VARIETIES | HOW TO USE |
|---|---|---|
| Amaranth | Tiny, mustard-colored seed with nutty, peppery flavor. Also available as flour. | Mix with other grains for any side dish. |
| Barley | Pearled. Somewhere between whole and refined. | Use in soups, risotto, salads, or any way you use rice. |
| Brown Rice | Brown rice flour<br>Long-grained rice<br>Short-grained rice<br>Brown basmati rice<br>Brown Texmati rice | Used in baked goods or noodles. Side dishes, rice pudding, stuffings, stir frys, rice and bean salads, soups, as base for creamed dishes, cooked cereal. |

| | | |
|---|---|---|
| Buckwheat | Flour | Pancakes, blini. |
| | Kasha or roasted buckwheat groats | Used in place of rice where earthy flavor will not overwhelm other ingredients. |
| Oats | Rolled or steel-cut oats | Cooked cereal, baked goods. |
| Quinoa | Mild-tasting, small, round ivory-colored grain. High protein and quick-cooking. | Side dish, stuffed bell peppers, chowders, bean/grain salads. |
| Wild Rice | Chewy texture, earthy flavor. | Side dishes, stuffings, mix with brown rice in pilafs, salads, and as accompaniment to main course. |
| Spelt | An ancient form of wheat, low in gluten. Good for people with gluten intolerance. | Use as wheat. |
| Wehani Rice | Mahogany-colored whole-grain with robust, nutty flavor and chewy texture. | Use as rice. |
| Whole Wheat | Flour | |
| | Bulgur or cracked wheat | Any time you use flour. As pilaf, stuffings, breakfast cereals. |
| | Wheat berries | As pilaf, stuffings, breakfast cereal. |
| | Wheat bran | Add to baked goods and cereal. |
| | Whole-wheat couscous | Use any way you use rice. |
| | Wheat germ | Add to baked goods, pancakes, waffles, bread dough, meatloaf or meatballs. Sprinkle on cereal. |

Soluble fibers, such as pectin in fruit, oat bran, and the fiber in cooked dried beans and peas, lower your risk for heart disease and diabetes. Both help you lose weight and maintain the loss.

No one food supplies all the soluble and insoluble fiber needed for health, so a wide variety of minimally processed, high-fiber foods is needed in the diet. In addition, it is the wide variety of fibers in natural foods, such as whole grains, vegetables, fruit, and legumes, that lowers disease risk. Other processed fiber foods, such as commercial bran muffins, often are high in sugar, fat, or salt.

In general, the less food is processed, the greater its fiber content. The average American woman consumes only 10 to 15 grams of fiber daily, which is half of the 27 grams to 35 grams considered optimal. On the other hand, eating too much fiber, i.e., 50+ grams daily, could irritate the intestinal lining, cause diarrhea, or even reduce the absorption of certain minerals. The recommended daily amount of fiber can be obtained from the following foods:

| | |
|---|---|
| 5–8 servings of fruits and vegetables | 12–23 grams |
| 6 servings of whole-grain breads/cereals | 13 |
| 1 cup cooked dried beans and peas | 9 |
| Total | 34–45 grams |

## Fats: Cholesterol, Triglycerides, and Lecithin

- What has more calories, a tablespoon of lard or a tablespoon of canola oil?
- Is the cholesterol in egg yolks the "good" (HDL) or "bad" (LDL) kind?
- Which contains a lower percent of calories from fat: a fast-food fish filet sandwich or a double-hamburger with cheese?
- Can you burn off cholesterol by exercising?

For decades, we have been warned to ferret out the fat from our diets. Although most of us know that fat is bad, many can't tell one fat from another, a calorie from a gram of fat, or whether blood cholesterol is different from that in an egg yolk. "Knowledge levels are so inadequate that they have to be considered obstacles to successfully implementing effective dietary change," say researchers at the Food and Drug Administration (FDA) who have assessed Americans' fat know-how.

Even among those who have taken the fat message to heart, misinformation is rampant. For example, in the FDA study, only one in every five people knew that a tablespoon of any fat, be it lard, canola oil, or margarine, contains the same calorie dose (i.e., approximately 110 calories).

---

**TABLE 1.2    Fat Finale**

Test your fat know-how with the following questions.

**True/False**

1. Egg yolks contain the "bad" cholesterol called LDL.
2. Mayonnaise made from canola oil has less fat than regular mayonnaise.
3. The more unsaturated fat a food has, the more it will raise blood cholesterol levels.
4. Polyunsaturated fats are converted to saturated fats when heated, such as in deep-fat frying.
5. A jar of peanut butter labeled as "cholesterol free" is better than regular brands.
6. A label that reads "95 percent fat free" means the food contains only 5 percent of its calories from fat.
7. The best way to decrease blood cholesterol levels is to eat less cholesterol.
8. Salad dressing is the number one source of fat in women's diets.
9. A label that reads "low cholesterol" means the food has fewer calories and no saturated fat.
10. Veggie burgers are low-fat alternatives to hamburgers.

**Multiple Choice**

Select the best answer to the following questions.

11. A product is labeled as containing only vegetable oils. It would contain
    a. only saturated fat
    b. only unsaturated fat
    c. either saturated or unsaturated fat
    d. unsaturated fat and cholesterol

12. A person has a total blood cholesterol level of 220 mg/dl and an HDL level of 60 mg. What is this person's ratio of total cholesterol to HDL cholesterol and is he/she at high or low risk for heart disease?
    a. 3.6 ratio and low risk
    b. 2.7 ratio and low risk
    c. 7.2 ratio and low risk
    d. 4.5 ratio and high risk

**13.** A 5-ounce serving of ground beef has _____ more fat than the same size serving of chicken breast.

   a. 50 percent

   b. 65 percent

   c. 75 percent

   d. 95 percent

**14.** There are 30 grams of fat and 309 calories in an avocado. What is the percentage of fat calories?

   a. 42 percent

   b. 62 percent

   c. 87 percent

   d. 97 percent

**15.** For every 7 teaspoons of fat consumed, _____ potentially can be stored as body fat.

   a. 6.9 teaspoons

   b. 5.7 teaspoons

   c. 3.5 teaspoons

   d. 2.3 teaspoons

**16.** A label on olive oil states the product is "extra light." This means

   a. it has a lighter color and taste

   b. it weighs less than other olive oils

   c. it is lower in calories

   d. it is lower in saturated fats

**17.** Whole milk is 48 percent fat calories. What percentage of calories comes from fat in 2 percent low-fat milk?

   a. 2 percent

   b. 15 percent

   c. 25 percent

   d. 35 percent

**18.** Experts recommend limiting saturated fat to no more than 10 percent of total calories. If you eat 2,000 calories, your saturated fat gram allowance would be

   a. 10 grams or about two teaspoons

   b. 22 grams or about five teaspoons

    c. 27 grams or about six teaspoons

    d. 36 grams or about eight teaspoons

## Answers

  **1.** F. LDL is a carrier of cholesterol in the blood. It is not found in food.

  **2.** F. They both contain similar amounts of fat and calories.

  **3.** F. The more saturated fat in the diet, the higher the blood cholesterol level.

  **4.** F. Frying, however, does expose these fats to oxygen and once they are "oxidized" they can increase heart disease risk.

  **5.** F. All peanut butters are cholesterol-free. Cholesterol is only found in animal products.

  **6.** F. The label only refers to fat content by weight. The product's fat calories could be much higher.

  **7.** F. Although dietary cholesterol is a consideration, reducing saturated fat intake is the most important dietary change for lowering blood cholesterol.

  **8.** T. Women guzzle more salad dressing than any other fatty food.

  **9.** F. A food can be cholesterol-free and still be high in calories or saturated fat.

**10.** F. The fat content of commercial veggie burgers ranges from 6 percent up to 66 percent fat calories.

**11.** c. Most vegetable oils are high in unsaturated fats. However, manufacturers also use tropical oils, such as palm or coconut oils that are as saturated as lard.

**12.** a. HDL is very important for women. Even if total cholesterol is more than 200 mg/dl, a high HDL can help curb the risk for heart disease.

**13.** d.

**14.** c. (30 grams X 9 calories/gram divided by 309 = 87 percent)

**15.** a.

**16.** a.

**17.** d. (the 2 percent on the label refers only to the fat content by weight, not by calories)

**18.** b. (2,000 calories X .10 = 200 fat calories divided by 9 calories/fat gram = 22 grams of fat)

---

    Despite the confusion, the fat issue is the most clearly defined topic in nutrition. Yes, most Americans should cut the fat. We need to do it now and for the rest of our lives. On the other hand, some fats are "good" for you and everyone needs a little fat in the diet to help absorb the fat-soluble vitamins, to supply the essential fat called linoleic acid and the omega-3s, and just for the pleasure, taste, and aroma of a good meal. Most people should aim for 20 to 30 percent fat calories.

*The Fat Primer:* The fats that supply calories and texture in foods, that float in your blood, and that accumulate in your thighs and hips are called triglycerides. They can be saturated or unsaturated, and the unsaturated ones can be either monounsaturated or polyunsaturated. Regardless of the type, all triglycerides supply 9 calories per gram (about the weight of a paper clip or raisin) and can contribute to weight gain and elevated body fat. The saturated fats are associated with numerous diseases, from heart disease to cancer.

In general, the harder a fat, the more saturated it is. Beef and milk fat (i.e., butter) and stick margarine are mostly saturated fats. Liquid oils are usually unsaturated fats and include the monounsaturated oils in olive and canola oils and the polyunsaturated oils in safflower, corn, soybean, and fish oils. Coconut, palm, and palm kernel oils are exceptions to the rule. These liquid vegetable oils are highly saturated fats. All foods are mixtures of saturated and unsaturated fats with one fat usually predominating, such as saturated fat in meat and monounsaturated fat in avocados.

Cholesterol is a no-calorie fat, so it can't be burned during exercise, sweated out, or used for energy. It is found only in animal products, including meats, chicken, fish, eggs, organ meats, and dairy products, and is used to make some hormones, the digestive juice bile, and other compounds in the body.

Two other fats are essential to health.

- Linoleic acid is a component of polyunsaturated fats and is the only fat the body cannot manufacture. It is called the "essential" fatty acid, and can be obtained from safflower or sunflower seed oils, nuts, seeds, and wheat germ. It is important for healthy skin.
- Lecithin is a type of fat called a phospholipid, which means it contains water-soluble and fat-soluble sides. It is a source of choline, is manufactured in the body, and does not supply calories.

*Why Do We Need Fats?* Thousands of years ago, fat came in handy. It was scarce in the diets of our ancient ancestors, but supplied a rich source of calories and came packaged with protein, vitamins, and minerals in meat, nuts, avocados, and other real foods. Fats, or more specifically saturated and unsaturated fats, are the most concentrated source of energy, supplying more than twice the calories of carbohydrate and protein, or 252 calories versus 112 calories per ounce, respectively.

For most of our history on earth, calories were in short supply, so our bodies evolved a system to store the calories as fat tissue to fend off starvation in times of famine. Consequently, the fats we eat are more likely to be stored as fat in the body, compared to lower-fat foods. Fat also is not very satiating, so it is easy to overconsume fatty foods before we feel full and stop eating. Today, fatty foods are abundant, but our appetites remain fine-tuned to a world where fat was in short supply. It's not surprising that the higher the fat content of the diet, the greater is a woman's likelihood of gaining weight. (See chapter 8 for more on how to lose weight and keep it off.)

Both the type and the amount of fat are important to a woman's health. Excess intake of saturated fats from dairy products, meats, and processed foods, and in a number of cases the unsaturated fats in certain vegetable oils, increase a woman's risk for cancer, heart disease, diabetes, and many other degenerative disorders. The ratio of fat also is important. Our bodies evolved on diets rich in omega-3s and low in saturated fat. But today we consume excessive amounts of saturated fats in meat and unsaturated fats in vegetable oils and very little omega-3s. This imbalance in the ratio of fats is suspected by researchers to increase our risk for most chronic diseases.

*Your Blood Fats:* Just as homemade oil-and-vinegar dressing separates into a watery pool with a fat-slick topping, so also would fats if they were dumped directly into the blood. To solve this dilemma, the body transports fats by coating them with a water-soluble "bubble" of protein called a lipoprotein (lipo = fat). Low-density lipoproteins (LDLs) carry cholesterol out to the tissues. This is the "bad" cholesterol since high LDL levels are linked to increased risk for atherosclerosis and heart disease. High-density lipoproteins (HDLs) carry excess cholesterol back to the liver where it is processed and excreted. HDLs are the "good" cholesterol; the more HDL you have, the lower your risk for developing heart disease. HDL and LDL cholesterol is not found in food (including egg yolks), only in your blood.

All of your blood cholesterol and triglycerides are packed into lipoproteins. Consequently, in a blood cholesterol test, your total cholesterol reading should approximate the sum of your LDL, HDL, and other lipoproteins. That is also why the ratio of total cholesterol to HDL cholesterol is so important. The ideal ratio is 4.5 to 1 or lower, i.e., for every 4.5 mg of total cholesterol, 1.0 mg is packaged in HDLs. According to the National Cholesterol Education Program, a person's total cholesterol should remain below 200 mg/dl (unless HDL is high), LDL should be lower than 130 mg/dl, and HDL should be 35 mg/dl or higher. (People under age thirty may want to shoot for an even lower total cholesterol of 180 mg/dl.)

*Fear of Frying:* A diet oozing with saturated grease from red meat and fatty dairy products raises the bad LDLs and drops the good HDLs, increasing the risk for heart disease. Cut the saturated fat and blood cholesterol levels and heart disease rates drop. Cancer rates also decrease. A low-saturated, high-polyunsaturated diet (i.e., little meat and fatty dairy products and more salad dressings) lowers total blood cholesterol levels, but unfortunately also drops HDL levels, so you lose both good and bad cholesterol. A diet too high in polyunsaturated vegetable oils also has another glitch; it increases the risk for cancer.

*The Good Fats:* Olive oil is another story. This oil lowers total blood cholesterol and LDL cholesterol just like the polyunsaturated fats. However, olive oil also maintains HDL levels, thus lowering the total cholesterol to HDL ratio and reducing heart-disease risk. Olive oil also is not as susceptible to damage by highly reactive compounds called free radicals that escalate atherosclerosis, heart disease, and cancer processes. Consequently, olive oil and other monounsaturated fats (avocado and canola oil to name two) are the oils of choice.

The omega-3 fatty acids also are good fats. They are found primarily in fish oils and are manufactured in the body, but possibly in insufficient amounts to sustain optimal health. Omega-3s are important components of cell membranes in the brain and eyes and might help boost immunity and lower the risk for heart disease, arthritis, depression, and other mental, emotional, and physical problems. Recent research shows that we need to boost omega-3 levels by including several weekly servings of omega-3-rich fish.

*Trans Fatty Acids:* Hydrogenated fats are liquid vegetable oils made creamy when manufacturers convert some of the unsaturated fats into saturated ones through a process called hydrogenation. This process also rearranges some of the remaining unsaturated fats so their natural "cis" form is converted into an abnormal Z-shaped "trans" form called trans fatty acids or TFAs.

While TFAs are found naturally only in minute amounts, they comprise up to 60 percent of the fat in processed foods that contain hydrogenated fats. TFAs, in amounts typically consumed by Americans, raise LDL levels and increase the heart-disease risk by as much as 27 percent. In short, these unsaturated fats act like saturated fats.

The Nurses' Health Study, conducted by Walter Willett, M.D., Dr.P.H., and colleagues at the Harvard School of Public Health in Boston, compared dietary intakes to disease rates in more than 85,000 women and found that as intakes of TFA-containing foods, including margarine, cookies, biscuits, and cakes, increased, so did women's risks for heart disease. Women with the highest intakes had nearly twice the risk of women who ate few hydrogenated fats; women who ate four or more teaspoons of margarine a day increased their risk of developing heart disease by 66 percent, compared to women who limited margarine to less than one teaspoon a month.

*The Bottom Line:* Eat less fat and what fat you do consume, make sure it is omega-3s, monounsaturated fats in olive or canola oil, and polyunsaturated fats in nuts and seeds. Limit your intake of any processed product that contains "hydrogenated vegetable oil" in the ingredient list. When it comes to choosing between the fish fillet or the double hamburger with cheese, you are better off going hungry. Although the fillet is higher in fat, both contain almost a full-day's allotment (more than 44 grams) of fat!

## *Vitamins and Minerals*

You eat platefuls of food, but only grams or micrograms of vitamins and minerals. Despite the tiny quantities, these nutrients are critical to your health and longevity. To qualify as a vitamin or as an essential mineral, a substance must be essential for normal body functioning and create deficiency symptoms when removed from the diet.

Vitamins are either fat-soluble or water-soluble. The fat-soluble vitamins include A, D, E, and K. The water-soluble vitamins include the B vitamins—vitamins $B_1$, $B_2$, $B_6$, $B_{12}$, folic acid, pantothenic acid, biotin, and niacin—and vitamin C. In the past, water-soluble vitamins were considered safe at any dose, while the fat-soluble vitamins were thought to be stored in the body and capable of reaching toxic levels if consumed in excess. This black-and-white view has changed; water-soluble vitamin $B_6$ can produce toxicity symptoms when consumed in excess for long periods of time, while fat-soluble vitamin E appears relatively safe at doses several times the recommendation.

## TABLE 1.3    A Summary of the Vitamins*

| NUTRIENT | FUNCTIONS | TOXIC EFFECTS |
| --- | --- | --- |
| Vitamin A (RDA[†]:4,000 IU) | Eyesight, healthy tissues, bone growth immunity, reproduction, anticancer agent, skin. | More than 50,000 IU causes joint pain, hair loss, itching, dry skin, weakness, fatigue, birth defects. |
| Beta carotene (RDA: none) | Same as vitamin A. | No toxicity symptoms except possibility of increased risk for lung cancer in smokers. |
| Vitamin D (RDA:200–400 IU) | Strong bones, muscles, nerves, hearing, immunity, possibly anticancer agent. | More than 10,000 IU causes nausea, vomiting, loss of appetite, headache, bone pain. More than 1,200 IU might cause kidney stones or calcification of soft tissue. |
| Vitamin E (RDA:12 IU) | Antioxidant against cancer, heart disease, eye disorders, aging, diabetes, arthritis. | No adverse symptoms with doses less than 800 IU. More than 1,200 IU might cause bleeding after surgery. |
| Vitamin K (RDA:55–65 mcg) | Blood clotting. | Large doses cause anemia, jaundice in infants. |
| Vitamin $B_1$ (RDA:1.0–1.5 mg) | Energy metabolism, nerve function, converts excess calories to fat. | No toxic dose has been established. |
| Vitamin $B_2$ (RDA:1.2–1.3 mg) | Energy metabolism, growth and development, hormones, red blood cells. | No toxicity symptoms reported. |
| Niacin (RDA:13–15 mg) | Energy metabolism, hormones, red blood cells, detoxification | Nicotinic acid: More than 100 mg causes flushing, tingling, itching. Long-term effects |

|  |  |  |
|---|---|---|
|  | of drugs, lowers blood cholesterol, improves some psychiatric disorders. | include nausea, diarrhea, ulcers at 100–300 mg. Niacinamide: More than 300 mg causes headache and nausea. More than 3,000 mg causes fatigue, hives, and sore mouth. |
| Vitamin $B_6$ (RDA:1.4–1.6 mg) | Energy, protein, and fat metabolism; asthma; improves depression, irritability, insomnia; carpal tunnel syndrome; premenstrual syndrome; heart disease; immunity; kidney disorders. | More than 250 mg, potentially irreversible nerve damage, including impaired walking, numbness, tingling, poor sense of touch. |
| Vitamin $B_{12}$ (RDA:2.0 mcg) | Energy, protein, and fat metabolism; nerve function; red blood cells; maintains genetic code. | No toxic effects reported. |
| Folic Acid (RDA*:400 mcg) | Maintains genetic code; red blood cells; growth and development of all cells; helps prevent cervical cancer, birth defects, memory and mood problems, heart disease. | Might mask a vitamin $B_{12}$ deficiency at doses of more than 1,000 mcg. Might interfere with anticonvulsant medications. |
| Biotin (RDA:30–100 mcg) | Energy, protein, and fat metabolism. | No toxic effects reported. |
| Pantothenic Acid (RDA:4–7 mg) | Energy, protein, and fat metabolism; helps manufacture cholesterol, bile, vitamin D, red blood cells, and some hormones; stimulates wound healing. | More than 200 mg might cause diarrhea, fluid retention, memory loss, nausea. |
| Vitamin C (RDA:60 mg) | Formation of collagen, antiallergy agent, | More than 1,000–2,000 mg might cause impaired |

| NUTRIENT | FUNCTIONS | TOXIC EFFECTS |
|---|---|---|
| | anticancer agent, anticataract agent, prevention of heart disease, boosts immunity. | glucose tolerance test or cause digestive tract upsets. |

*Values are for nonpregnant, non-breast-feeding women.
†RDA: Recommended Dietary Allowance.

---

Essential minerals are inorganic substances (i.e., they do not contain carbon) required in small amounts from the diet to sustain life and promote health. Twenty minerals and mineral-related compounds are recognized as essential. They include:

| | | |
|---|---|---|
| calcium | iron | selenium |
| chloride | magnesium | silicon |
| chromium | manganese | sodium |
| cobalt | molybdenum | sulfur |
| copper | nickel | vanadium |
| fluoride | phosphorus | zinc |
| iodine | potassium | |

These minerals are absorbed and work together, so should be consumed in the right balance to each other. For example, calcium, magnesium, zinc, and iron compete for absorption in the intestine, so overconsumption of one mineral could reduce absorption of another mineral and result in what is called a "secondary deficiency." Copper and iron work together in the formation of red blood cells. Magnesium and calcium work jointly in the regulation of muscle contraction, nerve function, and bone formation.

The bottom line is that food is the best source of minerals, since a wide variety of minimally processed real foods supply the best balance of minerals. If you decide to take supplements, they should be chosen wisely to maximize the benefits and reduce the risk of developing secondary deficiencies. (See chapter 6 for guidelines in choosing a supplement.)

**TABLE 1.4    A Summary of the Minerals\***

| NUTRIENT | FUNCTIONS | TOXIC EFFECTS |
|---|---|---|
| Calcium (RDA†:1,000–1,200 mg) | Bones and teeth, blood clotting, anticancer agent, lowers blood pressure, muscle contraction, nerve transmission. | More than 2,500 mg might cause nausea, diarrhea, calcification of soft tissue, reduced zinc and iron absorption. |
| Chromium (RDA:50–200 mcg) | Blood sugar regulation, lowers blood cholesterol, protein synthesis, possible weight loss aid. | No known toxic effects reported. |
| Copper (RDA:1.5–3.0 mg) | Enzymes, hormones, red blood cells, hair and skin color, antioxidant, possible anticancer agent. | More than 20 mg causes nausea, vomiting. |
| Iron (RDA:15+ mg) | Red blood cells, oxygen transport within cells, immunity. | More than 25 mg might cause constipation or diarrhea. Excess intake (more than 100 mg) causes iron overload, characterized by abdominal and joint pain, weight loss, fatigue, excess thirst, hunger, yeast infections. Women with underlying genetic predisposition or kidney disorders develop toxic symptoms at lower doses. |
| Magnesium (RDA:300mg) | Energy, protein, and fat metabolism; removes toxic waste products; muscle relaxation; nerve transmission; heartbeat; helps prevent | More than 600 mg might cause diarrhea. More than 1,700 mg might cause low blood pressure, drowsiness, slurred speech, nausea. |

| NUTRIENT | FUNCTIONS | TOXIC EFFECTS |
|---|---|---|
| | heart disease/high blood pressure; premenstrual syndrome; reduces pain of intermittent claudication. | |
| Manganese (RDA:2.5–5.0 mg) | Connective tissue, fat metabolism, blood clotting, protein formation, and digestion. | Excessive intake might cause secondary deficiency of iron. |
| Molybdenum (RDA:75–250 mcg) | Formation of uric acid, iron metabolism, normal growth and development. | Toxicity varies with age group. More than 10 mg might cause goutlike symptoms, including pain and joint swelling. |
| Selenium (RDA:50–55 mcg) | Antioxidant against cancer, heart disease, aging, and arthritis. | More than 2,400 mcg causes brittle hair and fingernails, dizziness, fatigue, jaundice, nausea, diarrhea, discolored skin. |
| Zinc (RDA:12 mg) | Numerous enzymes, detoxification of alcohol, protein synthesis, bone growth, protein digestion, energy metabolism, insulin regulation, genetic code, taste, wound healing, immunity, hormones, blood pressure, oil glands of the skin. | More than 80 mg might lower HDL (good) cholesterol. More than 50 mg might cause secondary deficiency of copper. More than 150 mg might impair immune function. |

* Values are for nonpregnant, non-breast-feeding women.
† RDA: Recommended Dietary Allowance.

# The Phytochemicals

Phytochemicals are not vitamins or minerals. They are not a type of fiber. They do not supply calories. Instead, they are health-enhancing compounds found in unprocessed foods that prevent cancer, possibly boost the immune system, and protect against aging and heart disease. They're found only in fruits, vegetables, garlic, soybeans, nuts, wheat germ, green tea, and other real foods. They are lost when foods are processed, such as when whole wheat is refined to make white bread.

"Phytochemicals have completely changed the way we view foods. It's no longer appropriate to evaluate a food solely on its vitamin, mineral, and fiber content," says Mark Messina, Ph.D., former head of the National Cancer Institute's Designer Foods Program. Preliminary evidence already shows, for example, that

- Sulforaphane in broccoli lowers cancer risk.
- Lycopene in tomatoes, along with beta carotene and other carotenoids, helps maintain normal cell communication and prevent free radical damage to cells, thus helping prevent cancer.
- Lutein in spinach reduces a woman's risk for age-related macular degeneration, a leading cause of blindness.
- Sulfur compounds in garlic lower risk for heart disease and cancer, while boosting a woman's natural immune system.
- Lignans in whole grains enhance fiber's protective effects against colon cancer.
- Phenolic compounds in grapes, saponins in beans, and phytoestrogens in soy are major players in protecting against heart disease.

These and thousands of other phytochemicals work as teams with nutrients and fiber to strengthen the body's defenses against disease.

*How Much Do We Need?* Since humans evolved on diets that contained pounds, not ounces of produce, it's likely a woman's body functions best on a high level of these phytochemicals. "The Dietary Guidelines suggest up to five servings of vegetables and four servings of fruit daily; that's nine servings a day from a very conservative recommendation," says Jeffrey Blumberg, Ph.D., professor of nutrition at U.S.D.A. Human Nutrition Research Center on Aging at Tufts University in Boston.

But what is an optimal intake? According to Winston Craig, Ph.D., R.D., chairman and professor of nutrition at Andrews University in Michigan, "We don't know what an optimal dose is when it comes to phytochemicals, but we do know that the more phytochemical-rich fruits, vegetables, and whole grains you eat, the more protection you get."

## *Water: The Most Important Nutrient*

Water is the most important—yet often most likely forgotten—nutrient. A woman's body is about 60 percent water. That means the body of a 135-pound woman contains 81 pounds of water, while the remaining 54 pounds come from a combination of fat, protein, carbohydrate, and minerals.

*Why Do We Need Water?* Water is essential for all body processes. It surrounds and fills all cells and tissues, lubricates the joints, and transports oxygen and nutrients to all the tissues. Water cushions the organs and protects them against injury, helps maintain the proper acidity of the body, and keeps skin moist. Drinking enough water helps prevent bloating by flushing excess water out of the body, prevent fatigue, and regulate body temperature.

*How Much Water Do You Need?* Women who are only moderately active should drink at least six to eight glasses of water daily. Women who exercise or live in hot climates should consume even more. If you are thirsty, you're already dehydrated and, since thirst is a poor indicator of water needs, you should consume twice as much water as it takes to quench thirst. Water, green tea, and diluted fruit juice are the best fluids.

## *Eating a Little, But Not Enough*

In the days of scurvy, beriberi, and goiter, the epitome of sound nutrition was the "balanced diet." Everyone thought that a diet based on the Four Food Groups— grains, vegetables/fruits, meat, and milk—would more than meet this minimum requirement. Nutritional status in those days was based primarily on a visual inspection. If a woman looked well, if her gums did not bleed, if the number and size of her red blood cells were normal, and if she did not suffer from severe dermatitis or hair loss, she was considered nutritionally healthy. Things have changed.

A wealth of evidence shows that consuming some, but not enough, of one or more nutrients can undermine your emotional, mental, and physical health.

Long-cherished beliefs about nutritional adequacy are changing. The amounts of nutrients known to prevent outright deficiency diseases, such as scurvy or anemia, are not necessarily adequate to maintain optimal nutrition and health, or prevent disease. The middle ground between optimal health and outright deficiency is called marginal deficiency, and it might be more common than many people once thought.

## Symptoms of Marginal Deficiencies

Nutritional depletion develops much like other disorders, such as cancer, arthritis, and the common cold—you start out well, one hopes, but slowly succumb to a deficiency over the course of days, weeks, months, or years. In other words, nutritional status is a continuum from optimal health to clinical deficiency, with marginal deficiencies being the middle ground. Symptoms of a marginal nutrient deficiency are vague and often progress undetected. You might feel "under the weather" or "not up to par." Often people complain of feeling tired, stressed, or irritable. They might suffer from insomnia, poor memory, or mood swings. They are more prone to colds and infections or they lose their appetites.

Take for example iron deficiency, which in its final and clinical deficiency state results in anemia. A woman can suffer from a marginal deficiency of iron for weeks, months, years, even decades, since routine tests for iron status (i.e., the hemoglobin and hematocrit tests) only check for anemia. Iron is the oxygen-carrier in the body, supplying vital oxygen to all tissues, from the brain to the muscles. As iron is drained from the body, tissue iron stores are depleted, oxygen-carrying enzymes that require iron are lost, and vague symptoms that reflect these changes develop. A woman feels tired, is more susceptible to colds and infections, doesn't think as clearly, underperforms at work, and has trouble improving if she exercises. All of this goes undetected unless she requests a more sensitive measure of her iron status—the serum ferritin test. A ferritin value below 20mcg/l means she's iron deficient.

## How Common Are Marginal Deficiencies?

National diet surveys repeatedly show that the American diet does not meet the Recommended Dietary Allowances (RDAs) for several nutrients. This likelihood of nutritional inadequacy is further compounded by the wide fluctuations in individual nutrient requirements that can vary as much as two hundredfold.

As with any disorder, it is best to treat nutrient deficiencies in the early stages before the quality of life has been threatened or a disease has progressed to more serious stages. For example, identifying and treating abnormal cell changes of the cervix from a routine Pap smear has almost a 100 percent cure rate as compared to the poor prognosis if cervical cancer is allowed to progress to life-threatening stages. The same holds true for nutrient deficiencies.

Many diseases once thought to be inevitable consequences of aging, such as osteoporosis, cataracts, and heart disease, are now suspected to be at least partially a result of marginal nutrient deficiencies. In short, a marginal deficiency of one or more nutrients could have far-reaching effects on a woman's health today and in the future. Taking charge of your health today by eating an excellent diet and supplementing responsibly is one of the most important actions you can take to look and feel great into your eighties, nineties, and beyond! The trick is knowing how much of what foods are best for your body.

## Nutritional Individuality

I had a friend years ago who swore if he cut back to less than a few grams of vitamin C a day, he'd get sick (the recommended vitamin C intake is under 100 mg). I argued that dose was several hundred times the recommended intake, but sure enough, he'd catch a cold every time he stopped taking supplements.

Hidden within the data of most research studies is this hint of individual nutritional variation. Researchers report on averages, but a hard look at the raw data shows people are responding all over the charts to the same dose. For example, chromium picolinate, on average, has little effect on weight loss. Yet, some people respond quite remarkably to this mineral, while others show no effect at all.

Individual variability was considered when developing the Recommended Dietary Allowances (RDAs), the standards for nutrient intakes. Age, gender, life stage (puberty, menopause, and reproductive status, such as pregnancy and lactation), body size, and lifestyle are the main variances that distinguish one group from another when establishing nutrient needs and the RDAs. An "Estimated Average Requirement" (EAR) is set based on the amount of a nutrient needed by most people to be healthy, then a safety factor is added. Thus, the RDAs are designed to exceed most people's requirements and aim to satisfy at least 97.5 percent of the population. (A percentage that is a guesstimate at best.) A "Tolerable

Upper Limit" (UL) for safety of a nutrient is more unclear, since even less is known about individual variability in UL than is known about variability in requirements.

Seldom are medical conditions, or even the genetic susceptibility to chronic disease, used as criteria for establishing nutrient requirements. And the concept of nutritional or biochemical individuality is still in the dark ages. Nutritional individuality was first proposed back in the 1950s. The thesis was that individual variation was potentially large and conceivably the solution to many "baffling health problems."

Current discoveries into mapping the human genome might well be the key to unlocking the mystery of nutritional individuality. The three billion nucleotides distributed sequentially among twenty-three pairs of chromosomes provide a staggering field for nutrient variations. If the metabolic pathway influencing nutritional requirements for each of the forty-plus nutrients (not to mention the 12,000 phytochemicals!) was affected independently on even two sites at a single genetic locus, we could expect that the number of variations in nutritional variability could be in excess of two hundred trillion!

Each of us is genetically unique in our nutritional needs. But, while each of us might not fit the "normal range," we haven't a clue as to what to do about that. Until human genome sequencing explains this topic, it's easy for the message to be misused to justify taking megadoses of vitamins, going on low-carb fad diets, injecting growth hormone, or other senseless, and potentially harmful, practices. Yes, you are unique. Just how unique is still a mystery.

So what is a woman to do? How can you devise a diet program tailored to your unique individual biochemistry? How do you know when you're getting enough, but not too much, of all the nutrients available in foods? Until we have more precise methods for assessing individual variation, your best bet is to use a little common sense based on a thorough review of the research. We have thousands of studies, spanning decades of research to show that the dietary guidelines spelled out in this book can do much more than just fend off diseases. For a start, they can lengthen your healthy middle years, improve your memory, help you look twenty years younger, and boost your energy. I guarantee if you follow the advice in chapter 2, you'll feel better than you ever thought you could feel! Use Table 1.5, "How Good Is Your Diet?," on pages 38–39, to get an overview of your current eating habits.

---

### TABLE 1.5     How Good Is Your Diet?

How can you tell if your diet is adequate? How do you know how many calories you're consuming, or how much fat? Answers to these questions might not be as complicated as you think.

#### First and Foremost

Assessing your diet is simple, just compare it to the Real Foods in the Healthy Woman's Diet on page 45. You're getting at least recommended amounts of all vitamins and minerals (with the exception of vitamin E) for less than 2,000 calories if you consume daily:

- 8 to 10 servings of fresh fruits and vegetables, including one citrus fruit and one dark green leafy vegetable.
- 6+ servings of whole grains, including bread, rice, cereal, or pasta.
- 3 servings of nonfat milk, plain yogurt, or fortified soy milk.
- 2 servings of legumes or extra-lean meat.

#### How Many Calories Do You Think You Eat?

Obsessing over calories is a waste of time. You are much better off listening to your body, eating when you are truly hungry, and choosing nutritious foods when you are. The best calorie guidepost is your weight: if you gain weight, you're eating too many calories, if you lose weight, you're not eating enough to maintain your current weight, and if you maintain a desirable weight, you're doing just fine.

Granted, you can measure calorie intake by using a calorie counter—either a book that lists foods and calories, a computer nutritional analysis program, or a specialized calorie calculator—to determine the exact calories. But watch out. You're likely to become calorie and food obsessed and lose sight of the real goal—choosing foods that look good, taste good, and are good for you.

#### How Much Fat Do You Think You Eat?

Fat has gotten a bad rap. Granted, we should cut total fat intake to about 20 to 30 percent of calories. However, not all fats are bad, just as not all fat-free foods are good. If you follow the guidelines in chapter 2 and accent these foods with small amounts of wholesome fatty foods, such as olive oil, nuts, seeds, nut butters, or avocados, your fat intake will remain low and you'll fuel your health as well without having to obsess over fat grams.

Like calories, you can write down your food intake, tally fat grams by using any number of fat-counting books or computer programs, or read labels and only choose foods that supply no more than 3 grams of fat for every 100 calories. But for those who can't be bothered with books, calculators, and label reading, your best bet is to develop a personalized eating plan based on wholesome, minimally processed foods.

## Are You Eating Too Much?

This is an easy one. Just compare your diet with the Healthy Woman's Diet in chapter 2. Short or inactive women should aim for the lower number of servings of whole grains, while tall or active women can consume more. Everyone should include at least eight, preferably up to ten, servings of fresh fruits and vegetables in their daily fare, but stick with the recommended servings for nonfat milk, low-fat meat, and beans, no more. No food should be consumed in such great amounts that it interferes with meeting at least these minimum standards.

## What Is Missing?

Again, return to the Healthy Woman's Diet. If you're like most women, your red flags will be fruits, vegetables, milk, and iron-rich foods. While you make an effort to improve your diet, consider taking a moderate-dose multiple vitamin and mineral that fills in the nutritional gaps.

# CHAPTER 2

# The Healthy Woman's Diet

**B**ehind my back I'm holding a dark chocolate truffle in one hand and a handful of broccoli in the other. Which hand do you choose? My guess is you're hoping for the chocolate; broccoli is the booby prize.

Why is that? "Duh Mom, because the chocolate tastes better," says my daughter Lauren—fifteen years old, already a chocolate lover, and wise in the ways of the world.

While you wipe away the drool from the thought of that missed truffle, let's take a look at this love-hate relationship we have with broccoli, or all vegetables, fruit, whole grains, and other healthful foods for that matter.

## Why We Don't Always Eat Perfectly

We all know vegetables, whole grains, fruits, and legumes are good for us. "Thousands of studies spanning decades of research consistently show that people who eat diets rich in these foods significantly lower their risks for most age-related diseases, from heart disease and diabetes to hypertension and cataracts," says Jeffrey Blumberg, Ph.D., professor in the School of Nutrition Science and Policy at Tufts University in Boston. Researchers estimate that at least 35 percent of cancer deaths could be avoided by diet alone, with fruits and vegetables leading the pack in cancer prevention, and cutting the fat reduces heart-disease risk by almost 50 percent in women.

Other studies show that heaping the plate with produce, whole grains, and legumes, as well as drinking three glasses of nonfat milk a day, helps sidestep stroke, reduce symptoms of non-Hodgkin's lymphoma, build bones resistant to osteoporosis, and boost the immune system. Hefty servings of vegetables and a few whole grains also are a must for lifelong weight control. Then there's the longevity factor. According to a study from the University of Naples in Italy, people who live more than a century also live the healthiest. Their secret? You guessed it—they eat the most fruits and vegetables.

We're talking about Mother Nature's perfect foods. Fruits and vegetables are the best dietary sources of antioxidants, such as vitamin C and beta carotene. Along with whole grains and legumes, they are major contributors of fiber, which lowers your risk for heart disease and breast cancer and helps satisfy your appetite on few calories. Yet even if you took supplements and ate bran cereal, you couldn't make up for a lack of real foods, since fruits, vegetables, legumes, whole grains, nuts, and other real food contain thousands of phytochemicals—from sulforaphane in broccoli, lycopene in tomatoes, and flavonoids in grapes to lutein in spinach, phyto-estrogens in soybeans, lignans in whole grains, and limonene in citrus—that boosts defenses against most diseases.

## Couch Potatoes

With the deck stacked so high in favor of eating real food, you'd think we'd be shoveling handfuls of carrots into our mouths, blending gallons of strawberries and yogurt into smoothies, heaping our plates with brown rice, stopping at every roadside produce stand, fighting over the last bite of lentils at the dinner table. We're not. In fact, it's just the opposite.

Every national nutrition survey dating back to the late 1960s repeatedly reports that Americans avoid healthy foods like the plague. Back in 1991, the National Cancer Institute established its "5-a-Day for Better Health" program to encourage Americans to eat more fruits and vegetables. Not that there is anything magical about five a day. It's just that we're eating so little fruits and vegetables that boosting intake to even a measly five servings seemed like a manageable first-step goal. Only one in every ten of us meets this goal. The rest of us average about four daily servings. More than half of us don't eat fruit at all, one in three turns her nose up at milk, and one in every five of us doesn't include even one vegetable on any given day.

Even when we nibble on real foods, the choices we make are mostly nutritional duds. We choose fried potatoes and iceberg lettuce over sweet potatoes and spinach, fatty muffins over whole-grain bread, ice cream over nonfat milk, and hamburgers over split-pea soup. The good choices—the colorful stuff chock-full of antioxidants, vitamins, minerals, phytochemicals, and fiber—barely ever make the plate. Dark green and orange vegetables, for example, make up less than 10 percent of our produce choices: in fact, the average American woman puts a leafy green on her plate less than once a week, eats about one salad every other day, and takes about three bites of carrots every day. Less than one woman in every ten regularly chooses oranges or cruciferous vegetables. In short, our children's guinea pigs put away more vegetables in a day than most women eat in a week.

## The Excuses We Use

We know we should eat 'em, so why aren't we walking the walk? There are all kinds of excuses given for women's lack of enthusiasm over real food.

- It is pricey. "Fresh produce, whole grains, and other healthful foods are expensive, so many people turn to cheaper foods that provide more calories per dollar, like fast food," says Adam Drewnowski, Ph.D., professor in the Departments of Epidemiology and Medicine at the University of Washington in Seattle. Granted, that might play a part, but price can't be the determining factor. A study from the University of California, Berkeley, found that only 14 percent of women with money to burn included even one green leafy on any four days. And, according to the U.S.D.A., Americans are spending a smaller percentage of their dollars on food than ever before.
- Healthy food is scarce. Wait a minute . . . availability can't be the main issue, since the variety of produce and whole grains has increased dramatically since the 1970s and many selections once only found in health-food stores are now regular inclusions on most supermarket shelves.
- No time. Hey, with so many quick-fix options available today, from bagged lettuce and precut vegetables to instant brown rice and fortified soy milk, this excuse is a bit lame. Besides, the time we save grabbing highly processed junk food is not worth the extra weight we gain on these foods.

One possible reason why we fail at broccoli is we don't realize how little we're eating. In studies from the University of Maastricht in The Netherlands, 88 percent of people who didn't include ample produce in their diets thought they were getting enough. Feeling the need to make a change is the number one motivator for cleaning up your diet, but people aren't likely to eat more broccoli if they think they're already doing just fine.

## Working against Your Genes

My daughter is right, the big reason why many women choose the chocolate truffle over broccoli is plain ol' immediate gratification—chocolate tastes better. But, since fruits, whole grains, legumes, vegetables, and other healthful foods are so good for us, why don't our bodies have a built-in system to ensure we get enough? In short, why don't we lust over cauliflower like we do Mrs. Fields' cookies? The answers to those questions are in your genes.

For hundreds of thousands of years, our bodies evolved to meet the demands of a harsh environment. To counter vigorous living and low-calorie supplies, the human body evolved complex systems to defend against weight loss and to maximize weight gain. Vegetables, and to a lesser extent fruits, were abundant throughout our evolutionary history, so our bodies had no reason to evolve a system for craving or storing them, but did develop a satiety button to protect against excess intakes. This explains why:

1. fiber-rich foods like vegetables or beans fill us up long before they fill us out,
2. our tissues don't store vegetable-derived nutrients like vitamin C, and
3. why we take vegetables for granted, i.e., foods our ancestors ate automatically to survive.

Vegetables and whole grains, with the exception of olives and avocados, contain no fat and little sugar, the two high-energy items for which our bodies evolved complex appetite systems to ensure we got enough. "We humans have a love affair with fat and sugar that dates back to our most ancient roots when these calorie-dense nutrients were in short supply," says Dr. Drewnowski. Our brains release a stew of appetite chemicals, from serotonin to the endorphins, to entice and even force us to eat sweet, creamy, and crispy foods like chocolate, ice cream, and chips. No comparable appetite controls are in place for produce. Today we live in a glut of sweet and greasy foods, so our bodies get more than enough calories and there's no reason to fall back on the old staples: leaves, roots, and berries. The bottom line: We need to use our highly developed brains to make sure we do consciously what our ancestors did automatically.

## *The Healthy Woman's Diet in a Nutshell*

Before you set your mind to eat better, you need to know how many servings of what foods to shoot for. Also refer to pages 7–9 in the Introduction for more information.

*Fruits and Vegetables:* There is no upper limit when it comes to vegetables and fruit. The research shows that the more we eat, the healthier we are. Aim for at least eight, and preferably ten, servings daily.

At first glance, that might seem like a lot, when you consider that it's two to three times what most Americans eat. But it's really not a monumental goal when you consider that a serving is only:

- One small piece (one small apple or carrot).
- One cup raw, such as lettuce or chopped fruit.
- One-half cup cooked vegetables or canned fruit.
- 6 ounces juice.

*Whole Grains:* Women typically average less than one serving a day. Instead, aim for at least six servings. If you exercise and can afford to eat more calories, your additional servings can come from more whole grains or from refined grains, such as white bread, white rice, egg noodles, and cereals and bakery items made from refined grains. See Table 1.1, "Whole Grains," on pages 18–19.

*Calcium-Rich Foods:* You are hard-pressed to meet your calcium needs without drinking milk or fortified soy milk. While many women think they are getting enough, the average intake of calcium is less than 600 mg a day. You need at least 1,000 to 1,200 mg daily. Each glass of milk supplies 300 mg of calcium, so you need at least three glasses daily to approach the daily recommendation. Select nonfat or low-fat choices when possible.

*Iron-Rich Foods:* Women in their childbearing years typically consume about half their iron needs, which explains why this mineral is the number one deficiency for women. Extra-lean red meat is the best source, but poultry breast, fish and shellfish, and legumes also are excellent sources. These foods also will supply high-quality protein. Select two of these each day and complement them with other iron-rich foods, such as dark green leafy vegetables. A three-ounce serving of meat or fish is the size of the palm of your hand or a deck of cards. It doesn't take much to meet your protein needs!

---

**TABLE 2.1    Real Foods in the Healthy Woman's Diet**

The main goals of the Healthy Woman's Diet are to eat enough "real food" to fuel your body and maintain a desirable weight. By "real food," I mean foods that are minimally processed, including fruits, vegetables, whole grains, legumes, nonfat milk and soy products, extra-lean meats, fish, chicken breast, nuts, and seeds.

Each day aim for the following:

8 to 10 fruits and vegetables. Make sure at least one is a vitamin C–rich citrus fruit and two are dark-green or deep-orange selections, such as oranges, apricots, sweet potatoes, spinach, or broccoli. (1 serving: 1 piece of fruit, 1 cup raw, ½ cup cooked)
6+ whole grains, including brown rice, whole-wheat breads, oatmeal, and whole-grain ready-to-eat cereals such as NutriGrain and Shredded Wheat. (1 serving: 1 slice of bread; ½ cup cooked pasta, rice, or noodles; 1 ounce ready-to-eat whole-grain cereal)
3 calcium-rich foods, including nonfat milk or yogurt, or fortified soy milk. (1 serving: 1 cup)
2 iron-rich foods, including legumes, seafood, white breast of poultry, extra-lean meats (less than 7 percent fat by weight). (1 serving: 3 ounces meat, ¾ cup cooked legumes)
8+ glasses of water. (1 serving: 8 ounces)

Several times a week include in your diet:

• Fish, such as salmon, herring, or mackerel. Preferably baked, grilled, or poached.
• Nuts, such as almonds, walnuts, cashews, or macadamia nuts, or nut butters.
• Tea, either green tea or black tea.
• Olive oil, avocados, olives, and other healthy fats.

Optional foods include:

• Eggs, limit to five per week or use egg substitutes to your heart's content.

---

**TABLE 2.2    Fifty Ways to Love Your Veggies**

 1. Open a bag of preshredded cabbage. Mix with a little light coleslaw dressing (chopped apples or canned pineapple chunks are optional).
 2. Add grated carrots or zucchini to spaghetti sauce.
 3. Mash green peas into guacamole. It reduces fat without changing taste or texture.
 4. Add chopped fresh tomatoes and cilantro to bottled salsa as a quick dip for chips, baby carrots, or pita bread, or pile it on as dressing for salads, tacos, burritos.
 5. Make pumpkin pie with fat-free canned milk and low-fat crust.
 6. Add lots of leaf lettuce, red onion, and thick tomato slices to a turkey sandwich.
 7. Pop frozen blueberries or grapes into your mouth for a sorbetlike treat.
 8. Top your morning cereal with dried plums or cranberries or a handful of fresh berries.
 9. Drink a travel-size box of orange juice on the way to work.
10. Stir fresh peaches or berries into frozen yogurt.
11. Add canned mandarin oranges to your spinach salad.
12. Skewer more vegetables (cherry tomatoes, carrot slices, mushrooms, eggplant, onion, squash, sweet potato, etc.) than meat on your shish kebabs.
13. Add frozen green peas to canned chicken noodle soup.
14. Never, *and I mean never,* leave the house without a snack stash (i.e., banana, orange, apple, baby carrots, raisins, grapes, and/or jicama).
15. Puree fresh fruit, sweeten with concentrated apple juice and freeze into ice cubes or pops. Add cubes to club soda for a refreshing drink.
16. Add fruit to your milk shake.
17. Make fruit or vegetable salsa and sauces with mango, papaya, peaches, or pineapple and use in place of creamed sauces on meats, fish, and chicken.
18. Purchase nonfat, plain yogurt and sweeten with fruit.
19. After dinner, place a platter of cut-up fruit on the table for snacking in the evening.
20. When eating out, order entrées that feature vegetables (grilled vegetable sandwich, salad, vegetable soup).
21. Ask your waiter to hold the potato and instead bring two side orders of vegetables (steamed) with your order.
22. Add grapes, mandarin oranges, or cubed apples to chicken salad.
23. Skip syrup, and top pancakes, waffles, or French toast with fresh fruit.
24. Puree vegetables, such as cauliflower, carrots, or broccoli, and add to soup stock and sauces.
25. Add dried fruit to stuffings and rice dishes.

26. Double your normal portion of any vegetable (except French fries or iceberg lettuce!).
27. Cut sweet potatoes into half-inch strips and roast for a tasty alternative to French fries.
28. Stuff an almond into each of five pitted dried plums for a sweet, chewy, crunchy snack.
29. Plan your dinner around the theme of "meat and three veggies."
30. Toss a bag of frozen stew vegetables (large hunks of carrots, potato, celery and onion) with a tablespoon of olive oil, dash of salt and pepper, and a few sprigs of fresh rosemary. Roast at 425 degrees for thirty minutes.
31. Toss chopped tomatoes, corn, red onion, salt, and rice vinegar for a quick and filling snack or lunch salad.
32. Add cilantro, chopped tomatoes, corn, grated carrots, or other vegetables to tacos and burritos.
33. When flying, ask for tomato or orange juice for your in-flight beverage.
34. Once a week, have a meal salad for dinner, such as Cajun salmon Caesar salad or grilled chicken spinach salad with mandarin oranges.
35. Take advantage of precut vegetables, prepackaged salads, supermarket salad bars, and exotic specialty produce.
36. Grill extra vegetables at dinner to use in a quick wrap for tomorrow's lunch.
37. Fill a halved cantaloupe with lemon-flavored yogurt.
38. Skip the fruit drinks, blends, and ades; go for the 100 percent orange, grapefruit, prune, and pineapple juices.
39. Add flowers, like dandelions, violets, daylilies, clover, and oxalis, to salads.
40. Add steamed asparagus or green beans to your favorite pasta dish.
41. Top pizza with extra quartered artichoke hearts (canned in water), roasted red peppers, red onions, sliced zucchini, and fresh tomatoes.
42. Order deli sandwiches with extra tomatoes.
43. Whip steamed, chopped collards or chard into mashed potatoes.
44. Buy produce at various stages of ripeness to avoid spoilage.
45. Stock up on frozen plain vegetables for last-minute meals.
46. Keep dried fruit on hand for a quick snack.
47. Plant a pear or apple tree, row of blueberry bushes, or vegetable garden in the backyard.
48. When eating out, order off the menu, ask for two sides of vegetables, or split an entrée and complement with a salad.
49. At parties, sip on orange juice, tomato juice, or a Bloody Mary mix.
50. Take a low-fat cooking class and share vegetable recipes with friends.

The days when meals revolved around pork chops or meat loaf are past. The Healthy Woman's Diet is planned around vegetables, whole grains, or bean dishes with extra-lean meat, chicken, or fish serving as a condiment. Examples include spaghetti with meatballs (made from extra-lean beef or ground turkey breast), Chinese or East Indian dishes of vegetables and grain with small amounts of meat, or stews and soups made with small amounts of meat.

*Water:* If you are thirsty, you are already dehydrated and suffering the fatigue associated with dehydration. Force fluids by drinking at least eight glasses of water daily.

*Fish:* Fatty fish are the best sources of the omega-3 fats, which lower the risk for heart disease, depression, osteoporosis, and even pregnancy complications. Several times a week include a serving of salmon, herring, or tuna in your diet.

*Healthy Fats:* The monounsaturated fats in olive and canola oils, avocados, nuts, and seeds lower disease risk and might even help manage weight. Include them sparingly in the weekly diet. In contrast, the saturated fats in meat and fatty dairy products like cheese, sour cream, and cream cheese increase your risk for heart disease and certain cancers. These should be limited in the daily diet.

## Beyond the Basics

If you focused on the above foods, all your diet concerns would be over. But in case there are any lingering questions, here are a few extra guidelines.

*What about Calories?* Base your diet on at least 2,000 calories of real foods. Never let your intake drop below 1,500 calories a day, unless supervised by a registered dietitian (R.D.) or physician (M.D.). If you can't lose weight on 1,500 calories, you need to exercise more, not further cut calories. Select less nutritious foods only after you have met all the recommendations in the Healthy Woman's Diet. Include a moderate-dose vitamin/mineral supplement when your intake drops below 2,000 calories. (See chapter 6 for guidelines on how to supplement.)

Fat is your biggest problem when it comes to calories, supplying more than twice the calories per teaspoon of protein or carbohydrates. Visible fats are easy to spot and include the marbling in meat, oil in salad dressing, and cream bases of sauces and soups. Hidden fats are more tricky. They make a bran muffin look shiny, or cause a potato chip to leave a slick feeling in the mouth, or a cheese cube and a French fry to leave a greasy feel on the fingertips.

**TABLE 2.3    Fast and Healthy Meals and Snacks**

**BREAKFAST**

- Top one-half whole-wheat English muffin with 1 ounce no-fat cheese and broil until bubbly. Serve with a glass of orange juice.
- One packet of instant, plain oatmeal with nonfat milk, raisins, and a banana.

**LUNCH**

- Whole-wheat pocket bread filled with garbanzo beans, tomatoes, sprouts, grated low-fat cheese, and green onions.
- A sandwich made with whole-wheat bread, 3 ounces of turkey, leaf lettuce, and a tomato slice. Serve with nonfat milk or fortified soy milk.
- Stuff a large tomato with water-packed tuna mixed with low-calorie mayonnaise and chopped celery. Serve with whole-wheat crackers.
- A whole-wheat tortilla filled with beans, low-fat cheese, tomatoes, and salsa. Serve with orange juice.

**DINNER**

- Reheat homemade soup. Serve with a whole-grain roll, carrot sticks, and nonfat milk.
- Fresh fruit slices on no-fat cottage cheese, a whole-wheat roll, a baked potato (cook in a microwave) seasoned with chives and Butter Buds, and a 3-ounce slice of lean beef or turkey.

**SNACKS**

- Fresh blueberries
- Fresh fruit and nonfat milk "milk shake"
- Three-bean salad, prepared with no-oil marinade
- One-half papaya filled with chicken salad or cottage cheese
- Peanut butter on a whole-wheat bagel topped with raisins or banana slices
- A slice of bread with apple slices and low-fat ricotta or no-fat cottage cheese

Besides added fats in foods, oils and fats can be eliminated from cooking methods with no loss of flavor or appearance by:

- Sautéing vegetables, chicken, fish, and other foods in wine, lemon juice, defatted chicken stock, or water and herbs.
- Removing the skin from poultry.
- Baking, broiling, roasting, grilling, or stewing extra-lean meats, poultry, and fish.

For other ideas on how to cut unnecessary fat calories from the diet, see Table 2.4, "Cut the Fat."

*What about Fast Food?* The biggest culprit in most American diets when it comes to fat and calories is fast food, which can supply up to an entire day's allotment for fat in one meal. If your only option is a fast-food restaurant, choose from the salads (go light on the dressing), low-fat milk, orange juice, and grilled chicken sandwiches (skip the mayonnaise dressings).

---

### TABLE 2.4    Cut the Fat

At a loss on how to cut the fat? Here are a few suggestions that maximize taste, while minimizing unnecessary fat and calories. Pick and choose which tricks will work for you. Remember, you need some fat in the diet, so there is no need to adopt all of these suggestions.

| INSTEAD OF . . . | USE . . . |
|---|---|
| Whole-milk ricotta cheese | Fat-free ricotta cheese. |
| Cream or whole milk | Low-fat or nonfat milk, evaporated nonfat milk or nonfat milk mixed with instant nonfat dry milk solids. |
| Preparing cream sauces with whole milk and butter | Use nonfat milk or evaporated nonfat milk and thicken with flour or cornstarch. |
| Using the full amount of cheese | Reduce portion in sauces of hard cheese to one-third to one-half. Sprinkle on top of dishes as garnish or grate. |
| Sour cream | Fat-free sour cream. |

| | |
|---|---|
| Whipped cream | Partially frozen evaporated nonfat milk, whipped into a foam or nondairy fat-free toppings. |
| Cream cheese | Fat-free cream cheese. |
| Heavy cream | Fat-free Half & Half. |
| Whole eggs | Egg whites, two per whole egg; egg substitutes. |
| Chicken breast with skin | Chicken breast with skin removed. |
| Tuna packed in oil | Tuna packed in water. |
| Preparing 4–8 ounce meat servings | Prepare 2–3 ounce servings and mix or serve with rice, whole-grain noodles, and vegetables. |
| Using fatty meats | Use ground round, extra-lean chuck, or ground beef or turkey breast: trim fat from meat. |
| Frying meat | Bake, roast, broil, steam, or stew; drain excess fat. |
| Flavoring soup with ham hocks | Use lean pork or one to two drops liquid smoke. |
| Using fatty meat stock, stews, gravies | Refrigerate and skim off hardened fat from surface. Invest in a defatting cup that pours from the bottom, leaving fat on the top. |
| Regular salad dressings | Low-fat or fat-free salad dressings, nonfat yogurt or buttermilk-based dressings flavored with rice vinegar, lemon juice. |
| Oil, margarine, and butter for sautéing | Nonstick pans, defatted chicken stock, or vegetable sprays. |
| Using the full amount of oil in a recipe | Reduce oil by one-third. Substitute up to one-half the oil with an equivalent amount of applesauce or baby food prunes in quick breads and muffins. |
| Margarine or butter on toast | Fruit butter, jam, or apple butter. |
| Mayonnaise on sandwiches and in salads | Reduced fat or fat-free mayonnaise, nonfat yogurt, or low-fat cottage cheese. |
| Pound cake | Angel food cake. |
| Ice cream | Sherbet, sorbet, fruit ice, nonfat ice cream. |
| Preparing French fries | Brush parboiled potato wedges with olive oil and spices (try chili powder and crushed rosemary) and bake until browned. |
| Popping popcorn in oil | Use a hot-air popper or fat-free microwave popcorn. |

*What about Cheese?* According to the U.S. Department of Agriculture, cheese has now replaced meat as the number one source of saturated fat in women's diets. Since this is the type of fat that clogs arteries and increases cancer risk, show some self-restraint when it comes to cheese. The dairy case now contains lots of low-fat cheeses, but looks sometimes deceive. Many of the "light," "reduced-fat," or "part-skim" cheeses still have a fat content comparable to conventional cheeses. To sift through the packaging and identify a truly low-fat cheese, ignore the label on the front and go straight to the grams-of-fat listing on the back. A low-fat cheese will have either 3 grams of fat or less per serving or no more than 3 grams per ounce. Moderate-fat cheeses have 4 to 5 grams of fat per ounce, while high-fat items contain 6 grams or more. Also, check the serving size; some packaged slices are "lighter" only because they weigh less than an ounce rather than the full ounce of other brands. Read labels and select only those low-fat cheeses that provide 3 grams or less of fat for every 100 calories.

*What about Sugar?* The average woman consumes her weight in sugar every year, or 158 pounds. As sugar intake increases, diet quality takes a nosedive, increasing the risk for nutrient deficiencies and a host of health problems, not to mention weight gain. Curtail your sweet tooth by limiting desserts and soft drinks. Also, read labels for hidden sugars in foods. Keep in mind 4 grams of sugar is a teaspoon. Avoid foods that list sugar as one of the top three items or mention several types of sugar in the ingredients list.

*What about Alcohol?* Alcohol is a double-edged sword. While a glass of wine lowers heart-disease risk, more than one alcoholic beverage a day increases some women's risk for cancer. There is no safe level of alcohol for pregnant women. Alcohol also interferes with weight-loss efforts by reducing willpower and by adding extra calories to the daily menu. You must decide, based on your health history, whether or not to include modest amounts of alcohol in your diet.

*What about Salt?* Some women are salt sensitive, which places them at high risk for developing hypertension. Few women know their tolerance level and susceptibility to high blood pressure, while typical American diets contain excessive amounts of salt (as much as twenty-five times the recommended dietary levels). Since reducing this excessive salt intake has no harmful side effects, national dietary recommendations agree that all Americans would benefit by limiting salt to no more than 6 grams/day (that is slightly more than a teaspoon). Further reductions to four grams or less are even better. Keep in mind salt (sodium chloride) is 40 percent sodium, so this recommendation is the equivalent of 2.4 grams of sodium.

*Does It Matter When I Eat?* Yes. Women who divide their food intake into little meals and snacks throughout the day, starting with breakfast, have lower risks for diseases such as heart disease, think more clearly and perform better at work and school, and have an easier time managing their weights compared to women who skip meals.

## Tricks for Eating Well

The two biggest steps for making diet changes are deciding to actively include more real foods in your daily diet and having a plan how you will do that. The following six rules can help you override your genes and meet your quota:

1. *Bring it:* "Always bring food with you," recommends Debra Waterhouse, M.P.H., a registered dietitian and author of *Outsmarting Female Fatigue* (Hyperion, 2001). "Stuff your purse, briefcase, backpack, gym bag, or diaper bag with apples, oranges, bananas, baby carrots, whole-grain crackers, yogurt, and boxes of raisins so you aren't caught short with the only option being a candy bar," she adds.
2. *Double it:* Turn one serving into two by doubling the amount you serve. Turn a salad into two or more servings by adding additional vegetables or fruits to that pile of lettuce.
3. *Hide it:* Disguise vegetables by grating them into sauces, pureeing them in soups, chopping them into pita sandwiches, stirring them (corn, carrots, blueberries) into muffins, or adding more vegetables to canned vegetable-beef soup. Cook oatmeal in nonfat milk or soy milk. Crumble tofu into lasagna. Stuff bell peppers with brown rice.
4. *Cross-dress it:* Please your appetite chemicals by disguising fruit as dessert, i.e., dunk strawberries in chocolate syrup, sprinkle crystalline ginger over mandarin oranges, or mix kiwi into strawberry-kiwi yogurt.
5. *Two-fer it:* Include two fruits and/or vegetables at every meal and at least one at every snack.
6. *Like it:* With hundreds of selections to choose from, there must be at least a dozen fruits and/or vegetables even the most ardent vegetable-hater is willing to eat. Also, try preparing the same vegetable or grain different ways. Use Table 2.5, "Record My Progress," page 54, to keep track of how well you are doing.

**TABLE 2.5    Record My Progress**

Use this sheet as a master copy to monitor your progress in following the guidelines in the Healthy Woman's Diet. Scores rank as follows: A: 90 to 100 points, B: 80 to 89 points, C: 70 to 79 points, D: 60 to 69 points, F: less than 60 points.

Date:_____

Long-Range Health Goal:_____

_____.

This Week's Minigoal:_____.

| | POSSIBLE POINTS | MY POINTS |
|---|---|---|
| **Healthy Food Choices** | | |
| **1.** Fruits, Vegetables, Whole Grains: Give yourself one point for every serving up to ten fruits/vegetables and six whole grains. | | |
| Subtotal | 1–16 | _____ |
| | | |
| **2.** Fat Consumption: | | |
| Avoided foods cooked in oil or fat. | 4 | _____ |
| Avoided adding butter, margarine, or other fats. to my food, and used olive oil or canola oil sparingly. | 3 | _____ |
| Consumed only extra-lean meats (less than 7 percent fat by weight), poultry breast without the skin, fish, and cooked dried beans and peas. | 4 | _____ |
| Avoided highly processed, convenience foods, such as potato chips, cookies, and granola bars. | 2 | _____ |
| Included a serving of fish. | 1 | _____ |
| Included nuts, seeds, or avocado. | 2 | _____ |
| Subtotal | 16 | _____ |
| | | |
| **3.** Calcium-Rich Foods: Consumed at least three servings of nonfat or low-fat milk or milk products, or the equivalent in other calcium-rich foods, such as fortified soy milk. | | |
| Subtotal | 5 | _____ |

**4.** Iron-Rich Foods:

Included two servings of iron-rich meat or legumes.    3   _____

Included several iron-rich vegetables, such as

spinach, chard, and broccoli.    2   _____

    Subtotal    5   _____

**5.** Sugar and Alcohol:

Limited sugar consumption to two teaspoons

(jelly, jam, table sugar, honey, candy, etc.).    2   _____

Limited desserts, sugary baked goods, and soda pop to

one small serving or less.    2   _____

Consumed no more than one alcoholic beverage (one

beer, one six-ounce glass of wine, or one ounce alcohol).    1   _____

    Subtotal    5   _____

**6.** Salt, Fluids, and Calories:

Avoided adding salt during food preparation and/or

at the table.    1   _____

Avoided high-salt snack items.    1   _____

Consumed at least eight glasses of water.    2   _____

Consumed the recommended number of servings of

all nutrient-dense foods in the Healthy Woman's Diet

or consumed a moderate-dose, balanced

vitamin-mineral supplement when intake was less than

1,500 calories.    1   _____

    Subtotal    5   _____

## Activity

**1.** Exercise:

25 points for the first 30 minutes and 1 point for every

2 minutes after that of low-to-moderate-intensity,

continuous activity. No points for less than 30 minutes.

40 points maximum.

    Subtotal    40   _____

**2.** Practical Activity:
Movement during the day, including climbing stairs,
gardening, vacuuming, etc. No points for less than
one hour.

|  |  |  |
|---|---|---|
| Subtotal | 6 | _____ |

**Healthy Behaviors**

| | | |
|---|---|---|
| I ate only when I was hungry and stopped eating when I was satisfied, but not overly full. | 2 | _____ |
| I ate at least three meals and snacks today. | 1 | _____ |
| I maintained my weight or, if I'm overweight, lost no more than two pounds per week. | 1 | _____ |
| Subtotal | 4 | _____ |

| | | |
|---|---|---|
| Total | 100 | _____ |

## *Stress and Your Diet*

Nutritional needs are at an all-time high during stress, but ironically, this is when many of us eat at our worst! Attempting to fuel your body with a poor diet is a stress in itself, since suboptimal amounts of even one or more nutrients, from vitamin A to zinc, place a strain on all the body's processes. Second, stress increases your body's need for some vitamins, minerals, and choline: consequently, you are more vulnerable to nutritional deficiencies when stressed than during almost any other time in life. Finally, how well your body is nourished prior to and during a stressful event affects how well you handle the stress. In short, a well-nourished person is more likely to cope better and rebound faster from stress than is a poorly nourished one.

A look at iron, the antioxidants, and magnesium demonstrates how stress and diet overlap. Low iron intake, especially in women, results in poor oxygen supply to the brain and tissues. This aggravates feelings of fatigue and poor concentration that accompany stress. On the other hand, low intake of the antioxidant vitamins

C and E weakens the immune system during stress and increases your risk of developing a cold or infection. Finally, magnesium requirements increase during stress and if you don't meet that increased demand by eating more magnesium-rich whole grains, soybeans, greens, or wheat germ, the low magnesium status can aggravate the stress response and possibly leave you feeling even more irritable.

Many women enter into stress already nutritionally compromised and stress is the straw that breaks the camel's back. The antioxidant nutrients, such as vitamins C and E, are important in regulating the immune system during stress. Daily requirements for the B vitamins also might increase. But minerals are important, too. For example, researchers at the U.S. Department of Agriculture studied the effects of work-related stress on mineral status and found that, despite adequate dietary intake, blood levels of several minerals dropped as much as 33 percent within five days of heavy deadlines at work. Actually, it is difficult to pinpoint any one nutrient, since most vitamins and minerals work as teams in the body and almost any nutrient can be in jeopardy during stress.

Can foods calm you down? Yes. Include a few all-carbohydrate snacks during the day, such as popcorn, graham crackers, a handful of cereal and raisins, or pretzels, to help boost a brain chemical called serotonin, which has a calming effect. Vitamin C helped people cope with stress in a study from the Center for Psychosomatic and Psychobiological Research. In this two-week study, 108 young, healthy adults took placebos or one gram of vitamin C three times daily, while researchers measured the subjects' blood pressure, cortisol levels, and subjective response to psychological stress. Results showed that the vitamin C–supplemented group had lower blood pressures, reduced reactions to stressful situations, and quicker recovery times in blood pressure and cortisol levels following stress compared to the nonsupplemented group. The researchers conclude that these improvements in coping ability were seen only at high-dose supplemental levels, not when people consume normal dietary intakes of vitamin C.

Why do we overeat when stressed? Sometimes the need to munch is more a need for either taste or for something to bite down on. If you need taste, try using salsa as a dip, having a spicy meal such as Thai food or curry, or adding new tastes like mustard or jalapeño relish to sandwiches. If it's crunch you need, then bite into baby carrots, raw broccoli, fat-free tortilla chips, red bell peppers dipped in fat-free sour cream dip, or cantaloupe strips.

Your best plan during stress is to follow these guidelines:

- Skip the caffeine, alcohol, and sugar. These quick fixes, from candy bars, cookies, and coffee to wine, beer, and colas, only aggravate stress. If you can't avoid them, then limit coffee to no more than three cups daily, alcoholic beverages to no more than one a day, and sugar to a small serving daily with meals.
- Eat small meals and snacks. Stress often interferes with appetite, so don't expect to sit down to large meals. Instead, spread your food intake evenly into four to six minimeals and snacks.
- Focus on unprocessed foods. Fuel your day with minimally processed whole grains, vegetables, fruits, and nonfat milk products. For example, have a piece of cantaloupe and yogurt for breakfast; an apple and graham crackers for a midmorning snack; half a turkey sandwich on whole-wheat bread and a salad for lunch; munch on crisp vegetables and dip instead of potato chips midday, then have at least two vegetables along with your entrée for dinner. That will guarantee you're getting the vitamins and minerals, especially the antioxidants, that are so important to keep you healthy during stress.
- Take a supplement. Find a moderate-dose multiple that supplies about 100 percent of the Daily Value for a wide variety of vitamins and minerals. This will fill in the nutritional gaps on those days when you can't eat perfectly. Don't waste your money on stress formulas; they are poorly formulated, supply a poor mix and too much of most nutrients, and are no more effective than a moderate-dose multiple. (If you don't drink at least three glasses of milk daily or consume lots of magnesium-rich greens, soybeans, and wheat germ, you might consider taking a calcium-magnesium supplement, too.)

The bottom line is that too much stress isn't good for you, but sometimes it is unavoidable. So, when you can't beat stress, join it, but go into battle nutritionally well armed.

## Vegetarian Diets

Vegetarian diets have moved from the sidelines into the mainstream in the past two decades. A well-balanced vegetarian diet is safe, healthy, and better for a woman's health and the prevention of diseases, such as arthritis, heart disease, cancer, and diabetes, than more typical American diets.

A well-balanced vegetarian diet easily meets the dietary recommendations for servings of fruits, vegetables, whole grains, and other foods of plant origin. By their nature, vegetarian diets also are high in complex carbohydrates and fiber and lower in saturated fats and cholesterol than diets containing meat. Studies show that women vegetarians consume more fiber, vitamins, and minerals, and less fat and cholesterol than do women who include meat in their diets.

There are several different types of vegetarian diets.

- A lacto-ovo vegetarian is one who eats fresh fruits and vegetables, whole-grain breads and cereals, cooked dried beans and peas, nuts and seeds, milk products, and eggs, but avoids meat, chicken, and fish.
- A lacto vegetarian avoids meat, chicken, fish, and eggs.
- An ovo vegetarian avoids meat, chicken, fish, and milk products.
- A strict vegetarian or vegan consumes only foods of plant origin and avoids all animal-derived products, including meat, chicken, fish, eggs, and dairy products.

People who avoid red meat, but eat chicken and/or fish, are not vegetarians.

## Dispelling the Protein Myth

The biggest myth about vegetarian diets is that they do not supply enough protein. Except for the vegan diet, most vegetarian menus contain ample protein from milk products, whole grains, beans, and nuts.

Protein is made up of building blocks called amino acids. Approximately twenty-plus amino acids are needed to build tissues, red blood cells, and the hundreds of other protein-rich molecules that sustain life. The body can produce all but eight to ten of these amino acids, which must be obtained from the diet. This cluster of amino acids is called the "essential amino acids," not because they are any more important than the other amino acids, but because it is essential that they are obtained from the diet.

Meat, chicken, fish, eggs, and milk products contain all the essential amino acids and are called "complete" or high-quality protein foods. Whole grains, dried beans and peas, nuts, seeds, and vegetables contain varying amounts of the essential amino acids, so are called "incomplete" proteins.

### Complementary Proteins

Nature, in its infinite wisdom, balances the amino acids in whole grains and cooked dried beans and peas, so that when the two are eaten together, the result is a complete or high-quality protein. For example, beans are low in the amino acid methionine and are high in the amino acid lysine, while whole grains are high in methionine and low in lysine. A bowl of baked beans and brown bread, lentil and rice soup, or a peanut butter sandwich combine two incomplete proteins to make a high-quality protein. In addition, combining a high-quality protein, such as cheese, with an incomplete protein, such as a whole-grain bagel, also produces a complementary protein-rich meal.

All the essential amino acids are not required at the same meal. The body maintains an "amino acid pool," so as long as complementary proteins are consumed sometime during the day normal protein metabolism is maintained. For example, an English muffin at breakfast and a bowl of lentil soup at lunch provides ample amounts of essential amino acids for normal body functions. Even vegetarian exercisers and athletes can consume enough protein to meet the extra demands of sports as long as three servings of milk products, two or more servings of cooked dried beans and peas, and at least 2,000 calories of nutrient-dense foods are consumed daily.

### More Important Nutritional Considerations

For all vegetarians, except vegans, complementing proteins is a minor issue, since numerous combinations of protein-containing foods are included in the daily diet. Other nutrients are much more likely to be low unless care is taken to ensure the right proportion and amounts of nutrient-rich foods.

For example, red meat, chicken, and seafood are the best sources of iron and zinc. In addition, a high-fiber diet, which is typical of most vegetarian diets, interferes with iron and zinc absorption. Finally, the iron in plant foods is poorly absorbed compared to "heme" iron in meat. Consequently, some vegetarians consume too little of these minerals and what is consumed is poorly absorbed. If a lacto-ovo or lacto vegetarian relies heavily on milk products for protein, it is almost a given that the diet will be inadequate in iron and zinc.

To ensure optimal intake of these minerals, at least three servings of cooked dried beans and peas, nuts, and seeds should be included in the daily diet. A woman might consider an iron supplement if intake is below 3,000 calories a day.

**TABLE 2.6     Guidelines for Vegetarian Diets**

The same guidelines in the Healthy Woman's Diet apply to vegetarians, except more servings of cooked dried beans and peas replace the recommendations for meat. Ovo vegetarians also must consume more dark green vegetables, tofu, and calcium-fortified soy milk to meet their calcium and vitamin $B_2$ needs, and must find a supplemental source of vitamin D.

1. Limit empty-calorie foods high in sugar or fat, and choose a variety of fresh or frozen plain fruits and vegetables (five servings or more).
2. Replace meat with eggs, cooked dried beans and peas, nuts and seeds (occasionally), and meat alternatives (four servings or more).
3. Use low-fat or nonfat milk products, such as yogurt, cheese, cottage cheese, kefir, and buttermilk (three servings or more).
4. Select whole grains, rather than refined or "enriched" grains (six servings or more).
5. Include several servings daily of iron-rich and zinc-rich foods, such as dark green leafy vegetables and legumes.

## A Closer Look at Vegans

A woman who chooses a vegan diet is most susceptible to vitamin and mineral deficiencies, especially vitamin $B_2$, vitamin $B_{12}$, vitamin D, calcium, iron, and zinc. Every day she must consume foods rich in these nutrients or take a well-balanced vitamin/mineral supplement.

The only reliable plant sources of vitamin $B_{12}$ are fermented soy products (i.e., miso or tempeh) and vitamin $B_{12}$-fortified soy milk. Vitamin D is obtained from exposing the skin to sunlight, fortified soy milk, or supplements.

## *Simple Changes*

Making changes in what and how you eat takes time. Don't try to change everything at once. Make small changes, like switching from white bread to whole-wheat bread, adding an additional serving of calcium-rich milk or soy milk, or adding one extra serving of fruits or vegetables to your daily menu. These little steps accumulate over time slowly adapting your eating to fit the Healthy Woman's Diet guidelines.

---

**TABLE 2.7    The Vegan Diet**

The daily food guide for women on strict vegetarian diets includes:

**Vegetables:** five or more servings. At least two servings should be dark green leafy vegetables and 1 raw salad.

**Fruits:** four or more servings. At least one iron-rich selection, such as strawberries or watermelon, and one vitamin C–rich selection, such as oranges or grapefruit.

**Grains:** six or more servings. Whole-grain varieties only.

**Cooked dried beans and peas:** three or more servings. Beans are preferable to nuts and seeds as a low-fat protein source.

**Soy milk:** three servings. Choose varieties that are fortified with calcium, vitamin D, and vitamin $B_{12}$.

---

# CHAPTER 3

# *Supermarket Savvy*

Half the battle of changing eating habits is learning how to shop and bring only foods on the Healthy Woman's Diet into your home. Becoming familiar with the best food choices, getting to know where to find them at the store, figuring out how to decipher marketing hype, and learning to read food labels might take a little extra time at first, but I guarantee it will pay off in the future and eventually become second nature.

## *Plan Ahead*

Careful planning prior to shopping saves time and helps to avoid impulse shopping (for all the wrong stuff!). A list based on a thorough check of the cupboards, refrigerator, and freezer for needed items, and a plan for the week's meals and snacks help you stay on track. A list posted on the refrigerator is handy for jotting down needed items and organizing the shopping list according to the sections of the grocery store.

At the store, the most important rule is to be fat and sugar conscious. Shop primarily around the periphery of the grocery store, where most of the minimally processed, low-fat foods are located. The produce department, dairy case, meat and fish department, and bakery usually line the side walls and back of the store. Other nutritious foods, such as whole-grain cereals, noodles, canned and frozen vegetables, and dried beans and peas are located on a few aisles, while the greatest percentage of shelf space is devoted to processed and convenience foods. If the grocery store does not carry some nutritious items, such as baby food prunes to use as a fat substitute in baking, soy milk, or the sugar substitute Splenda, ask the grocery-store manager to stock these items or purchase them from a health-food store.

Planning ahead helps you get in and out of the store in record time. The longer you shop, the more likely you'll succumb to marketing tricks that entice you to purchase unnecessary or high-priced items. Impulse foods are often placed at eye level, at the end of aisles, out of place, or at the checkout stand. Hunger reduces your resistance to these impulse foods, so never go to the store hungry. Mothers be aware that shopping with small children also can result in unnecessary food purchases, unless you plan ahead what foods are nutritionally acceptable.

Take advantage of advertised sales, coupons, and specials only if they are compatible with the guidelines of the Healthy Woman's Diet. Check unit pricing and buy economy-sized items only if they really save money. Some people also find it useful to bring a calculator to estimate the cost per serving, the fat content of foods based on label information, or to maintain a running total of the food bill.

---

**TABLE 3.1    Your Shopping List**

Use the following shopping list as a guide for purchasing low-fat, nutrient-dense foods.

### Produce: Fruits, Vegetables, Tofu

All fresh fruits and vegetables
Fruits canned in own juices
Juices: Orange, grapefruit, prune, vegetable (canned, bottled, or frozen concentrate)
Tofu: Firm, silken, regular
Dried fruit

### Bakery/Grains/Cereals

100 percent whole-wheat bread, bagels, English muffins, pita bread, rolls, and tortillas
Corn tortillas
Whole-wheat crackers: Akmak, Ry-Krisp, or other low-fat whole-wheat crackers
Popcorn, air popped
Brown rice (instant or regular), brown basmati or Texmati rice, Wehani rice, wild rice
Hot cereals/grains: Rolled oats, Kashi, bulgur, quinoa, barley, and other whole-grain cereals
Whole-grain ready-to-eat cereals: Shredded Wheat, NutriGrain, Post Whole Wheat Raisin
        Bran, Grape-Nuts, low-fat granola, Puffed Kashi
Wheat germ

Pasta: Whole-wheat noodles, spinach noodles, enriched noodles

Flour: Whole-wheat, rye, oat, unbleached white flour (less nutritious than the whole-grain varieties)

## Other Canned and Packaged Goods

All dried beans and peas, including kidney, black, garbanzo, navy, soybean, lentils, split peas, and lima

Canned cooked dried beans and peas (beans in dishes such as chili or baked beans should be chosen on an individual basis by their fat content)

Packaged bean mixes, such as hummus and lentil pilaf

Nut butters, including peanut, almond, soy, and cashew (choose major brand names to ensure low levels of aflatoxin)

Tomato sauce, tomato paste, canned tomatoes

Low-fat marinara sauce

Salsa

## Dairy Case

Nonfat or 1 percent fat milk, plain yogurt, buttermilk, and cottage cheese

Low-fat cheeses

Fat-free or low-fat ricotta cheese

Fat-free cream cheese, sour cream, Half & Half, whipped cream

Eggs or egg substitutes

## Meat and Fish

Chicken or turkey breast, remove the skin before cooking

Extra-lean beef, i.e., 7 percent fat or less by weight

Extra-lean pork

All fresh and frozen fish and shellfish

Canned or packaged tuna, packed in water

## Oils and Fats

Low-calorie margarine

Fat-free or low-calorie salad dressing

Fat-free or low-calorie mayonnaise

Safflower oil, olive oil, canola oil

Dry roasted nuts, such as almonds
Sunflower seeds

**Sweets and Desserts**

Jam (preferably all-fruit, no-sugar variety)
Honey
Sugar-free pudding mixes
Sugar substitutes: aspartame, Splenda
Baby food prunes (as fat replacement in recipes)
Angel food cake mix
Sherbet
Vanilla wafers
Frozen fruit bars and fruit ices
Low-fat ice creams, sorbets

---

# Read Labels

A label provides information on the nutrient composition of a food, including the calories and grams of protein, fat, and carbohydrates per serving, which is helpful in determining the percentage of calories supplied by fat (i.e., the fat calories). The Healthy Woman's Diet contains less than 30 percent fat calories. Although some foods can be higher in fat than others and still meet this quota, in general, when purchasing foods, choose items that are within this allotment.

*The 3 Grams of Fat Rule:* Look for foods that contain no more than 3 grams of fat for every 100 calories. (Each gram of fat supplies 9 calories, so the grams of fat in a serving multiplied by 9, divided by the total number of calories, and multiplied by 100 equals the percentage of fat calories.) A serving of yogurt that supplies 5 grams of fat for 150 calories would be the equivalent of 30 percent fat calories (5 grams × 9 calories = 45 fat calories divided by 150 total calories × 100 = 30 percent fat).

Labels are confusing when it comes to fat. Comparing grams of protein or carbohydrate to grams of fat is deceptive, since a gram of fat has more than twice the calories of a gram of carbohydrate or protein. Consequently, a product that contains fewer grams of fat than grams of carbohydrate and protein still might be a high-fat item.

In addition, often foods are labeled according to the percentage of fat by weight, not by calories. Ground beef labeled "less than 22 percent fat" is actually as high as 60 percent fat calories. Whole milk labeled as 3.5 percent fat (by weight) is actually 50 percent fat calories. In short, seldom do foods disclose the fat calories, the shopper must calculate this from information provided on the label, i.e., the number of fat grams and the calories per serving.

*Calories on Labels:* If you are weight conscious, use the calorie information provided on a label to compare different foods or to tally daily calorie intakes. For example, a one-cup serving of whole milk supplies 160 calories, while the same serving of nonfat milk contains only 90 calories. They both contain equal amounts of all other nutrients, including calcium, protein, vitamin $B_2$, vitamin D, and magnesium, but the whole milk has a higher fat and calorie cost.

*How Much Sugar Is in a Food?* The sugar content and nutrient density of a food sometimes can be determined by information on a label. Some labels provide detailed information on the sugar and complex carbohydrate content of the food item. For easy reference, 4 grams of sugar equal 1 teaspoon, 12 grams of sugar equal 1 table-spoon. A ready-to-eat cereal that contains 13 grams of sugar (more than 1 table-spoon) could contain more than 50 percent of its calories from sugar. Most labels, however, only disclose the total carbohydrates, which lumps all starch and sugars into one category. If this is the case, turn to the ingredient list to estimate sugar.

*Use the Ingredients List:* The ingredients list on a label provides a general indication of the nutrient content of a food. Foods are listed in descending order according to weight, so the ingredients listed first are present in the greatest amount. A food is likely to be high in calories and low in nutrients if fats or sugars are listed in the first three ingredients. All fat—whether it is polyunsaturated, monounsaturated, saturated, or a fatty acid, or listed as vegetable oil, milk fat, or hydrogenated vegetable oil—contains the same amount of calories.

Sugar is disguised by a variety of names, such as dextrose, sucrose, fructose, "natural sweeteners," honey, brown sugar, corn sweeteners, and corn syrup, and often appears more than once in an ingredient list. It is the total amount of all sugars that is important to note. Any food with more than one source of sugar is probably too high in sugar.

## Label Lingo

The language on labels is designed to promote sales, not nutrition. Labels have become so deceptive and confusing that in 1990 Congress passed the National

Labeling and Education Act (NLEA), which attempted to simplify label lingo and protect the consumer against fraud. Despite this law, beware of the following:

- "Wheat flour" does not mean whole-wheat flour. Most breads are made from wheat flour; however, most of this flour is *refined* wheat flour, which is white flour. A product must state "100 percent whole wheat" or it probably contains primarily refined flour.

- An ingredient list on a label that reads "vegetable oil" could contain either saturated fats, such as coconut oil or palm oil, or unsaturated fats, such as safflower oil or corn oil. Hydrogenated vegetable oils found in shortening, margarine, crackers, French fries, and many snack foods also contain saturated fat and trans fatty acids. These altered polyunsaturated fats act more like saturated fats in the body and are linked to an increased risk for heart disease and possibly cancer.

- Products that claim to be low in cholesterol still might be high in fat, salt, or other unhealthful ingredients. For example, a peanut butter that claims "no cholesterol" is deceiving, since no peanut butter contains cholesterol. The product contains the same amount of fat and calories as any other peanut butter on the grocery-store shelf.

- Note the wording of ingredients. "Beef flavoring" is flavoring, not beef. A soup titled "Noodles and Chicken" contains more noodles than chicken; whereas another soup titled "Chicken and Noodles" contains more chicken.

- The words "diet" or "dietetic" do not necessarily provide fewer calories. A diet product is defined as any food that is lower in sodium, cholesterol, protein, or other food components; calories may be the same, higher, or lower than a comparable product.

- The word "sodium" in the title of any ingredient, such as monosodium glutamate (MSG), bisodium carbonate, or sodium nitrite, is the same sodium found in sodium chloride or table salt.

- More than half of all Americans think "natural foods" are more nutritious than other foods. Terms, such as natural, organic, and health food, are, in many cases, meaningless. The most important considerations when choosing nutritious foods are that they are fresh, wholesome, and minimally processed.

- "Fruit flavored drinks" and "fruit drinks" contain little or no real fruit juice. "Fruit juice" is 100 percent fruit juice. However, many mixed fruit juices contain concentrates of apple, pear, or white grape juice, which is deceptive, since these highly refined juices are just sugar water.

- "Sugar-free" or "sugarless" means the food contains no sucrose (table sugar); however, other sugars, such as high-fructose corn syrup or brown sugar, can be included.
- Foods that claim "no preservatives" still can contain sweeteners, fat, emulsifiers, stabilizers, flavorings, colorings, and other additives. Foods flavored with "natural flavors" also may contain synthetic flavor enhancers.

## *"Enriched" and "Fortified" Foods*

Many convenience foods, from bread and rice to milk and "fruit" drinks, are either enriched or fortified with vitamins or minerals.

"Enriched" refers to the addition of vitamins or minerals to the level previously found before the food was processed. For example, bread made with white flour is enriched with three vitamins (vitamin $B_1$, vitamin $B_2$, and niacin) and one mineral (iron) to replace the loss of these nutrients during the refining process. The term "enriched" is deceiving, since it implies extra nutritional benefits when in reality many more nutrients and fiber have been removed than are replaced. "Enriched" products are actually poor nutritional substitutes for their original, unprocessed, wholesome foods, which are higher in magnesium, vitamin E, vitamin $B_6$, fiber, chromium, selenium, and phytochemicals.

The term "fortified" means that one or more vitamins or minerals have been added to levels greater than were originally found in the unprocessed food. Fortifying some foods has been beneficial, such as the fortification of milk with vitamin D, which reduced the risk of rickets in children, or grains with folic acid, which helps lower birth defects. The fortification of salt with iodine reduced the risk for developing goiter.

Fortification is misused when random amounts of nutrients or herbs are added to otherwise nutrient-poor, highly processed foods, such as high-sugar breakfast cereals, fruit drinks, soft drinks, or granola bars. Usually these nutrients make an otherwise junk food look nutritious. In all cases, the original, minimally processed food is more nutritious than the processed and fortified product, since convenience foods never are fortified with all the nutrients, fiber, or other essential dietary factors at the same level as found in the original food.

## *Convenience Foods: What Is the Nutritional Cost?*

Foods prepared at home from scratch have given way to convenience foods, or foods partially or entirely manufactured outside the home. The number of convenience foods has rapidly increased since the 1940s and includes everything from ready-to-eat cereals and frozen waffles to gravy packets and powdered fruit punch.

Some convenience foods are minimally processed versions of natural foods, such as 100 percent whole-wheat bread or pure frozen orange juice. These selections retain most of the original nutrient content, while supplying relatively few calories. Most convenience foods, however, are highly processed, refined, fabricated, canned, packaged, enriched, fortified, engineered, condensed, tenderized, powdered, flaked, freeze-dried, or precooked to varying degrees. They often contain additives, synthetic vitamins, or have lost much of their original vitamin, mineral, and fiber content.

In general, the more processed a food, the higher its content of fat, salt, sugar, calories, and/or cholesterol and the lower its content of vitamins, minerals, phytochemicals, and fiber. For this reason, fresh broccoli is better than frozen broccoli with cheese sauce, rolled oats are better than a granola bar, a baked potato is better than potato chips, and nonfat milk is more nutritious than ice cream.

When purchasing convenience foods, choose minimally processed products that contain whole grains, plain fruits and vegetables or canned versions packaged in their own juice, nonfat or low-fat milk products, chicken, fish, legumes, or lean cuts of meat. Ignore the label claims and go straight to the nutrition information on the back. Only purchase convenience foods that follow the "3 grams of fat" rule. For example, many luncheon meats labeled as 80 percent fat-free actually contain as much as 12 grams of fat in two slices, or the equivalent of almost three teaspoons of fat!

**TABLE 3.2    Shopping Cart Face-Lift**

Here are some suggestions to filling your cart with healthful alternatives to your favorite foods.

| OUT WITH THE OLD | IN WITH THE NEW | THE BENEFITS |
| --- | --- | --- |
| Granola bar | Bite-size frosted Shredded Wheat | 94 percent less fat |
| Vanilla ice cream | Low-fat vanilla ice cream | 83 percent less fat |
| Ground beef (15 percent fat) | Ground beef (5 percent fat) | 58 percent less fat/ounce |
| Cinnamon roll | Cinnamon-raisin bread | 50 percent less fat/2 slices |
| Potato chips and dip | Baked tortilla chips and salsa | 95 percent less fat |
| Ranch dressing | Light ranch dressing | 50 percent less fat |
| 2 percent milk | 1 percent milk | 45 percent less fat/cup |
| Frozen broccoli in cheese sauce | Fresh broccoli | 100 percent less fat |

# Artificial Sweeteners

If you're like most women, you could cut your sugar intake in half and still be overdoing it. Averaging 20 to 40 teaspoons of sugar every day, we would do well to tame our sweet tooths. But there is no reason to cut out sweets, just because you're cutting back on sugar. You often can cut sugar in recipes by up to a third without altering the taste. Also, several no-calorie substitutes are available that would make any sugar freak proud. All of these substitutes can be found at your local grocer on the same aisle as sugar and baking goods.

*Aspartame (NutraSweet or Equal):* This no-calorie sweetener has been more intensely studied than almost any other additive. No, it doesn't cause brain tumors, and yes, it is safe, except for people with a rare genetic disorder called PKU and for a few people who develop headaches when they go overboard. Aspartame works particularly well in drinks or desserts that require minimal cooking. It does have an aftertaste.

*Splenda:* Also called sucralose, this sugar substitute is derived from sugar but is altered so the digestive tract doesn't recognize it as sugar. It is much sweeter than sugar, and has no calories and no effect on digestion, nutrition, or blood-sugar levels, so it's safe for diabetics. You can cook with Splenda; it's great for cakes, pies, and cookies, like oatmeal cookies. Because Splenda doesn't brown, you can't use it for sugar cookies or a cobbler that needs a golden crust. It's safe for pregnant women, too. It has very little aftertaste.

*Stevia:* This sugar substitute is an herb with an active ingredient called stevio-side that is two hundred to three hundred times sweeter than sugar, yet is calorie-free. No adverse effects have been reported in Japan, where Stevia has been used for the past thirty years. However, it is not allowed in Canada or some European countries and has not been approved by the U.S. Food and Drug Administration (FDA) because of some unresolved concerns about its effect on fertility and other health issues. For this reason, you won't find Stevia at your local grocery, but you can find it in powdered and extract forms at the health-food store. Stevia has a bitter aftertaste, so you'll have to experiment using it in recipes or mixing it with some sugar for desserts.

*Saccharin:* Don't forget good old saccharin, which was taken off the cancer-causing substances list in May 2000 when officials announced there was no clear association between saccharin (Sweet'N Low) and cancer in humans. It also has an aftertaste, so it takes some getting used to.

## Functional Foods

Forget the pharmacy. Now you can boost brain power with chewing gum. Curb depression with potato chips. Lower risk of heart disease with salad dressing. Strengthen bones with orange juice. Even get your vegetables in candy. Welcome to functional foods, the latest trend to hit your supermarket.

A functional food, according to the Institute of Medicine's Food and Nutrition Board (the same people who develop the Recommended Dietary Allowances), is any food or food component that provides a health benefit beyond traditional nutrients it contains. Calcium-fortified orange juice qualifies as a functional food because calcium is not found naturally in this food, but calcium-rich yogurt doesn't. Other functional foods range from fiber-enhanced potato chips and energy bars laced with antioxidants to omega-3-enriched eggs and herb-fortified drinks.

Functional foods are now the number one trend in the food industry, according to Clare Hasler, Ph.D., executive director of the Functional Foods for Health Program, the nation's leading center of research into medicinal benefits of foods and food extracts. They also are as controversial as they are profitable. The FDA has yet to impose guidelines on these new items, allowing manufacturers free rein and few restrictions. The impressive health claims attached to these products also blur the line between food and medicine. "Scientifically, herbs are drugs, so to add them to processed foods makes as much sense as adding aspirin to soup or diazepam to potato chips," says Varro Tyler, Ph.D., Sc.D., former distinguished professor emeritus in the School of Pharmacy at Purdue University. On the other hand, some functional foods could improve your diet and health. Here are the questions to ask when sifting hype from health in the realm of bionic foods.

## Does It Do the Job?

A wealth of evidence supports adding calcium to orange juice or soy milk to prevent bone loss or folic acid to grains to prevent birth defects. There's also reason to find alternative sources of omega-3 fatty acids, fats shown to lower heart-disease risk but found primarily in seafood. But what about a fruit juice that claims its ginseng will "jump-start your day" or a snack bar with gingko promising to boost mental function? "The research on many of the herbs added to functional foods is sketchy at best, and even then are only useful for people with serious health concerns. There's no evidence that these herbs help healthy people with routine forgetfulness or fatigue," says David Schardt, associate nutritionist for the Center for Science in the Public Interest in Washington, D.C.

## What Are You Getting?

Even if a functional food contains beneficial ingredients, does it supply enough to do the job? Foods fortified with vitamins and minerals, such as milk with vitamin D, must list amounts on the label. That's not the case with phytochemicals or herbs. "You don't get a therapeutic dose of any herb in any product I'm aware of," says Dr. Tyler. "Often we're not told how much is in the food and even the manufacturer doesn't know."

The same concerns go for phytochemicals, the thousands of nonnutrients in plants that lower our risk for disease and boost immunity. Even if stated, no one knows optimal doses for lycopene, the sulfur compounds from garlic, or any of the other 12,000 phytochemicals. Most people don't know when a herbal dose is too much or too little. For example, an energy bar with ginkgo biloba says it supplies 20 mg of the herb. How many people snacking on this bar know that it would take six of them, for a total of 1,200 calories, to get an effective dose of the herb?

These companies counter by saying their products are meant to supplement a consumer's regular supplements, not to supply an entire day's requirement. But adding up the dosages from drinks, foods, and supplements makes it difficult to keep track of how much you're taking. To be on the safe side, avoid any product that doesn't list how much of the herb or active ingredient is in each serving.

## Is It Safe?

Some experts argue that tinkering with uncharted food territories is blindly messing with a good thing. "We know so little about optimal doses, interactions, or long-term consequences of most phytochemicals and herbs that to begin adding them haphazardly into foods could produce any number of potential toxic effects," warns Winston Craig, Ph.D., R.D., chairman and professor of nutrition at Andrews University in Michigan.

Beta carotene taught us the importance of whole foods over single components. For years, studies showed a diet high in beta carotene–rich foods reduced cancer risk. So supplement and food companies added this phytochemical to supplements and cereals. Subsequent studies using beta carotene supplements found that, at best, beta carotene had no effect and might even raise cancer risk in smokers.

When it comes to herbs, you shouldn't take them lightly. "Herbs are drugs and like other drugs, they can have side effects or can interact with other medications," warns Dr. Tyler. Saint-John's-wort should not be taken with antidepressant drugs, kava might interact with antianxiety medications, and echinacea produces allergic reactions in some people.

It's also a crapshoot whether or not you'll know the functional food is harming your health. "It's relatively easy to identify harmful side effects from medications, but how will we make the connection between symptoms like heart palpitations or headaches and a varied diet that contains a functional food?" questions Cyndi Thomson, Ph.D., R.D., spokesperson on functional foods for the American Dietetic Association.

## It Glitters. Does That Mean It's Gold?

We have an age-old belief that foods have medicinal properties, which explains why nine out of ten people believe that certain foods have health benefits beyond just basic nutrition. That must be the reason we're willing to wolf down nutrient-fortified snack bars that taste like sweetened dog chow or herb-laced cereal with the texture of cardboard under the guise that they're good for us.

You don't see Mother Nature's functional foods, like broccoli or strawberries, touted as mood boosters and energizers at the supermarket. It's the processed items, in many cases gilded junk food, that are fortified with a handful of nutrients to create the false impression of a product that is somehow valuable. Since when did sugar-laden products become health foods? Fortified or not, these products are not as nutritious as wholesome real food.

## Can You Get It Cheaper Elsewhere?

Most functional foods are costly. So, if you have your heart set on taking Saint-John's-wort, flaxseed, or some other health food, find out if there is a more economical way to get it. For example, a fruit beverage with ginkgo might cost more than two dollars a day for the recommended herbal dose of 120 mg, while you can buy ginkgo supplements and get the same standardized dose for fifty-one cents a day. An energy bar that supplies your daily vitamin C needs for about a dollar is costly compared to a glass of orange juice that does the same thing for pennies.

## Can You Overdo It?

Just picture it. It's late, you're tired, but before you can drop like deadweight into that inviting bed, you have one more task at hand: Total up your functional food intake. For calcium, you poured milk on your cereal this morning. That's about 300 mg. Then there was the glass of calcium-fortified orange juice—another 350 mg. You snacked on an energy bar at lunch (the label says it supplies 35 percent of the Daily Value for calcium so that's about 350 mg), and quenched your thirst with a glass of sparkling juice with calcium. That added another 100 mg. You tallied about 1,100 mg of calcium without adding the yogurt you had for lunch, the calcium-fortified rice at dinner, and the bowl of ice cream in the evening. Besides, it's late and you've got twelve other functional foods to tally. Skip it, you're going to bed.

Should you be concerned about getting too much nutrition from functional foods? With herbs, you could be getting too much if you take supplements plus munch on too many herb-laced products. Children are a particular concern here, according to Dr. Thomson. "We haven't a clue how these herbs affect kids, but we do know that children's bodies are likely to be more sensitive to effects compared to adults," adds Thomson.

Most nutrition experts agree that it is difficult to overdo it when it comes to nutrients in foods. "A person is not likely to overdose on a nutrient like calcium from foods for the very reason that we are limited by how much we can eat," says Fergus Clydesdale, Ph.D., in the Department of Food Science at the University of Massachusetts. Besides, these nutrients are often added for the very reason that we don't get enough. Just use some common sense and supplement a great diet with a few of these fortified foods.

Functional foods aren't magic bullets. Some improve our health or reduce our risk for disease. But they are not the answer to dysfunctional diets, so don't lose your incentive to drink orange juice or eat broccoli just because you got your vitamin C from a soft drink.

---

### TABLE 3.3    Five Functional Foods Worth Trying

The following functional foods really deliver on their promise, are backed by solid research, and taste great!

**1. Tropicana Pure Premium Orange Juice with Calcium (and Vitamin C)**

*Active Ingredient:* One cup supplies 350 mg of calcium as calcium citrate malate, a very absorbable form of calcium.

*How Much Do You Need?* Children and adults need between 1,000 mg and 1,300 mg of calcium daily from a variety of sources.

*Comments:* Most people don't get enough calcium, which places them at increased risk for osteoporosis. For those who can't get enough of this bone-building mineral from milk, calcium-fortified orange juice is a great alternative.

**2. Benecol and Take Control Margarines**

*Active Ingredient:* Sterols and stanol esters, extracts from pine tree bark.

*How Much Do You Need?* 1 packet of Benecol (contains 1.5 grams of plant stanol esters) three times daily or 1 to 2 tablespoons of Take Control.

*Comments:* Stanol esters prevent the body from absorbing dietary cholesterol and also help remove cholesterol from the body, thus lowering blood cholesterol levels and potentially reducing heart-disease risk. Only useful when combined with a low-saturated fat, high-fiber diet and exercise. Benecol also comes as salad dressings; two tablespoons of full-fat Ranch dressing is equivalent to 1 packet of Benecol margarine.

### 3. 8th Continent Soymilk

*Active Ingredient:* Calcium and vitamins A, $B_2$, $B_{12}$, and D.

*How Much Do You Need?* Three glasses supply the same amount of these nutrients as is found in three glasses of milk.

*Comments:* Fortified soy milk is the best alternative source of calcium and vitamin D for people who do not drink enough milk.

### 4. Vitamin E and/or Omega-3-Rich Eggs

*Active Ingredient:* The antioxidant vitamin E and/or omega-3 fatty acids.

*How Much Do You Need?* Amounts vary, with most brands containing about 3 mg of vitamin E and anywhere from 100 mg to 500 mg omega-3 fatty acids per egg. (Daily recommended amount for the omega-3s is 1 gram or more.)

*Comments:* Depending on the brand, contains 20 to 50 percent of the Daily Value for vitamin E, which means you still must take a supplement to reach the 100 IU to 400 IU of vitamin E recognized to lower heart disease. However, these eggs provide an alternative to fish as a source of omega-3 fatty acids that might lower risk for numerous health problems, such as heart disease, cancer, and depression. Most companies feed hens only natural, all-vegetarian diets.

### 5. Viactiv Soft Calcium Chews

*Active Ingredient:* Calcium.

*How Much Do You Need?* Each chew packs in 500 mg of calcium and 100 IU of vitamin D, to aid in calcium absorption. One to two chews will meet your total day's need for calcium.

*Comments:* Each chew is sweetened with a teaspoon of sugar (as corn syrup) and they're a bit pricey, but this supplement tastes so good you'll look forward to tomorrow's dose. (Keep out of the reach of children, who might overdose on these tasty treats!)

## CHAPTER 4

# *Healthy, Quick-Fix Cooking*

As a nutritionist, I've promised people for more than two decades that it won't cost any more to eat well—or take any more time—than it does to eat poorly. I'm also convinced you don't need to sacrifice taste or enjoyment to save your waistline or heart. Most people don't believe me. Typical responses are "Come on, how can it cost less to eat California plums and imported olive oil?" or "You mean to tell me a home-cooked meal from scratch takes no more time than takeout? Come on!"

OK, fresh raspberries out of season are pricey, grilled salmon and a spinach salad outcost a Happy Meal, and some health-conscious recipes take what seems like weeks to prepare. Yet my promise holds true: If you make smart choices, shop carefully, and adopt some cheap-shopping and quick-fix cooking tricks, you can boost your health and shave enough off your food bill and food prep time to afford and find time for a trip to the Caribbean next year!

## *Will It Cost More to Eat Well?*

Surprisingly, very little research has been done on how eating well affects your pocketbook. Adam Drewnowski, Ph.D., professor in the Departments of Epidemiology and Medicine at the University of Washington in Seattle has investigated the subject and says I should start telling people the truth. "It does too cost more to eat well. It's low-quality food that's cheap and comes in supersized portions. You don't see anyone giving away extra servings of arugula or Belgian endive," says Drewnowski. A study from the Rowett Research Institute in Scotland supports Dr. Drewnowski's findings, concluding that fruits and vegetables added to the daily diet jack up the grocery bill.

On the other hand, a study at the Research Institute at Bassett Health Care in Cooperstown, New York, found that a person following a heart-healthy diet reduced the shopping bill by up to $8 a week. For a family of four, that could mean about $1,664 in annual savings. Dietitians at the 5-A-Day program also made a few healthful changes in a typical menu and saved almost $1 a day. Why the discrepancy in the findings? "It's a difficult subject to study, since people can eat poorly on a tight or loose budget, just as they can eat well for more or less," says Susan Krebs-Smith, Ph.D., research nutritionist for the National Cancer Institute in Bethesda.

## Hidden Costs of Cheap Eating

Even if humongous Big Gulps and football-sized hamburgers and doughnuts provide the most calories for the least cost—known in the trade as the "cal-a-buck ratio"—there are hidden costs of eating poorly. "Supersized portions of cheap food appear to be a great deal, but when you factor in the added costs of wardrobes, weight-management programs, health-care costs, and lost days of work due to complications of being overweight, it's not such a bargain," says Barbara Rolls, Ph.D., at Pennsylvania State University in University Park. More than one in every two of us is eating too much, with the extra pounds costing a person more than $5,000 in added health-care bills, plus the more than $33 billion spent annually in this country on weight-loss products and services. Obviously, getting the most calories for your buck—i.e., a good cal-a-buck ratio—isn't cost effective, while getting the most nutrients for your buck is.

## Who Wants to Be a Millionaire?

You don't need to spend freely to eat well. After all, pound for pound, health-boosting oatmeal, beans, and apples are a whole lot cheaper than eggs and bacon, steak, or even chips. Even the prices at a fast-food restaurant can be deceiving. A grilled chicken sandwich is only 20 cents more than a double cheeseburger and, as you'll see in the meal comparison in Table 4.1, "See for Yourself," if you bring a few items from home to complement the sandwich, you even underprice the cost of those meal deals.

*Meat Tricks:* The first place to start is with meat, which accounts for a third of our food bills. You can save money by redefining this one item as a complement, not the main attraction. For example, instead of steak, serve beef stew made with extra-lean meat, carrots, potatoes, celery, mushrooms, and onions, and cut your dinner bill by up to one half. Not only that, but while the steak gets 66 percent of its calories from fat, the stew gets only 29 percent.

---

**TABLE 4.1    See for Yourself**

Still not convinced that you can eat well and save money? Take a look for yourself. You not only can eat healthily, but you'll shave calories, and still save yourself up to $7 a day! That's more than $2,500 during the year . . . enough to pay for a cruise! And that's using bagged salad greens (which are more pricey than regular lettuce, but hey, who's got the time to wash and trim?). You could save even more dollars if you used coupons, bought in bulk, and purchased sale items.

**HEALTHY DAY**

**Breakfast:**

⅔ cup oatmeal cooked in I cup I percent milk
I tablespoon brown sugar
I cup orange juice
Cost: $1.13

**Snack:**

I banana
I cup low-fat, fruited yogurt
Cost: $1.00

**Lunch:**

Grilled chicken sandwich, hold the mayo
I carton I percent milk
I orange (from home)
I cup carrot sticks (from home)
Cost: $4.66

**JUNK FOOD DAY**

**Breakfast:**

Coffee shop special:
I large Café Mocha
I cranberry-orange scone
Cost: $5.60

**Snack:**

I Power Bar
I bottle Fruitopia fruit drink
Cost: $3.25

**Lunch:**

Double cheeseburger
I regular order French fries
I medium chocolate shake

Cost: $5.47

## Snack:

1 cup grapes

Ice water with lemon

Cost: $1.00

## Dinner:

Pork stir-fry:

3 ounces lean pork, sliced thin

1 cup frozen stir-fry vegetables

1 tablespoon hoisin or soy sauce

1 teaspoon minced ginger

½ cup steamed instant brown rice

1 cup Italian-blend salad greens (prebagged)

1 tablespoon creamy bacon dressing

Cost: $3.08

## After-Dinner Snack:

1 baked apple

Cost: $.50

## Nutrition Information:

2,003 calories; 21 percent fat

(47 g fat; 14 g saturated fat),

59 percent carbs (297 g),

20 percent protein (102 g), 30.5 g fiber,

10.5 mg iron,*

1,329 mg calcium.

Total Cost: $11.37

Savings: $7.46

## Snack:

1 ounce potato chips

12-ounce cola

Cost: $1.68

## Dinner:

1 pork chop

½ cup broccoli with cheese sauce

½ cup packaged rice mix

1 cup iceberg lettuce tossed salad

1 tablespoon creamy bacon dressing

Cost: $2.39

## After-Dinner Snack:

2 apple-cinnamon-filled cookies

Cost: $.44

## Nutrition Information:

2,794 calories; 44 percent fat

(138 g fat; 60 g saturated fat),

45 percent carbs (317 g),

11 percent protein (80 g),

12.4 g fiber; 12.4 mg iron,

1,178 mg calcium.

Total Cost: $18.83

*Make sure your multiple vitamin and mineral supplement contains iron.

*Skip the Processed Stuff*: The less processed a food, the more nutritious and less costly it is. A potato costs almost half what a serving of frozen hash browns or Tater Tots costs. You can cut the cost of breakfast in half by switching from cinnamon-flavored oatmeal to plain instant oatmeal. Frozen plain vegetables also tend to be cheaper than canned and are much cheaper than frozen vegetables in sauce.

*Snack on Fruits and Vegetables*: Highly processed snack items aren't as cheap as they look. A small bag of potato chips seems cheap at only 40 cents, but price those chips by the pound and they add up to $6.40—that outprices steak! If you're a typical American, you consume about 5.64 pounds of potato chips a year (or 1,579 chips). Switch to the same pounds of oranges and you'll save more than $32 alone on snacks! Check out Table 4.2, "Cheap Tricks," for more ways to cut costs and boost nutrition without sacrificing enjoyment.

*Skip the Organic*: It is tempting to purchase foods that promise to be pure, void of contaminants, and pesticide free. But these fruits, vegetables, milk products, and others are much more expensive than conventional foods. Wash and peel produce and you eliminate most chemicals, and save yourself a bunch of money.

---

**TABLE 4.2    Cheap Tricks**

Want to get the biggest nutritional bang for your buck? Follow these tried-and-true cost-saving tips and you might just shave enough money off your yearly food bill to afford a trip to Paris!

1. *Buy less expensive produce.* Apples, oranges, bananas, carrots, cabbage, and onions are usually less expensive year-round. Use the expensive mangos, arugula, or papaya to garnish an occasional dish.

2. *Look for specials/use coupons.* Buy discounted foods in quantity and store or freeze. For example, purchase pounds of bananas when they go on sale for 33 cents a pound. Peel and freeze to use in smoothies later.

3. *Buy in bulk.* Oatmeal, rice, nuts, tea, dried fruit, seasonings, sugar, and many other dry goods are now available in bulk bins at supermarkets, health-food stores, discount groceries, and food co-ops. You can buy the exact amount you need *and* cut costs.

4. *Shop at warehouse clubs.* You buy in large quantities at these stores, but comparison shopping can save you big bucks. No place to store the box of apples or case of water-packed tuna? Shop with friends and split the food.

5. *Buy in season.* Raspberries might cost $10 a basket in March, but be patient and enjoy them for a fraction of the price in July.

6. *Bean it up.* Americans average more than eight ounces of meat per person per day, accounting for a third of your food dollars. Follow the Healthy Woman's Diet and switch to beans a few times a week and you'll save hundreds of dollars over the course of the year! A bag of kidney beans costs less than a dollar and provides twelve servings, not to mention fiber, B vitamins, minerals, and protein! Even canned beans are well under a dollar a pound!

7. *Think quantity.* Make extra servings of that stir-fry, stew, soup, or grilled chicken and freeze them in individual containers for future quick-fix instant dinners. Freeze batches of basic sauces, such as tomato-based sauce or low-fat creamed sauces that can be thawed and seasoned (add Italian spices or clams for pasta dishes, peppers and cumin for enchiladas, tuna or shrimp for a creamed dish over rice) for instant meals.

8. *Grow your own.* If you have the space and the time, there is nothing fresher and more rewarding than lettuce, carrots, corn, or other vegetables straight out of your garden. You're also likely to eat more produce when you grow your own. If your family eats a lot of whole-grain bread, consider investing in a bread-making machine, make weekly batches, and save a dollar or more on every loaf.

9. *Visit farmers' markets.* Locally grown produce often is less expensive and fresher than store bought.

10. *Bring food with you.* Stuff your purse, briefcase, glove compartment, diaper bag, or desk drawer with low-fat cheese, peanut butter, whole-wheat breads, oranges, apples, carrot sticks, and other nutritious, low-cost foods so you're less tempted to put a dollar in the vending machine for a candy bar or pull up to a drive-through window for a cheeseburger.

11. *Beware of impulse buying.* That sushi from the deli looked good, but you never got around to eating it. How many bags of lettuce were tossed after sitting in the fridge for a week? Eat before you shop and bring a list to cut back on these wasted food dollars.

12. *What will you really eat?* Take a hard look at your food wastes. If you buy fresh pineapple or peaches but throw out more than you eat, then purchase canned fruit (in its own juice), which can sit on the shelf longer. Bottled lemon juice might be more cost efficient than the real thing if you usually end up throwing out the moldy lemon.

13. *Price compare.* Sure, the whole chicken appears cheaper than the boned and skinned chicken thighs, but when you factor in the amount that is thrown away—a third to half the weight is skin, bones, and unusable parts—you might find that the more expensive cut is actually cheaper. When purchasing produce, consider which fruits and vegetables give you the most edible food for your buck.

**14.** *Eat in more.* We're spending almost half of our food dollars in restaurants these days, where food choices are higher in calories, fat, saturated fat, cholesterol, and cost than homemade food. Limit dining out and you'll be healthier *and* pocket money for that white-water rafting trip or spa vacation.

**15.** *Store it right.* Store vegetables, such as peppers, broccoli, carrots, cauliflower, green onions, and lettuce, in the crisper bin. Artichokes, asparagus, Brussels sprouts, corn, and mushrooms should be stored in the refrigerator, but not the crisper. Keep in mind that even the freshest produce stored under perfect temperatures and humidity conditions maintains best quality for only a few days.

**16.** *Buy generic.* Store brands of frozen vegetables, canned fruit, milk, and other items usually cost less than brand names. Quality can vary, so pick and choose which brands are worth the extra cost.

---

### BOX 4.1    Is Organic Worth the Price?

Organic will cost you. Organic produce is half again and up to three times more expensive than conventional produce. Is it worth the price? The answer depends on what you're after.

If you want more nutrition, then skip organic. Decades of research comparing organic with conventional produce has found only small differences in nutritional quality (organic has slightly more vitamin C). The time of year, the variety of produce, the amount of rain and sunlight, handling, storage, etc., have a far greater impact on a plant's vitamin and mineral content. In short, you'll get more nutrition for your dollars buying vine-ripened, very fresh produce than buying organic.

A better reason to go organic is to reduce intake of pesticide residues, which are lower (but not absent) in organic than in conventional foods. In 1995 alone, United States farmers dumped 566 million pounds of pesticides on our food crops. Pesticide use is even more rampant in other countries. Whether this causes health problems is unknown, but it's probably wise to avoid these contaminants when possible. Some produce, such as strawberries, corn, bananas, green beans, peaches, and apples, because it typically has especially high levels of pesticide residues, might best be bought organic or at least United States grown. Organic baby food also might be a consideration.

## *Will It Take More Time to Eat Well?*

For the past fifteen years, I have been perfecting the art of the quick-fix meal. The search for the twenty-minute meal was a survival thing after my daughter was born. All of a sudden, those leisurely dinners by candlelight and Sundays spent trying new recipes were gone. I didn't have time for a social life, let alone complicated gourmet meals.

The time crunch has hit most of us. We grab a bag of chips while filling the car with gas and zip up to a drive-through window to grab a hamburger on our way to the next appointment. Then we race in the door at 6 P.M. with the family starving and only a half hour before someone's softball practice. Trying to fit a diet into an already overbooked schedule might seem like a no-win situation. Who has time to cut up vegetables, boil beans, or make a salad, when it's so much easier to order Chinese takeout?! I didn't, especially after my second child was born and my work schedule picked up. It seemed the choices were either to choose high-fat foods that fit into my high-speed life or quit my job and spend all day preparing nutritious foods.

I've learned that time isn't the issue when it comes to eating well, especially with the wealth of new, healthful convenience foods. "You don't need to eat a hot meal or even cook to be healthy," says Evelyn Tribole, M.S., R.D., author of *Eating on the Run* (Leisure Press, 1992). In fact, with a well-stocked kitchen, it takes less time to prepare a low-fat, nutritious meal than it does for that takeout order to arrive. It does take a change in mind-set and a little planning up front.

If you think that eating healthy or losing weight requires a total revamp of your eating habits, think again. More often, all it takes are a few minor changes in what, when, or how you eat. I've seen people lose up to thirty pounds by including two fruits or vegetables at every meal or snack. Others are successful when they take the time to eat a five-minute breakfast, which boosts energy and curbs uncontrollable hunger cravings later in the day. For some, paying closer attention to portion size might be all it takes to drop those last five pounds. Many people agree that once they started bringing healthy foods with them, they found it easy to lose weight and stay well.

**Plan Ahead**

For the time-challenged woman, the solution to eating well might not be a lecture on calories or whole grains but a lesson in planning. Getting organized starts in the kitchen. Keep healthful staples on hand, such as pasta, frozen vegetables, and green peppers, onions, and carrots—fresh vegetables that will wait for you. With a well-stocked kitchen you can prepare a tasty and healthful meal with little or no planning.

This weekend, take the one hour you would have spent reading the paper and go grocery shopping. This first shopping spree will be time-intensive, but shopping time will shorten as you familiarize yourself with the options. Basically, you're looking for foods that give you the most nutritional punch for the least calorie bang. These foods are outlined in Table 4.4, "The Supermarket Survival List." Also, think quantity. Shop with the week in mind to avoid extra minitrips during the week.

When shopping, look for no-fuss healthy fast food. You can buy boxes of hummus (all you do is add water and you have a dip or sandwich spread filled with fiber, minerals, and vitamins), fat-free Half & Half, cans of beans, bottled lemon juice, bottled marinara sauce, egg substitutes, minced garlic or ginger, roasted red peppers in a jar, instant brown rice, precooked polenta, de-skinned and boned chicken breast, frozen whole-wheat waffles, and frozen plain vegetables, just to name a few.

To save even more time, prepare extra amounts of foods that are used frequently. For example, cook extra chicken, chop extra celery or green onions, grate extra carrots, or squeeze extra lemon juice and store in the refrigerator to use later in the week. Many dishes—from spaghetti, lasagna, and stew to soups, casseroles, and sauces—can be made in bulk and frozen in individual containers for later use.

**Bring It with You**

Never, *and I mean never,* leave the house without packing your briefcase, purse, backpack, or diaper bag with healthful, quick-fix snacks. Select healthful snacks from Table 4.5, "No Time to Snack? Get a Life!," page 89, to keep in your desk at work, your glove compartment, or your purse, then plan to eat regularly throughout the day to avoid uncontrollable cravings. You wouldn't dream of starting the day without brushing your teeth or combing your hair; in the same way, think of packing this snack survival bag as an essential habit to practice every day.

---

**TABLE 4.4    The Supermarket Survival List**

Your grocery list will vary from week to week, but in general, these are the quick-fix foods that should fill your cart. Use this list along with the shopping list in chapter 3.

- In the produce section (consider this your snack aisle), load the cart with fresh fruits and vegetables, in particular, precut vegetables and bagged salad fixings. Don't forget the minced garlic and bottled lemon juice!
- At the dairy case, choose fat-free or 1 percent low-fat milk, yogurt, and cheese. Also look for fat-free sour cream, Half & Half, whipped cream, and cream cheese.
- In the refrigerated section, pick corn tortillas, fresh pasta, egg substitute, fresh salsa, orange juice in cartons, and premixed hummus.
- In the freezer, load up on whole-wheat waffles, all-fruit sorbet, light vegetarian pizza, frozen plain vegetables and fruit, and low-fat frozen entrées.
- In the bakery section, choose 100 percent whole-wheat bread, bagels, and pocket bread.
- In the aisles, read labels and choose foods that contain no more than 3 grams of fat for every 100 calories. Foods that fit this criteria include canned beans, fat-free whole-wheat crackers, water-packed tuna, low-fat soy milk, whole-grain pastas, whole-grain ready-to-eat cereals, fat-free chocolate syrup, fat-free vinaigrette dressing, low-fat canned soups, Boboli pizza crust and sauce, boxes of couscous, rice pilafs, low-fat pancake mix, instant mashed potatoes, pretzels, dried fruit, canned fruit, and some bottled spaghetti sauce (to name only a few).

---

## *Will Healthy Foods Taste Good?*

How often do you fall victim to your taste buds? You find yourself craving a greasy hamburger, a pepperoni pizza, or a chocolate-frosted doughnut? Have you ever nibbled out of the refrigerator in search of just the right taste? You even might have grazed on hundreds of calories but never felt satisfied.

Taste is one of the most powerful urges to eat, yet many of us ignore the finer flavors, opting for the same old familiar foods. Day in and day out we season our foods with salt. In an effort to eat healthier, we grab baby carrots or an apple, forgetting that food's greatest qualities—it's supposed to taste scrumptious, look appetizing, and smell like heaven—is critical to whether or not we feel satisfied at the end of a meal or snack.

If you think eating healthy means giving up taste, think again. Flavorful, satisfying food doesn't depend solely on fat, salt, and sugar. It's a myth that food has to be dripping in fat and sugar-coated to taste good. You can cut fat, sugar, and salt and never even miss them. Better yet, it doesn't take any more time to prepare low-fat, low-sugar foods. For example, most people know to remove the skin from chicken before cooking, to use broth and wine for sautéing instead of oil, to use broth instead of butter in stuffing, and to use cornstarch and broth instead of butter and flour for a roux when making creamed sauces. We also know we can cut fat by adding more vegetables and salads to the center stage. But you might not know that you can:

- Use potatoes instead of cream to make a rich creamed-vegetable soup.
- Use fruit puree, such as baby prunes, applesauce, apple butter, or Sunsweet Lighter Bake prune puree in place of all or part of the fat in baked goods, such as breads and muffins. (You also can puree 1⅓ cups pitted prunes with 6 tablespoons water until smooth to make your own puree.) One tablespoon of any of these purees replaces 2 table-spoons fat.
- Use kitchen gadgets, such as a fat-separator cup to separate the fat from the liquid in turkey drippings. Combine chicken bouillon granules, flour, salt/pepper, and nonfat milk to make an out-of-this-world gravy that is essentially fat-free. Compare that to traditional turkey gravy, which is almost 50 percent fat calories!
- Take advantage of the fat-free products on the market, such as fat-free Half & Half, cream cheese, cottage cheese, sour cream, whipped cream, and evaporated milk.
- Take advantage of sugar substitutes on the market, such as aspartame (sold as Equal or NutraSweet), Splenda, or saccharin. (See chapter 3 for more information on these sugar substitutes.)
- Take advantage of salt substitutes found in the seasoning section of your grocery store.

You will find that nutritious food has more flavor and is more satisfying than anything you can get at a fast-food restaurant!

**TABLE 4.5     No Time to Snack? Get a Life!**

The following snacks take less time to prepare than grabbing a soda pop from the vending machine. Just remember to bring them along! For each snack, pick at least two items from Group A and one or more items from Group B.

**Group A:**

Fresh fruit (the easiest to carry and eat include apples, oranges, bananas, grapes, peaches, nectarines, or tangerines)

Applesauce or fruit cocktail packaged in individual containers

Single-serving packages of dried fruit, such as boxed raisins or minibags of dried cranberries

A mixture of raisins (or other dried fruit), almonds, and your favorite cereal

Raw vegetables (buy the precut versions or the baby carrots and save even more time!)

A tomato

100 percent juice in a box (orange juice is the most nutritious)

Minicans of tomato juice, V8, or carrot juice

Salsa, preferably fresh

**Group B:**

Fat-free cottage cheese or ricotta cheese

Low-fat or nonfat yogurt, plain or fruited

8-ounce carton of low-fat milk (regular or chocolate)

1 ounce extra-lean sandwich meat

⅓ cup hummus

1 tablespoon peanut or almond butter

Fat-free whole-wheat crackers

Microwave fat-free popcorn

Minibagels

Graham crackers

Oven-baked tortilla chips

Low-fat bran muffins (from bakery)

Whole-wheat bread sticks

Premade crepes (some grocery stores carry these in the produce section)

Fat-free dips, such as salad dressings or fat-free sour cream dips

## Lip-Smacking Rules

"The taste of food is an important part of whether or not we feel satisfied after a meal," says Zoe Warwick, Ph.D., professor of psychology at the University of Maryland. Dr. Warwick found that depending on the flavor of foods, people reported they felt more satisfied and ate less. Studies from the Pennsylvania State University found that the most filling and satisfying foods are stews, soups, vegetables, whole grains, fruits, and legumes. Women also are most likely to lose weight when they eat small, frequent meals, rather than three big square meals. The trick is to make these minimeals and filling foods satisfying by following these guidelines:

1. *Know Your Favorite Flavors.* "Think about the tastes, smells, and textures of food that are most satisfying to you," recommends Dr. Warwick. Are they hard and crunchy foods like hard candy, creamy foods like ice cream, sweet and salty foods like Hawaiian pizza, or spicy foods like a bean burrito? Then incorporate these foods, or find low-fat alternatives, into your diet. "I used to crave Doritos and potato chips, now I'm happy with pretzels," confesses Dr. Warwick.

2. *Think Quality, Not Quantity.* Adding flavor and savoriness to your meals tantalizes the taste buds and accents the sensuous side to food—its color, texture, and aromas. The more you combine flavors, the more interesting the meal. Experiment with sweet, spicy, and sour tastes by adding fruit, red pepper flakes, and arugula to a salad; combining lemon and mint in a marinade; or blending roasted red peppers and cayenne and drizzling it over a creamed vegetable soup. Then serve yourself small portions of the best flavors.

3. *Pay Attention.* You are likely to overeat if you eat too fast. Instead, eat slowly and pay attention to each bite. Listen carefully and try to "hear" the subtle flavors, taste the colors, and experience the aromas. Take one bite at a time to avoid mixing foods and masking individual flavors. Listen to your hunger signals; stop periodically during a meal and sit back, then return to eating only if you are truly enjoying the food and are still hungry.

4. *Eat Only the Best.* So many times we take a bite of something that doesn't really taste all that good, yet we eat it anyway. If we just stop and ask ourselves, "Is this satisfying?," we might stop eating foods that aren't

good for us before the eating even begins. See Table 4.6, "How to Make Foods Tasty," for ways to flavor food with healthy ingredients.

Changing eating habits, exploring new foods and cooking methods, investigating new products, and trying new ways of eating are an adventure. Approach them with an open mind and a bit of excitement, just as you would if you were starting out on any of life's adventures. Eating well may take a little extra time up front, but with practice, you'll find it takes no more time and effort, and possibly less money to give your body the best fuel possible.

---

**TABLE 4.6    How to Make Foods Tasty**

Do you need an inspirational boost when it comes to flavoring your meals? Stock your kitchen with flavor-enhancing ingredients and you can muster a tasty meal even in a pinch. Here are twenty items that pack a taste punch for little or no calories:

1. *Fresh Cilantro:* Add to bottled salsa, a bean burrito, a summer soup, fruit or vegetable salads, vinaigrette dressings, black beans, or rice dishes.
2. *Canned Roasted Red/Yellow Peppers:* Add to a grilled cheese sandwich; blend with some cayenne and drizzle over a creamed vegetable soup, egg dishes, pasta sauces (cold and hot), or add as a topping with cheese for crackers.
3. *Canned Chilies:* Add whole chilies to a grilled chicken sandwich or diced chilies to soups, scrambled eggs, pita sandwiches, or on tortillas.
4. *Horseradish:* Use in potato dishes, vegetable dips with dill, vegetable or chicken wraps with sour cream, spicy soup like gumbo, turkey burgers (ginger is good here, too), cold potato salad, or cold green beans.
5. *Fresh Ginger:* Combine with curry to flavor chicken, add to hot or iced tea, season steamed vegetables such as pea pods or carrots. Use as a topping along with green onions on roasted fish. Add to stir-frys, tofu dishes, or salad dressings.
6. *Balsamic Vinegar:* Mix with olive oil for a bread-dunking dip, drizzle over steamed broccoli, or use instead of other vinegars in salad dressing. Add to soups or cold rice or pasta salads.
7. *Sun-Dried Tomatoes:* Use in pasta salads, sandwich spreads, vegetable dips, or as an extra topping on pizza. Mix into sautéed zucchini or as an accompaniment to grilled eggplant. Blend with olives, garlic, and balsamic vinegar to make a spicy spread for grilled vegetable sandwiches.

8. *Lemon:* The grated rind (called lemon zest) can be added to sorbets, frozen yogurts, or fruit salads. The juice can put a tangy taste to couscous, gazpacho, dressings, and as marinade for fish.

9. *Cloves:* Add whole cloves to a bouquet garni in stews or soups, add a pinch of ground cloves to chili or glazed carrots, mix into coffee-cake batter, or flavor your sugar bowl by adding a few cloves.

10. *Crushed Red Pepper Flakes or Tabasco:* Sprinkle on pizza, pasta dishes, salads, or soups. Add to olive oil or sour cream dips, rice dishes, or bean salads. Mix into corn-bread batter or bread dough.

11. *Apricot Preserves:* Roll into a crepe with sour cream, use with rice vinegar and soy sauce or oranges and garlic in marinades for chicken or lamb, mix into fruit salads or couscous, add to batters for scones, muffins, or tarts.

12. *Black Peppercorns:* Add to pasta, salads, eggs, fish, and beef dishes. Grind some into brown-bread batters, stewed fruits, hot chocolate, or spiced cider. White peppercorns are good on grilled meats, shish kebabs, and creamed soups. Or mix black, white, and green peppercorns in your mill.

13. *Fresh Herbs:* Fresh always tastes better than dried. Add fresh basil to pasta, tomatoes or other vegetables, bread dough, or even mango slices (basil and lemon are a good match). Fresh rosemary accents any meat, as well as pasta dishes, roasted vegetables, lima beans, peas, or squash. Fresh dill is an excellent flavorant for fish, chicken, omelettes and other egg dishes, salads, beets, cabbage, potatoes, or cucumbers. Fresh oregano is excellent in Italian, Greek, or Mexican dishes.

14. *Salsa:* Make your own by experimenting with grilled corn, vine-ripened tomatoes, garlic, red onions, and chilies. Or try fruit salsa made from mango, jicama, and black beans. Try adding rice-wine vinegar, fresh mint, lime juice, fresh herbs, avocado, or cilantro.

15. *Fruit:* Add fruit to unusual dishes. Cook chicken with mangos or grapes. Add pears, fresh berries, or peaches to a tossed salad. Accent a marinade with mandarin oranges.

16. *Gourmet Lettuce:* Throw out the iceberg and toss a great salad using radicchio, endive, escarole, baby lettuce, arugula, treviso, puntarelle, frisee (curly endive), purslane, watercress, young spinach, and large red oak leaf lettuce. Add pineapple, plums, or other fruit, or grilled vegetables or meats as a topping.

17. *Fresh Mint:* Flavor iced tea. Toss with new potatoes, fresh peas, or steamed carrots. Mix mint and basil for pesto sauces. Use as an accompaniment to any fiery foods, such as Southwest Asian dishes. Add to fresh fruit or citrus salsa or chutneys.

18. *Nut Oils:* Use walnut or hazelnut oils instead of olive oil in vinaigrettes. Drizzle over potato salad instead of using mayonnaise. Try on hot steamed vegetables, such as

asparagus, broccoli, or green beans, or use almond oil and sherry vinegar on a wild rice salad.

**19.** *Honey:* Drizzle over fruit salads. Use with fresh herbs in a glaze for roasted meats. Coat slices of sweet potato and roast. Blend with olive oil, vinegar, and mustard for a vinaigrette. Mix with soy sauce, ginger, orange juice concentrate, and rice wine for a marinade.

**20.** *Chipotle Peppers:* These spicy peppers give a smoky taste to dishes and are great mixed with hoisin sauce, ginger, cilantro, or other ingredients as a sauce for fish or chicken.

## CHAPTER 5

# *Eating Out*

You might have no trouble sticking with your new healthy diet plan during the week. But, oh my, what happens on the weekends!? Or on vacation? At a dinner party or social engagement? In fact, almost any change in routine can topple the best of intentions.

You have several options when approaching these slip-prone periods.

1. You can plan them into your weekly nutrition menus by eating more low-fat foods during the week and planning for impulse eating (in moderation) on special occasions.
2. You can plan your weekends, social engagements, or vacations to include precisely determined amounts of higher fat foods.
3. You can anticipate slip-prone situations and plan ahead how you will handle them to stick with your nutrition plan.
4. You can splurge on special occasions but also include more exercise and exercise-related activities to offset the additional fat, sugar, and calories. (See chapter 8 for more information on how to handle slips and relapses.)
5. You can read the next few pages and adopt a few of these tips for handling any type of eating-out occasion.

## *The Restaurant Challenge*

Americans are eating out more than ever before, and it's not doing our health or our waistlines much good. Here are just a few of the hard facts:

- Compared to our dining habits in the late 1970s when we ate around the dining room table about 85 percent of the time, we now gobble about a third of our meals at restaurants.

- Perhaps because we still consider a night without having to clean dishes as a special treat, we also tend to splurge when we eat away from home, averaging more calories, fat, sugar, and salt than if we'd prepared the exact same meal at home. Eat out frequently and expect to pack in about 17 percent more calories and 30 percent more fat than if you'd stayed home.

- Fat supplies one-fifth more calories in restaurant or takeout meals than at-home meals, according to the U.S. Department of Agriculture (U.S.D.A.).

- Meals eaten out also are usually 20 to 30 percent lower in fiber, calcium, and iron, to name only a few forgotten nutrients.

- A study from the University of Tennessee found that women who eat out more than five times a week consume about 300 calories more each day than women who eat out less often. Unless those women are walking an additional four miles every day, at a brisk pace, they will gain about two pounds a month!

- It's no wonder that studies from Purdue University and U.S.D.A. found that people who eat frequently tend to weigh more than those who eat in.

## The Restaurant Survival Guide

It's a sure bet that order of onion rings packs in a few too many calories and fat grams (up to 114 grams to be exact). And you probably know to order grilled chicken breast instead of a double cheeseburger. But, without food labels, recipes, and other necessary decision-making tools, who knows what you're getting when you eat out! At home you might use fat-free milk, olive oil, or sauté with chicken broth. It's likely those fat-conscious methods are not used at your favorite restaurant. Whether it is a fast-food hamburger joint or a gourmet delight, it's impossible to know how much fat (or what kind?), salt, sugar, cholesterol, and calories are in any menu item. Don't despair. You can survive a restaurant experience having enjoyed the food (and the company) without sacrificing your health.

You can

- Choose to eat anything you want and budget the calories and fat by eating less and exercising more that day.
- Choose to doggie-bag it by scooping half of your plate into a take-home bag for tomorrow's lunch. You even can ask the server to bring half your entrée already packaged, so you are less tempted to eat it all.
- Use a little self-restraint and choose healthy fare in reasonable portions.

Restaurants that help a woman order a healthful meal are usually small, privately owned restaurants or restaurants that prepare meals to order and, therefore, can accommodate special requests. Cafeterias and restaurants that buy preprepared frozen entrées are less likely to accept special requests, but even fast-food restaurants can accommodate by leaving off mayonnaise, fatty sauces, or by packing in more tomatoes or lettuce. Call the restaurant ahead of time and ask if food can be specially prepared. Be specific. Ask if the chicken can be dry broiled rather than sautéed, sauces can be made without oil, or the food can be cooked without MSG.

Know your meal plan or carry a copy of your plan to the restaurant. Decide ahead of time what you will order based on that plan. Mentally rehearse ordering low-fat foods. Prepare for possible stumbling blocks. If you plan to order a side of vegetables, remember to ask that they be served plain, otherwise it is likely they will be dripping in butter. Rehearse ordering salad dressing served on the side, butter and bread removed from the table, or mineral water with a twist of lime rather than a cocktail. Bring foods with you that are not offered at the restaurant, such as fat-free salad dressing, fruit or vegetable juices, or a favorite low-sodium seasoning. Try ordering off the menu; tell your server what you would like and see if the restaurant can make it ("I'd like grilled salmon with a huge portion of steamed vegetables; can you do that?").

### How Much Will You Eat?

Restaurant portions are deceivingly huge, especially when it comes to refined grains and meat. For example, a serving of pasta is defined by the U.S.D.A. as a half cup cooked, or about four fork twirls. But a typical takeout portion of spaghetti contains about eight cups. Served with two slices of garlic bread, this dinner packs in eighteen-plus servings of refined grain!

Practice with serving sizes to help recognize proper portions at the restaurant. Measure and weigh your food at home for two days, so you can accurately judge a reasonable serving. Plan to leave at least one half of the food on your plate or ask for a half order. Many restaurants serve more food or larger servings than designated by your meal plan. Plan to split an entrée with a friend, give the extras to someone else, ask the waiter/waitress to remove the plate, or request a doggie bag.

Finally, if it is likely there will be a wait at the restaurant, eat a low-fat snack or drink two glasses of water before leaving to avoid excessive hunger that can lower resistance to temptation.

## Ordering in Restaurants

At the restaurant, do not hesitate to ask questions about how the food is prepared or ask for foods not listed on the menu. In addition,

- Park several blocks away and walk to the restaurant.
- Introduce yourself to the owner or waiter/waitress of a local restaurant. They are more likely to work with people who are frequent customers.
- For a premeal drink, order wine spritzers or sparkling water as low-calorie alternatives to higher calorie alcoholic beverages.
- Order from the à la carte section of the menu.
- Eat slowly and enjoy the company. Put down the fork between bites to allow time for the brain to catch up with the stomach and correctly register the level of fullness.
- Select soup *or* salad, but not both unless that is the entire meal, or order a salad and share an entrée with a friend.
- Ask that foods be prepared without oils or fat; salad dressings, gravies, or sauces be served on the side or not at all; butter be removed from the table; or the dessert menu not be brought to the table.
- Check foods when they are served to make sure your requests were fulfilled. For example, steamed vegetables that are served with droplets of oil in the juice probably were sautéed. The breading can be removed from chicken if an order for baked chicken arrives having been fried.

- Make special requests for whole-wheat rolls, nonfat milk, vegetable platters (no cheese sauce or butter), fresh fruit for dessert, or plain oil-and-vinegar dressing (you can add mostly vinegar and little or no oil).
- Request low-fat or nonfat milk for coffee or tea, rather than nondairy creamers or whole cream.
- Send back orders that are prepared incorrectly and don't hesitate to leave a restaurant if there are no low-fat items on the menu and the establishment is unable to prepare a special order.
- If you do overeat, eat less and exercise more the rest of the day and the next day.

---

### TABLE 5.1    Ordering Low-Fat

**APPETIZERS**

Vegetable, bean, or tomato-based soups; vegetable juice; raw vegetable plates; fresh fruit cocktail; steamed seafood; shrimp cocktail; vegetables with dip on the side; low-fat dips such as salsa, yogurt-based spreads, or dips made from pureed vegetables.

**SALADS**

All tossed salads and most salad bar items. Use lemon juice, low-calorie dressing, or plain oil and vinegar served on the side.

**ENTRÉES: AMERICAN**

2- to 3-ounce portions of extra-lean meat broiled; fish poached, broiled dry, grilled, baked, stewed, barbecued dry, or roasted; poultry without the skin; sauces on the side; vegetable and grain dishes; pasta with vegetable sauce (not cream sauce); and entrées served with wine sauces.

**ENTRÉES: MEXICAN**

Send back the chips, but save the salsa to top salads (no cheese), chicken fajitas (skip the guacamole and sour cream), chicken enchiladas (again, no cheese), or grilled/baked fish dishes.

**ENTRÉES: CHINESE**

Dilute calories by heaping the plate with rice and using all entrées as condiments. Order items steamed (most fried dishes contain the fat equivalent of sixteen strips of bacon). Szechwan shrimp, dishes made with hoisin or plum sauce, and steamed fish dishes are low-fat.

**ENTRÉES: ITALIAN**

Order appetizers such as shrimp cocktail or grilled calamari for an entrée. Order half portions of pasta with a large side salad (dressing on side). Tomato-based sauces typically are lower in fat than creamed sauces or pesto. Grilled fish also is a good choice.

**ENTRÉES: THAI**

Thai salads and salad rolls, steamed mussels, broth-based curries (coconut-based curries contain up to 48 grams of saturated fat per cup), Pik Pow dishes, and grilled fish.

**SIDE ORDERS**

Plain baked potato served with chives, cottage cheese, or nonfat yogurt; mashed or boiled potatoes; plain noodles or rice; beans, rice pilaf, or grain salads, such as tabouli; steamed or raw vegetables, such as artichokes, mixed vegetables, or sliced tomatoes; or mushrooms cooked in wine.

**DESSERTS**

Gelatins, fruit ices, sorbet, fresh fruit, angel food cake, sherbet, frozen low-fat yogurt, or fruit juice.

**BEVERAGES**

Nonfat milk, coffee, herbal teas, sparkling water, fruit or vegetable juices.

Avoid high-fat foods described as: refried, creamed, cream sauce, au gratin, à la mode, marinated, prime, pot pie, *au fromage, au lait,* Parmesan, in cheese sauce, escalloped, basted, casserole, hollandaise, crispy, sautéed, béarnaise.

## Salad Bar Rules

Salads are often the answer to everything from waistlines to health. But are those big bowls of rabbit food really calorie-free answers to a ravenous appetite and a sure-fire way to beat the odds on cancer and heart disease?

Yes and no. Crispy greens are one of life's little fat-free pleasures. However, many fatty concoctions are guzzled under the guise of salad fixings. The fact that salad dressing is the number one source of fat in women's diets attests to the confusion over what is really a healthful salad and what is a fat-laden disaster. I did a segment for ABC's *Good Morning America* where I analyzed the salads people had prepared from a salad bar. Guess what! Some salad plates had more calories, fat, and saturated fat than five double cheeseburgers! Here are a few survival skills for surviving the salad bar minefield that can help you cut the fat, sodium, and sugar, yet keep the taste, nutrition and pleasure of the meal.

First, heap your plate with greens, the greener the better. Spinach is better than leaf lettuce, which is better than iceberg. Other raw-and-crispy "freebies" include grated carrots, mushrooms, raw broccoli florets, alfalfa sprouts, tomatoes, radicchio lettuce, purple cabbage, cucumber, and sweet red pepper. Use avocado slices, sunflower seeds, and olives sparingly.

Second, add one-half to two-thirds cup of beans, such as kidney, garbanzo, or black beans, or black-eyed peas, lentils, or split peas. Other low-fat protein sources include sliced, plain chicken or turkey breast or cooked egg white (whole egg contains more than a teaspoon of fat, while the white is fat- and cholesterol-free). Avoid the luncheon meats, such as salami, ham, and pepperoni, which contain up to 60 percent fat calories and too much salt. Low-fat cottage cheese is another healthy option and can be mixed with a low-calorie dressing to make less dressing stretch farther. Avoid the creamy cottage cheese that contains more than a teaspoon of fat for every half cup.

Third, skip anything mixed with oil, mayonnaise, cheese, or whipped cream. This includes potato or pasta salads, Mexican meat or cheese sauces, tuna mixed with mayonnaise, egg salad, macaroni and cheese, tartar sauce, and Waldorf salad. A one-ladle serving of these foods could contribute up to three tablespoons of fat to the meal. Grated Parmesan is a tasty alternative when used sparingly (one tablespoon contains about a half teaspoon of fat).

Fourth, complement your salad with soup and bread. Vegetable, split-pea, Manhattan clam chowder, or chicken noodle soups are usually low fat, although they also often are oversalted. A slice of whole-wheat bread or a plain bagel can add flavor without fat to the meal, but limit your intake of muffins or any baked item that has a shiny appearance, which is a red flag for too much fat and/or sugar.

Fifth, approach the salad dressing with a wary eye. Remember that one small ladle drizzles two tablespoons of dressing onto your plate, or up to four teaspoons of fat and 170 calories. In essence, too much of the wrong dressing can transform four cups of low-fat vegetables into a 70 percent fat-calorie lunch! Choose low-calorie dressings and use them sparingly. Select watery versions, such as Italian and French, rather than thicker blue cheese and Thousand Island dressings, since they spread more evenly over the salad. Better yet, portion out a half to one scoop serving into a separate container and lightly dip your fork into the low-calorie dressing first and then into the salad.

## Road Warrior: Food and Air Travel

Air travel is where killer PMS meets food hell. That frightening image came to mind when I was frantically racing through Chicago's O'Hare Airport. I was in major stress (I'd been away for a week, my kids were living on potato chips, and I was sure if I didn't get home they'd be in full-blown scurvy by morning). I was exhausted, panicked that I'd miss my connection, and starved. I needed a treat to calm me down after sitting for four hours like a canned sardine squeezed into a shoe-box-sized seat between the fat man from the circus and a lovely lady with the plague. Any otherwise sane woman battling the emotional roller coaster of PMS will tell you that any of those emotions can lead to a food binge.

Now, mix bad mood with bad food. As my roll-on rammed into a pizza box, I looked around and realized, like a bad dream, I was surrounded by every pound-packing food you could imagine, from double cheeseburgers, French fries, quarter-pound muffins, 32-ounce sodas, doughnuts, and ice cream bars to cinnamon rolls, chocolate chip scones, candy bars, and chili dogs. Not a sprig of broccoli, a steamed carrot, a spinach leaf in sight. It felt like a food horror movie. Welcome to air travel!

### All Tray Tables in the Upright Position

Airports are microcosms of our everyday toxic environment. Boy, do I know. I chalked up more than 170,000 frequent-flyer miles last year. At Dallas–Fort Worth, San Francisco International, JFK, Sea-Tac in Seattle—you name the hub—I've paced out the distance between eateries and found you walk only twenty to thirty steps, expending about a third of a calorie, to get from one greasy spoon to the next sugar-coated counter. "At airports, you negotiate food courts packed with fast food, newsstands selling candy bars and Fritos, vending machines stocked with sodas, Starbucks pastry counters, and ice cream shops," says Evelyn Tribole, R.D., author of *Stealth Health* and a frequent flyer. Don't think you're home-free when you reach your gate. Here a roll-cart attendant flings nuts and popcorn as you duck down the jetway. If you ate at each opportunity, you'd gain about ten pounds just making a connecting flight.

I've learned a few healthy-eating tricks—you might even say I'm a road warrior. You can eat well anywhere, even in an airport, on an airplane, in a hotel room, and at a train station. Of course, no one is saying it's easy. The healthy choices are there; it's making them that's the challenge. So, while you pack your bags, also muster your self-discipline, vigilance, and nerve.

## Baby Carrots, Come to a White Courtesy Telephone Please

In our country, food temptations are everywhere. But at airports, they've upped the ante. Regardless, the same rule applies: Choose only those foods that reduce your stress *and* boost your health—that means only foods on the Healthy Woman's Diet. You might savor a tasty burrito at the Albuquerque airport or a cup of chowder at the Boston airport, but there is nothing special about that Big Mac, and it isn't the energy-boosting meal you need to successfully survive three time zones!

Ask yourself, "Am I eating because I'm hungry, or because I'm stressed?" If you don't have hunger pangs, then burn off stress hormones with a brisk walk down the concourse and save the calories for the family feast. "An hour layover means you can log at least forty minutes of your day's workout by walking. And, unlike the mall where merchants get irritated when you don't saunter, people are accustomed to race walking at the airport," adds Vince Nistico, M.S., ACE-certified personal trainer in Salem, Oregon.

Let's say you're killing time while waiting for a flight. Do you risk the airplane food or grab a bite now? If you haven't ordered a special flight meal ahead of time, you might want to take the edge off by eating something at the airport. But watch out for impulse eating. It appears that nowhere else do we indulge so well as in preparation for flight.

## TABLE 5.2    At The Airport: From Den of Calorie Iniquity to Healthier Choices

| INSTEAD OF . . . | HAVE A . . . | YOU'LL SAVE . . . |
| --- | --- | --- |
| Chinese spicy chicken with peanuts/cashews | Chinese chicken with mushrooms | 340 calories and 20 fat grams |
| 2 Chinese entrées with rice | 1 Chinese entrée with rice | 400+ calories |
| Cheese pizza, 1 slice, with an orange and apple | Spinach and broccoli pizza | 107 calories, 12 fat grams, and increase fiber, vitamin C, and folic acid |
| Large deli tuna sandwich | Chicken breast sandwich with mustard | 670 calories, 22 fat grams, 1.7 grams sodium |
| Soft glazed raisin pretzel with butter | Soft whole-wheat pretzel | 160 calories, 3 fat grams, 7 tsp. sugar |
| Caramel dip for pretzel (1 oz.) | Marinara dip for pretzel (1 oz.) | 125 calories, 3 fat grams, 5 tsp. sugar |
| Café mocha (16 oz.) | Nonfat café latte (16 oz.) | 260 calories, 22 fat grams, 4 tsp. sugar |
| Chocolate chip cookie (3 oz.) | Kiddie cup TCBY chocolate frozen yogurt | 170 calories, 11 fat grams |
| Cinnabon (8 oz.) | Au Bon Pain triple berry muffin | 400 calories, 31 fat grams, 5 tsp. sugar |
| Plain hamburger | Junior hamburger | 80 percent fewer calories, 40 percent less fat |

The number one rule for staying healthy, avoiding jet lag, and boosting fortitude for travel is to bring food with you. You wouldn't dream of forgetting your toothbrush or clean underwear. Well, don't forget your travel K rations. Pack your briefcase, roll-on, backpack, purse, or even a paper bag with:

- Unsalted nuts, fresh fruit, cut-up veggies, string cheese, and/or boxed juice.

- Even an energy bar is a better bet than an airport muffin, saving you 160 calories and 14 grams of fat.
- Freeze-dried vegetable soups come in handy (you can find hot water in any airport).
- Starkist Charlie's Lunch Kit comes with tuna, crackers, and its own dish; just go light on the mayo and complement the snack with an apple or grapes.
- Toss berries, cottage cheese, and nuts into a washed yogurt container that you throw away after eating.
- Lettuce makes a great wrap for leftover chicken, beans, and other goodies.

In a few isolated instances you can get real food at an airport, say Rubio's fish tacos in San Diego or Macheezmo Mouse low-fat Mexican food at Portland International. But those are exceptions, not the rule. At some airports, you'll be hard-pressed to find a water fountain, let alone a decent meal. So focus on the Five Airport Food Groups: fruit, lettuce, bread (whole wheat when possible), chicken, and water. Keep in mind that any of the following can serve as a takeout meal for the airplane! Here are some tips:

- You always can find a fruit basket with apples, oranges, or bananas.
- Think only grilled or baked, from grilled chicken sandwiches and salads to a plain baked potato.
- Make an open-faced sandwich (and save up to 150 calories) by throwing out the top piece of bread.
- Go for a fast-food salad. Toss out the croutons, thick dressing, and cheese, and complement the meal with a glass of orange juice or low-fat milk.
- Be vocal. Ask for the burrito without cheese and sour cream. Send it back if they ignore your request.
- Go easy on salty foods that compound dehydration and traveler's fatigue.

### In Case of a Diet Emergency, an Oxygen Mask Will Appear

Eating right on the flight is another matter. Avoid deciding what to eat when you're in emergency starvation mode 35,000 feet above the ground. Instead, preorder a special meal no later than twenty-four hours before the flight. Most airlines offer a variety, including low-fat, low-cholesterol, Kosher, Hindu, seafood, and vegetarian options. These meals often taste better and are fresher than the typical fare, and there's no additional charge.

If you forgot to plan ahead, then follow these last-minute rules:

- Water is your best friend. The humidity in the airplane is as low as 2 percent, which leads to major dehydration, fatigue, and jet lag. Bring a water bottle, order three glasses of water every time you're offered a drink (drink at least two glasses per hour), and skip the salty snack, alcohol, and caffeinated beverages such as coffee and cola, since they aggravate dehydration.

- Board the plane with ready-made K rations. Those same snacks you had at the airport serve you well in a pinch on the plane. And a long trip that connects could mean that you miss being fed on both flights, while some airlines serve little more than peanuts. Pack water, fruit, and other nutritious snacks as a back-up for inedible plane food. Some flight attendants will even microwave your home-cooked meal—just make sure you let them know when you board. (Of course, there are those occasional attendants who won't even allow you to bring food on board, so be discreet.) Complement these rations with healthy plane food, such as tomato juice or Bloody Mary mix, orange juice, nonfat or low-fat milk, or grapefruit juice.

- Eat light on the flight. Airline portions might be small, but that doesn't mean they're low-cal. A smoked turkey and cheese sandwich with chips and a cookie packs up to 950 calories and 50 grams of fat! (A 150-pound woman burns only about 84 calories every hour she sits in a plane, so it will take an 11-hour plane ride to burn off that "light" meal.) Ask the flight attendant to remove anything you don't want, like the chips, cookie, mayo, and one slice of the bread.

- Eyeball the trays as they are served to fellow passengers. If the entrée is chicken cleverly disguised as a rubber duck smothered in congealed gravy or the pocket calzone is a grease wad in a tinfoil bag, say no to the meal. "We Americans are so concerned about eating enough that we sometimes forget that it's OK to just skip a bad meal entirely," says Adam Drewnowski, Ph.D., professor in the departments of epidemiology and medicine at the University of Washington in Seattle.

- Don't use the butter or cream cheese and use less than half the salad dressing.
- If you plan to eat upon arrival, then refuse the airplane food. You won't starve, even on a transcontinental flight.

Stretching is critical to your flight success. Sit in a cramped seat like a pretzel for four hours then sprint down the jetway; now there is a one-two punch to your health and vitality. As you deplane with muscles cramped, blood flow sluggish, and fluids pooled in the extremities, you feel like you've been tackled by a sumo wrestler. Moving can solve this problem. Get out of your seat for at least five minutes every hour of the flight. "Request an aisle seat in the middle of the plane, so it's easy to get up and walk back and forth without overdisturbing people up and down the aisle," says Vince Nistico, M.S. He adds that stretching frequently at the back of the plane and all kinds of isometric exercises at your seat (like squeezing your butt or abdominal muscles) can help circulation.

Think of eating well as an adventure when traveling. Like a scavenger hunt, you're determined to find something that will fuel your body, mind, and soul. Equipped with that attitude, you can turn a war zone into a game, and save your health and your waistline in the process.

## Social Situations: Parties, Dinners, Picnics, and More

Entertaining friends and family on the weekends while maintaining healthful eating habits is easy, and even fun. As hostess, you control the food supply and can offer foods that are enjoyable and low-fat. The secret to successful entertaining is not how rich the entrée is or how sweet the dessert, but rather how creative and entertaining is the presentation of food and how enjoyable is the company.

Gourmet cooking from the Healthy Woman's Diet can be nutritious and taste good, too. Guests probably won't even know the food is low-fat! The meal can be planned around favorite low-fat recipes or a light dinner can be followed by a sinful dessert served in small portions. Portion control is also useful. For example, a favorite cheesecake can be cut into twenty thin slices, rather than eight thick pieces. A lavish serving of an all-fruit topping increases the serving size and nutritional content without adding fat.

## TABLE 5.3    What to Eat When Traveling by Rail or Road and in Hotels

**Rule 1.** Avoid the major pitfall of traveling: skipping meals. Eat regularly, starting with breakfast to avoid the inevitable binge that comes from being so hungry you'll eat one hundred bags of peanuts, your entrée and that of the fellow next to you on the plane.

**Rule 2.** Watch out for alcohol. Combine a little alcohol with travel and hunger and it's an all-out throw-caution-to-the-wind blowout by dinnertime. Make predinner drinking nonalcoholic and have a glass of wine with your meal.

*In the Hotel:* Vow not to open the minibar in your hotel room. Better yet, don't accept the key when you check in. There's nothing worth eating and you'll only regret the one billion calories you inhale from the chips, candy bar, and jar of roasted nuts.

*Room Service:* Order off the menu. Sweet-talk the server by asking, "I'd like scrambled eggs with sliced tomatoes, a glass of orange juice, and whole-wheat toast dry. Can I get that?" Most will comply. Be specific. Tell them not to bring hash browns, butter, sausage, the bread basket. If you don't, you'll get and eat what you don't want.

*Hotel K Rations:* The poor-woman's alternative to room service is to carry individual boxes of cereal or instant oatmeal, purchase a little carton of nonfat milk and a banana the night before, keep the milk cold in the ice bucket overnight, and feed yourself in the morning.

*Other Hotel Accommodations:* When you book in at an airport motel the night before a flight, you can cash in on a growing trend of "grab and go" breakfasts and meals offered by motels, such as some Holiday Inns and Radisson Hotels.

*On the Road:* Your options increase when you drive. Pack a cooler with yogurt, sandwiches, fruit, low-fat cheese, water, minicartons of nonfat milk, cans of juice, cherry tomatoes, bags of baby carrots, whole-wheat crackers and peanut butter, small boxes of raisins, homemade snack mixes made with popcorn or pretzels and nuts, fig bars, and a few energy bars.

*At the Train Depot:* Vending-machine food is your last resort and might be all you have to choose from at a train depot. Your best bets here are pretzels, diet soft drinks, or nuts.

### Dining at Friends' Houses

Socializing at friends' homes also can be enjoyable without compromising nutrition goals. The more you plan ahead, the more likely you will stick with your healthy nutrition plan. Obtaining the following information prior to the event can help a woman plan:

- Will the meal be a sit-down meal or buffet? (Buffets allow more control over portion size and food selection.)
- Can guests bring anything? (If so, bring a low-fat, nutrient-dense food.)
- Will it be a formal or informal event? (Informal events allow more flexibility for meal selection.)
- You also can ask for support depending on how well you know the host or hostess.

With this information in mind, you can decide to eat modest-sized servings of everything or to decline certain foods, such as sour cream on baked potatoes, sauces on meats, or salad dressing. A modest serving should be clearly defined so that the decision is made easily at the time of greatest temptation. For example, a moderate portion might be one scoop, one piece, one slice, one-half slice, or one small bowl. Mentally rehearse the evening before you get there. How will you gracefully say, "No thank you"? (Eating slowly avoids an empty plate and the repeated offerings of more food.) Remember that saying no to food is not a personal rejection of the host or hostess.

During the meal, refrain from taking seconds, eat slowly, avoid dressings, and leave sauces, gravy, meat fat, breading, or other fatty foods on your plate. Decline alcoholic or sugary beverages and ask for water or sparkling water with a twist of lemon or lime. Take large portions of low-fat foods and small servings of high-fat foods.

### Picnics, Cookouts, and Other Outings

Summer picnics and cookouts or packing foods for a camping trip can fit easily into a low-fat, nutrient-dense nutrition plan. From chili, corn-on-the-cob, and chicken at a picnic to instant oatmeal, raisins, and nonfat dry milk powder packed for a hiking trip, the choices for low-fat nutritious foods are endless. A picnic can be planned around a salad bar that includes a variety of textures, colors, and shapes. Salads for a picnic can be made with anything from fruit and vegetables to beans and pasta and can be accompanied by a low-fat meat and no-fat cheese plate and bowl of whole-grain breads.

Since many of these foods will be exposed to air and high temperatures, the biggest concern when planning picnics and cookouts is to keep the food safe from contamination and spoilage. Foods should be refrigerated immediately after preparation and never should be set out to cool. Hands should be washed before handling foods at home and at the outdoor event. A clean utensil should be used to prepare and serve each dish. Foods that spoil easily, such as egg dishes, cream desserts, chopped meats, and potato salads, should be avoided or special care should be used to ensure they are kept at cool temperatures (i.e., at or below 40° F). Blocks of ice, freezer packs, and dry ice are useful for maintaining low temperatures. Finally, salad dressings should be stored in separate containers in the cooler and added to salads immediately before serving.

## *Brown-Bag Lunches*

You needn't fall prey to the vending machine or stale doughnuts at work. It takes only ten minutes to pack a healthy lunch, and that's including snacks.

- *Sandwiches:* For sandwich fillings, use two ounces or less of extra-lean meats, chicken, fish, low-fat or no-fat cheeses, water-packed tuna, no-fat cream cheese, or homemade bean spreads, such as hummus. Generously garnish sandwiches with leaf lettuce, tomatoes, cucumbers, grated carrots or zucchini, sweet bell peppers, apple slices, sprouts, scallions, shredded cabbage, spinach, or mandarin oranges. Serve on whole-wheat bread, pita bread, or roll into a whole-wheat tortilla.
- *Your Calcium Fix:* Choose nonfat milk and yogurt (plain), or vanilla, plain, or chocolate low-fat soy milk.
- *Hot Lunch:* Take a thermos of homemade chili, stew, or soup (for example, bean soup or vegetable soup).
- *Snacks:* Choose whole-grain pasta, cereals, breads, fresh fruits, and vegetables; for instance, potato salad with nonfat yogurt or sour

cream dressing, whole-wheat crackers, raw vegetables, a piece of fruit, or a fruit salad.

- *Salads:* Make pasta salads with no-fat or low-calorie dressing or mayonnaise. Use spinach and leaf lettuce, which contains more vitamins and minerals than iceberg lettuce.
- *Be Adventurous:* Try new vegetables and vegetable combinations such as broccoli, carrots, cauliflower, celery, cherry tomatoes, Chinese pea pods, Jerusalem artichokes, jicama, mushrooms, radishes, spinach leaves, turnips, or zucchini. Dip in nonfat yogurt or no-fat sour cream–based dressing.
- *Leftovers:* Leftover casseroles, chicken, turkey, fish, pasta dishes, soups, stews, or meat loaf are great brown-bag lunches. Pack leftovers for tomorrow's lunch while cleaning up the kitchen the night before.
- *Breakfast Leftovers:* Leftover pancakes can serve as tortilla-like wrappers for ricotta cheese and fresh fruit snacks.

---

**TABLE 5.4    Brown-Bag Snacks**

The following snacks supply approximately 100 calories each and are great snacks to accompany your brown-bag sandwich or soup.

- 10-ounce glass of vanilla soy milk
- 6 ounces nonfat plain yogurt
- ¾ cup nonfat milk warmed and mixed with 1 packet sugar-free cocoa mix
- 1 cup fresh-squeezed orange juice
- 1½ cups fresh blueberries
- 2 cups cantaloupe cubes, drizzled with lime juice
- 2½ cups fresh strawberries
- 1 banana, sliced and sprinkled with nutmeg
- 1 slice whole-wheat toast with 1 teaspoon apricot preserves
- ½ whole-wheat bagel (small) with 1 teaspoon fat-free cream cheese
- ½ cup raspberry sorbet
- 2 cups fresh spinach sautéed in 1 teaspoon olive oil with 2 minced garlic cloves
- 1 medium sweet potato, sliced into strips and baked until crispy
- 2 cups asparagus sautéed in 2 teaspoons soy sauce and 2 tablespoons chicken broth

- 2 cups tossed salad greens with 1 medium sliced tomato, 2 tablespoons kidney beans, and 1 tablespoon oil-free dressing
- ½ cup steamed corn kernels mixed with ⅓ cup chopped sweet red peppers
- 1 cup carrot circles steamed and mixed with 2 teaspoons orange marmalade
- 1 slice French bread
- ½ cup frozen nonfat chocolate yogurt
- 1 small slice angel food cake with ½ cup fresh red raspberries
- ⅓ cup custard (made with 2 percent milk)
- 3½ cups air-popped popcorn
- 1 cup mango slices
- 1 tablespoon crunchy peanut butter (94 calories)
- 3½ cups slightly steamed yellow zucchini, cut into rounds and salted
- 26 baby carrots
- 1¼ cups chicken noodle soup
- 1 cup tomato soup made with ¼ cup 1 percent low-fat milk and ½ cup water
- 2 ounces water-packed tuna, drained and mixed with 2 teaspoons fat-free mayonnaise, and served on 2 wheat Saltine crackers
- 1 cup shredded cabbage and 1 ounce firm cubed tofu sautéed in 2 teaspoons peanut sauce (just until warmed, 2 minutes), topped with 2 tablespoons chopped cilantro
- ¼ whole-wheat pita dipped in ⅓ cup fat-free refried beans with 1 teaspoon salsa
- 1 tablespoon orange juice concentrate, ½ banana, and 2 apricot halves blended to make a smoothie
- ½ cup cooked brown rice mixed with 3 tablespoons cooked black beans, seasoned with cumin, salt, and pepper to taste

## CHAPTER 6

# *Everything You Need to Know about Supplements*

A day without my supplements is a day destined for some unknown health disaster. I just don't feel completely safe without them! I make my family take them, too. Not too long ago, my daughter's friend told her mom that "If parents discipline their kids because they care, then Lauren's mom (that's me) must really love her, because she makes her take those nasty vitamins every day!"

Hmmm. Well, at least I'm not alone in my overzealous concern for my family's health. According to the Council for Responsible Nutrition (the professional branch of the supplement industry), about one in every two women take nutritional supplements—that makes supplements the most popped pills in America. Half of all nonsupplementers would pop a vitamin pill if someone could provide convincing evidence that it would do some good.

How do we know if the billions of dollars' worth of supplements sold in this country every year is doing us any good? Would we be just as well or better off without them, or would everyone benefit from a daily vitamin pill? Even if supplements are a good idea, how do you know what and how much to take, what to avoid, and even how to read those labels? What's "USP" anyway? Is natural better than synthetic? What about time released and chelated?

## *The Not-So-Perfect Diet*

Ask most nutrition experts and they will tell you to turn first to food to meet all your nutritional needs. According to this belief, you eliminate all nutritional worries if you eat a variety of healthy foods. Sounds reasonable, but there's one small problem—finding women who do that is like finding the proverbial needle in a haystack.

As far back as the 1960s, reports on Americans' eating habits repeatedly show that few women choose the balanced diet. Instead, we're eating too much fat and too few fiber-rich fruits, vegetables, whole grains, and legumes. The U.S. Department of Agriculture's (U.S.D.A.) Continuing Survey of Food Intakes by Individuals (CSFII) found that ninety-nine out of every one hundred women fail to meet even minimum standards for dietary adequacy: Only about one-third of us meet the recommendations for grains (and hardly ever are they whole grain); we average only two to three servings of vegetables not the more optimal five, and only 1½ servings of fruit compared to the recommended 2 to 4 servings. Three out of every four women consume far too few milk products; many don't consume any at all. According to the National Health and Nutrition Examination Survey (NHANES), which has gathered information on Americans' eating habits for decades, women are more likely to go for doughnuts than whole-wheat bread, colas than soy milk, hot dogs than skinned chicken breast, and iceberg lettuce than broccoli. "It's possible that women's diets could be nutritionally adequate if they ate really well at every meal; unfortunately, most women aren't doing that," says Walter Willett, M.D., Dr.P.H., professor of nutrition at the Harvard School of Public Health in Boston.

## Are You Willing to Eat Eight Cups of Almonds?

Even if you ate perfectly every day, your diet probably would come up short for a few nutrients. For example:

*Folic Acid:* "To reach the daily goal of 400 mcg women must double or even triple their current intakes of fruits and vegetables, which is not likely to happen in my lifetime," says Dr. Willett. That means at least two servings of dark green leafy vegetables a day. But when Gladys Block, Ph.D., at the University of California, Berkeley, analyzed data from three major national surveys that provided information on 3,529 women between the ages of 15 and 44, she found that 86 percent of women fail to eat even one dark green leafy vegetable, the best dietary source of folic acid, on any one of four days! Granted, folic acid intakes have gone up since manufacturers started fortifying highly refined grains with this B vitamin, but intake still falls short of optimal.

*Calcium:* The latest calcium recommendations for women are 1,000 mg to 1,200 mg daily, which is easy enough if you drink three to four glasses of milk

---

### TABLE 6.1    Do I Need a Supplement?

You probably have a pretty good idea whether or not your diet is perfect. But just in case you're still in a quandary as to whether or not to take a multiple, here's a quick test to assess what, if any, nutrients might be lacking in your daily intake.

| **Yes/No** | **If no, your diet could be low in:** |
|---|---|
| Every day do you consume | |
| _____ 1. at least 1 citrus fruit? | Vitamin C |
| _____ 2. at least 2 dark green leafy vegetables? | Folic acid, vitamins A and K, iron, calcium |
| _____ 3. an additional 5 to 8 fruits and vegetables? | B vitamins, trace minerals |
| _____ 4. at least 3 glasses of milk or fortified soy milk? | Calcium and vitamin D, possibly vitamins $B_2$ and $B_{12}$, magnesium, zinc |
| _____ 5. at least 2 servings of extra-lean meat or legumes? | Iron and zinc, B vitamins |
| _____ 6. at least 6 servings of whole grains? | Trace minerals, such as chromium, selenium, and copper, B vitamins |
| _____ 7. several servings of nuts, seeds, avocados, olives? | Vitamin E |

---

daily. If you shun milk, meeting this quota means consuming six ounces of tofu, a can of salmon with the bones, and 2 cups of black bean soup every day. Not likely for most women.

*Vitamin D:* Frankly, I don't know where women get their vitamin D if they don't drink two to four glasses of milk or fortified soy milk every day or spend time in the sun (without sunscreen lotion). It would take an eight-egg-yolk omelette to meet even minimum amounts of this bone-building nutrient.

*Iron:* Women struggle to get even two-thirds of their daily need for this important trace mineral. According to Fergus Clydesdale, Ph.D., professor and head of the Department of Food Science at the University of Massachusetts in Amherst, a well-balanced diet averages about 6 mg of iron for every 1,000 calories. To meet the RDA of 15 mg (women who menstruate heavily or use the IUD for birth control might have even higher iron requirements—between 18 mg and 25 mg), we must consume at least 2,500 calories daily. No wonder most of us get closer to 10 mg of iron, while somewhere between 11 and 80 percent of us are iron deficient. Iron supplements help. In a study from the University of Newcastle in Australia, women who supplemented with iron showed improved mental health, reduced fatigue, and increased vitality.

*Vitamin E:* You need at least 100 IU of this vitamin daily to lower heart-disease risk and pump up your immune system. It would take eight cups of almonds, three-quarters of a cup of safflower oil, or sixty-two cups of fresh spinach every day to meet this need.

## Are Supplements Helpful?

Despite the wealth of research showing that women's diets are anything but balanced, many nutrition experts still resist recommending supplements. "Many people think they are under a vitamin security blanket because they take supplements; consequently, they are more likely to let their eating habits slide," says JoAnn Hattner, R.D., M.P.H., spokesperson for the American Dietetic Association and clinical nutritionist at Stanford University in Palo Alto, California.

But Jeffrey Blumberg, Ph.D., at U.S.D.A. Human Nutrition Research Center on Aging at Tufts University in Boston counters by saying there is no evidence that this happens; in fact, just the opposite is true. Compared to nonsupplementers, women who supplement also are more health conscious, take better care of themselves, eat better, and maintain better overall health. Preliminary evidence also shows they might be at lower risk for developing heart disease, cancer, osteoporosis, hypertension, memory loss, diabetes, and birth defects. They have stronger immune systems and might even be less likely to die prematurely compared to people who don't supplement.

In addition, supplementation with some vitamins, such as folic acid and vitamin $B_{12}$, could save Americans billions of dollars in health-care costs. According to an analysis by researchers at the University of California, San Francisco, these B vitamins lower homocysteine levels in the blood, an independent risk factor for heart disease. An analysis of the cost-effectiveness of vitamin fortification and supplements of grains in both individuals at high risk of heart disease and the general public found that a combination of eating fortified grains and taking supplements would save more than $2 billion in health costs and save more than

300,000 quality-adjusted life years. For women without heart disease, vitamin supplementation would save more than 140,000 quality-adjusted life years for every ten-year period.

## *The Best Approach: Good Diet, Responsible Supplements*

The supplement issue isn't black-and-white. Like all areas of nutrition science, some studies show no effect on health. Some studies falsely assumed the vitamins or minerals in food protected against disease, when it might be other compounds or a combination of food substances that are most beneficial. On the other hand, some nutrients, such as folic acid, vitamin $B_{12}$, and vitamin K, are better absorbed or used by the body in supplement form than from food, and some nutrients, such as vitamin D, are needed in increasing amounts as we age. "We need more definitive research, but even without conclusive evidence it makes sense to eat well *and* supplement," recommends Dr. Willett.

Dr. Blumberg agrees: "The 'balanced diet' is increasingly recognized as narrow-minded. Nutrition and supplements are not an either/or issue, but rather the two enhance each together. You can't always get optimal amounts of all the vitamins and minerals from food, just as pills don't contain everything that food has to offer."

For one thing, supplements can replace the handful of vitamins and minerals otherwise found in food, but they never will supply the right balance of the thousands of other health-enhancing phytochemicals in real foods like fruits, vegetables, whole grains, and legumes. A well-balanced vitamin and mineral supplement also improves some of the nutritional shortcomings of a good diet, but it can't make up for bad eating habits. "You can't live on doughnuts and hot dogs, then take a vitamin E supplement and think you're doing fine," says Dr. Blumberg.

The bottom line? Eat well and take a moderate-dose multiple, a little extra calcium and magnesium, and/or the antioxidants. As Dr. Willett says, a well-chosen supplement is a "nutritional safety net" for those days when you eat well, but not well enough.

## *Designing Your Supplement Program*

For healthy people, a multiple vitamin and mineral is best. Nutrients are supplied as teams in food, so if your diet is low in one nutrient, it's a sure bet it's low in others, too. A multiple is a convenient, cost-efficient way to supply a balance of nutrients, while avoiding secondary deficiencies that result when you take too much of one nutrient and crowd out another. For example, many of the minerals compete for absorption, so taking a large dose of one, such as iron, could result in a deficiency of another, such as copper or zinc.

Most one-pill-a-day multiples don't contain enough calcium or magnesium. The pills would be the size of a Ping-Pong ball if they did. These minerals are important in the prevention of osteoporosis and possibly high blood pressure, colon cancer, and heart disease. Unless you include at least three servings daily of calcium-rich milk products or fortified soy milk and lots of magnesium-rich soybeans, nuts, and wheat germ, you might consider an extra supplement of these two minerals.

### How Much?

In general, 100 to 200 percent of the Daily Value for each nutrient as listed on the label is sufficient. Megavitamin-mineral therapy—consuming ten times or more of the Daily Value—implies more is better or therapeutic, but usually is a waste of money.

The body can only use so much of any one nutrient. At best, excesses are excreted; at worst, they are stored to potentially toxic levels. In some cases, consuming too much can backfire. For example, taking a moderate dose of zinc enhances the body's immune system and its defense against disease, but taking large doses of zinc actually suppresses immunity. The exception to this rule is vitamin E, which might be beneficial in doses several times current Daily Value levels.

### Avoid the Glitz

Although the debate rages over what is best, when it comes to supplements, your best bet usually is to stick with the basics and avoid the glitz. Here's a crash course on label lingo.

---

**TABLE 6.2     Frequently Asked Questions**

Selecting a good supplement might seem overwhelming when faced with a wall of pills, powders, and potions. But it's really not that complicated. Most women just need a well-balanced multiple vitamin *and* mineral, a calcium-magnesium supplement, and possibly extra antioxidants.

**1.** How can I cut down on cost without sacrificing quality?

First, steer clear of supplements that contain extra ingredients, such as lipoic acid, enzymes, primrose oil, or inositol, to name only a few. These extras only add cost, not value, to a product since they are either worthless or supplied in amounts too low to be of use. Also, avoid the natural products; they're costly and usually provide no added benefit over other supplements.

Purchase bigger or economy-size bottles when the unit price saves you money. However, make sure you can use the supplements before the expiration date on the label to ensure they retain their potency. Also, consider purchasing store-brand multiples. Often these generics are manufactured by the same companies who make the brand-name products.

**2.** When's the best time of day to take a supplement?

The time of day has no effect on how well the nutrients in a supplement are used by the body, according to a study from the University of Helsinki in Finland. What is more important is what you take them with. Most nutrients are best absorbed when taken with meals and when taken in small doses throughout the day. But the inconvenience of taking divided doses might make a one-pill-a-day product more appealing. For maximum absorption, take a multiple with iron at a different meal than your calcium supplement, since these two minerals compete for absorption.

**3.** How much should I pay for a supplement?

You shouldn't pay more than $10 a month for any or all your supplements. You can find quality multiple vitamin and mineral supplements that cost under 10 cents a day, or $3 a month. Add another $1 to $3 a month for a good calcium-magnesium supplement, and about the same for an antioxidant or vitamin E capsule.

**4.** What do the letters USP mean on a supplement label?

United States Pharmacopeia or USP is a nongovernmental standard-setting body. This seal of quality means the supplement should dissolve within the digestive tract, is made from pure ingredients, and contains the amount of nutrients listed on the label. While the USP seal is definitely a plus and is found on supplements such as Essential

Balance, not all companies who follow high standards, such as One-A-Day, choose to put this seal on their products.

**5.** Are "women's" formulas better than a general multiple?

Women's nutritional needs are different from men's, so theoretically a special formula would more closely match their needs. But every product I researched was formulated more on marketing than on science, falling far short of optimal and costing much more than well-formulated multiples. You're better off following the above guidelines than you are selecting a supplement because of its name.

**6.** Where's the best place to buy my supplements?

In terms of quality, it doesn't make much difference. Most supplement companies purchase the raw ingredients from the same national manufacturers, like Hoffman LaRoche or Eastman Chemical Company. You'll probably pay less at a pharmacy or grocery store, because supplements here are less likely to contain expensive frills, such as herbs or bioflavonoids, which are more often found in products at health-food stores or through mail order.

**7.** Can I trust the claims on the label?

Usually not. Claims that a product is "complete," "balanced," "high potency," or specially formulated, or that it contains "extra antioxidants" or is a "multivitamin or multimineral" have little to do with the real formulations. Claims that a supplement will cure, treat, or even prevent any health condition are more hype than fact. Ignore the packaging and go straight to the nutritional information on the back of the label. Again, the USP seal on a label is the only accepted guarantee of quality.

**8.** The ingredients list of my supplement contains starch, methylcellulose, FD&C yellow No. 5, and other extras. Are any of these harmful and why are they there in the first place?

Vitamins and minerals are basic ingredients, but a useful supplement is a work of art. Nutrients don't just stick together, so manufacturers use binders, stabilizers, fillers, and other so-called inert substances to make a product that not only stays together in the bottle, but flows through the machinery at the manufacturing plant, protects ingredients from rancidity, keeps a pill from sticking to your throat, and makes the tablet or pill a recognizable size. According to David Kropp, manager of Regulatory and Legal Affairs at Pharmavite Corporation, the parent company of NatureMade vitamins, "There are a relative few additives in supplements and most of these inert ingredients, including the most common one, dibasic calcium phosphate, have safely been used in pharmaceuticals for a long time."

Even the ones that on rare occasions cause side effects, such as FD&C yellow

No. 5 dye, lactose, or fructose, are unlikely to be a problem at the minuscule doses found in a supplement. For example, the possibility of an allergic reaction to the refined starch used as a filler is extremely rare; the amount of lactose in a supplement is a few milligrams, but it takes grams of lactose to produce a reaction.

---

*Chelated Minerals:* A chelated mineral is chemically bound to another substance, usually an amino acid (the building blocks of protein). Examples include iron/amino chelate or chromium proteinate. Although manufacturers propose that chelation improves the absorption of a mineral, there is little proof that chelated minerals are any better absorbed than other supplements.

*Time-Released Vitamins:* Theoretically, these supplements should raise and maintain blood levels of a vitamin better than regular supplements. In reality, most time-released tablets dissolve too slowly to be completely absorbed. Time-released forms of niacin are well absorbed but might be more toxic to the liver than a similar amount of a non-time-released brand.

*Natural versus Synthetic Vitamins:* The wholesome aura of "organic" and "natural" does little more than increase the cost of most supplements. First, the body cannot distinguish a natural from a synthetic nutrient. Second, many products labeled as natural are actually synthetic vitamins laced with small amounts of natural vitamins. For example, a natural vitamin C supplement often contains mostly laboratory-made ascorbic acid with a small amount of vitamin C from rose hips.

Selenium, chromium, and vitamin E are exceptions to the rule. The organic forms of selenium (selenium-rich yeast or L-selenomethionine) and chromium (chromium-rich yeast, chromium nicotinate, and chromium picolinate) are the best absorbed and used and, therefore, are your best bets. Body tissues prefer the natural form of vitamin E, called d-alpha-tocopherol to the synthetic counterpart, called dl-alpha- or all-rac-alpha-tocopherol, which is a mix of d-alpha-tocopherol plus seven less potent forms of vitamin E. However, these natural supplements are more expensive. If you can't afford the extra cost of natural, don't worry. A wealth of research has shown great results with synthetic vitamin E in lowering heart-disease risk and boosting immunity.

*Collodial Minerals:* Save your money and skip this scam. There is no evidence that minerals in suspension are better absorbed or used by the body than conventional minerals. Worse yet, some of these supplements contain toxic metals, such as silver, lead, and arsenic.

---

### BOX 6.1    Supplements Worth a Try

*Flax:* Flaxseed is one of the richest dietary sources of lignans. Lignans are converted to weak estrogen-like compounds in the digestive tract, which have anticancer and weak estrogen properties that help lower the risk for breast and colon cancer. Isoflavonoids in flax also fight cancer. The fiber in flaxseed might help lower blood cholesterol levels, while a type of fat called alpha-linolenic acid in flax is low in people suffering from depression. No optimal dose has been established. To get the full benefits of flaxseed, choose the seeds or meal over the oil.

*Zinc:* Zinc lozenges might not prevent the common cold, but a handful of studies show that it might shorten the duration and severity of some symptoms, such as coughing, headaches, hoarseness, congestion, and sore throat. So taking one or two of these daily is worth a try. However, watch out for overdoses here. More than 35 mg to 50 mg of zinc daily over time actually suppresses the immune system and could interfere with your body's efforts to get well.

*Echinacea:* This herb appears to stimulate naturally your immune system by turning on blood chemicals that regulate the duration and intensity of the immune response. Thus, either the capsules or the drops taken several times during the day might curb cold and flu symptoms. Make sure the product contains a standardized amount of the herb, or you're likely to see little or no results. Don't take echinacea for more than two to three weeks at a time, however, since its protective effects might wear off with prolonged use.

*Coenzyme Q10:* Also called ubiquinone, coenzyme Q10 (CoQ10) helps convert food and oxygen into energy. Produced in the body and obtained from the diet, CoQ10 might improve heart function, boost immunity, and function as an antioxidant, much like vitamin E and selenium, in protecting the blood vessels, heart, brain, and other tissues from free radical damage. No optimal dose has been established.

### The Eight-Step Plan

The following Eight-Step Plan will minimize waste and maximize benefits when choosing vitamin-mineral supplements.

*Step 1.* Choose a multiple vitamin-mineral preparation, rather than several single supplements, unless prescribed by a dietitian or physician.

*Step 2.* Choose a preparation that provides approximately 100 percent of the Daily Value for the following:

> *Vitamins:* beta carotene; vitamins D, E, C, K, $B_1$, $B_2$, $B_6$, and $B_{12}$; niacin; folic acid; and pantothenic acid. (Avoid large doses of vitamin $B_1$, vitamin $B_2$, and niacin. A supplement manufacturer adds hefty amounts of these nutrients only because they are inexpensive, not because extra is better.)

> *Minerals:* copper, iron, and zinc, and 50 to 200 mcg of both chromium and selenium, 5 mg of manganese, and 75 to 250 mcg of molybdenum.

*Step 3.* Vitamins C and E can be consumed in amounts greater than the Daily Value. Safe and potentially beneficial amounts of these nutrients are 250 mg to 500 mg vitamin C and 100 IU to 400 IU vitamin E.

*Step 4.* Consider a second supplement with 1,000 mg calcium and 500 mg magnesium, if your multiple is low in these minerals.

*Step 5.* Ignore the minute amounts of starch, sugar, or preservatives in a supplement, since they are relatively harmless. Avoid supplements that contain useless substances, such as inositol, vitamin $B_{15}$, PABA, or nutrients in amounts less than 25 percent of the Daily Value. The following nutrients are adequately supplied in the diet and are not needed in a supplement: biotin, phosphorus, chloride, potassium, sodium.

*Step 6.* Avoid the unsubstantiated claims of "natural," "organic," "therapeutic," "high-potency," "chelated," "time-released," "women's formulas," or "stress-formulated" supplements. They also tend to cost too much.

*Step 7.* If you are willing to put up with the inconvenience, select a product that can be taken in several doses throughout the day, since nutrients supplied in small doses throughout the day are better absorbed than are one-shot supplements.

Multidose multiples also provide flexibility; you can adjust the dose to meet your needs.

*Step 8.* Except for iron, which is best absorbed on an empty stomach, take your supplement with food and without coffee or tea.

---

**TABLE 6.3     A Crash Course on the Vitamins and Minerals in Your Supplements**

Here's a brief glance at some of the nutrients needed for health and what you should look for when choosing a supplement.

**Vitamin A/Beta Carotene**

*How much?* The Daily Value of 5,000 IU is a safe dose, especially for women who might become or are pregnant; higher amounts might cause birth defects in fetuses. Better yet, choose beta carotene, which is relatively nontoxic at doses of 10 mg to 30 mg, and can be converted to vitamin A in the body. Smokers should consult their physicians before supplementing with beta carotene.

*What should you look for?* A mixture of vitamin A and beta carotene. Most forms of vitamin A, such as retinyl palmitate or acetate, are well absorbed.

**Vitamin D**

*How much?* The Daily Value of 400 IU is a safe dose. Only seniors might need more than this (600 IU to 800 IU).

*What should you look for?* Vitamin D or cholecalciferol.

**Vitamin K**

*How much?* The RDA* is 65 mcg, but you're lucky if you find 25 mcg in most multiples.

*What should you look for?* Usually listed as vitamin K, vitamin $K_1$, or phylloquinone.

**Folic Acid**

*How much?* The Daily Value is 400 mcg (or 0.4 mg). Don't take more than 800 mcg without physician approval.

*What should you look for?* Folic acid or folate.

### Vitamin C

*How much?* The RDA is 60 mg. Smokers need at least 120 mg a day. You might need up to 250 mg to saturate your body's tissues.

*What should you look for?* Vitamin C, ascorbic acid, or calcium ascorbate.

### Vitamin E

*How much?* The Daily Value is 30 IU, but doses of 100 IU to 400 IU are safe and possibly beneficial. Few multiples contain this much, so a separate supplement is worth considering.

*What should you look for?* D-alpha tocopherol is the natural form of vitamin E and appears to be slightly better used by the body than the synthetic dl-alpha-tocopherol; however, the extra cost might not be worth the minor benefit.

### Vitamin $B_6$

*How much?* The Daily Value is 2 mg. Women on birth control pills might need slightly higher amounts. Excessive doses of 100 mg or more might cause neurological problems, such as tingling in the hands and feet.

*What should you look for?* Vitamin $B_6$ or pyridoxine hydrochloride (HCl).

### Vitamin $B_{12}$

*How much?* The Daily Value is 6 mcg.

*What should you look for?* Vitamin $B_{12}$ or cobalamine.

### Boron

*How much?* No RDA or Daily Value has been set for boron. Typical daily intakes range from 0.5 mg to 7.0 mg, and studies showing a health benefit often use 3 mg daily.

*What should you look for?* Boron, sodium borate.

### Calcium

*How much?* The Daily Value is 1,000 mg. No one-tablet-daily multiple contains this much, so you might consider taking a separate supplement, such as a combination calcium and magnesium. An Upper Limit (UL) for safety is 2,500 mg.

*What should you look for?* Most forms of calcium are well absorbed. Calcium carbonate and calcium citrate contain the most calcium per tablet. Calcium gluconate or lactate contains less calcium, so more tablets must be taken. Natural calcium from oyster shell, bone meal, or dolomite might contain unacceptable levels of lead.

## Chromium

*How much?* The Safe and Adequate Range[†] is 50 mcg to 200 mcg. There's no evidence that amounts greater than this are of any health benefit.

*What should you look for?* Chromium nicotinate, chromium-rich yeast, or chromium picolinate appear to be absorbed better than chromium chloride.

## Copper

*How much?* The Daily Value is 2 mg.

*What should you look for?* Copper gluconate, oxide, or sulfate, or cupric oxide.

## Iron

*How much?* The Daily Value is 18 mg, which is a safe amount for premenopausal women. Men and postmenopausal women should not take supplemental iron or limit intake to 10 mg.

*What should you look for?* Iron is best absorbed in the ferrous form, such as ferrous fumarate or ferrous sulfate.

## Magnesium

*How much?* The Daily Value is 400 mg. No one-tablet-daily multiple contains this much, so you might consider taking a separate supplement, such as a combination calcium and magnesium. Doses of 600 mg or more might cause diarrhea.

*What should you look for?* Magnesium oxide, citrate, or hydroxide.

## Selenium

*How much?* The RDA is 55 mcg for women. Don't take more than 200 mcg, since this mineral can be toxic.

*What should you look for?* Selenomethionine or selenium-rich yeast is possibly better absorbed than the inorganic forms, such as sodium selenate or selenite.

### Zinc

*How much?* The Daily Value is 15 mg. Doses greater than 50 mg might suppress immune
function.
*What should you look for?* Zinc gluconate, picolinate, oxide, or sulfate.

*No RDA has been established for this mineral, only a range of intakes considered both safe and probably
adequate. These values won't appear on labels.
†The Recommended Dietary Allowance (RDA) is used here when no Daily Value has been established.
These values won't appear on labels.

# CHAPTER 7

# Staying Slim: Losing Weight for Good

A h, to be a shrew. Those furry little critters eat their body weight in food every day, yet remain lean, mean machines. That's the equivalent of 200,000 calories daily for the average woman, or twenty-five double cheeseburgers, ten gallons of French fries, twenty-nine gallons of chocolate milk shake, thirty-five pieces of chocolate cheesecake topped with ten cups of whipped cream, and a big apple. OK, so that's excessive even on a high-binge day (say the week before your period, for example). Still, the gluttony of a shrew is enviable.

Alas, our metabolisms are more like that of a slug than a shrew, leading one in every two of us to try the latest weight-loss diet, while shaving our average daily intakes to a measly 1,600 calories even when we're not dieting. Despite our herculean diet efforts, we continue to gain weight, averaging seven pounds more today than we did ten years ago. Granted, we're experts at how to lose weight. The average dieter has lost several hundred pounds during her lifetime. It's keeping the weight off that eludes ninety-five out of every hundred dieters.

You can't eat like a shrew, but you needn't throw in the diet towel either. There's hope. Lots of it. That 95 percent failure rate is far too dismal and is based on studies of chronically obese people who turn to university research programs as a last resort—just the type of people you'd expect to fail. A much larger percentage of women outside these programs have successfully dropped the pounds and kept them off without feeling deprived, exercising like madwomen, or obsessing over calories, fat grams, or their weight.

## *Success Stories*

The National Weight Control Registry (NWCR), an ongoing project at the University of Pittsburgh and the University of Colorado, is brimming with thousands of success stories from people who have maintained a thirty-pound or more weight loss for more than one year. The registry and numerous studies show that successful dieters are no different than you and me. Like most dieters, they spent years at the win-lose weight game before they finally found success. Many were overweight as children, have one or more overweight parents, or have gained weight gradually over time. So why do they succeed when the rest fail? The answer is simple: They prepare themselves for the after-the-diet phase, while the diet duds don't.

According to Mary Lou Kelm, Ph.D., assistant professor in the Department of Psychology and lead researcher in the NWCR, success has little to do with how people lose weight. "It doesn't seem to matter whether people lose weight by joining a structured weight-loss program or just doing it on their own. More important, registry members say they finally succeeded when they became more committed to changing their behaviors, losing weight, and being physically active," says Klem. One common theme, however, is that none of the success stories used fad diets—from food combining or low-carbohydrate to eating for your body or blood type—to lose weight for good.

Anne Fletcher, M.S., R.D., who studied 280 successful weight maintainers or "Masters" for her book *Eating Thin for Life* (Chapters/Houghton Mifflin, 1997), agrees and adds, "The big difference between those who keep the weight off and those who don't is that the Masters stop drawing the arbitrary distinction between dieting and their normal lives." To reach your weight-loss goals, and more importantly keep the weight off, you must be willing to revise your life for good, adopting weight-loss strategies you can live with forever. If all you want is to lose weight fast and go back to your old ways, then forget it.

## *Strategies for Success*

But what are those strategies? According to all of the reviews on weight-loss success, including one from Duke University, our weight-loss heroes follow some very consistent guidelines: They are rigorous planners, developing strategies ahead of time to avoid pitfalls. They closely monitor their eating and exercise often by

---

**TABLE 7.1    Am I Ready to Make a Change?**

Is this the best time to attempt weight loss and become more fit? On a scale of 1 to 5 (1 = not at all, 5 = more so than ever), answer the following questions:

_____ **1.** Compared to dieting attempts in the past, how motivated are you to stick with it this time?

_____ **2.** How determined are you to stick with it until you reach your weight or fitness goals?

_____ **3.** Long-term weight management requires effort. How willing are you to take the time and make the effort to reach your goals?

_____ **4.** Weight loss should be gradual (no more than two pounds per week) to ensure permanent fat loss. How realistic are your plans to lose weight in a given amount of time?

_____ **5.** How much support for your weight-management efforts can you expect from friends, family, coworkers, and other people in your social support network?

_____ **6.** Learning weight-management skills is like learning any new skill, it requires time. How much time do you have to make permanent changes in your life?

**Add up your scores.**

6 to 16 points: Reflects a low commitment to weight management and a high likelihood of failure in losing weight or keeping it off. Wait and try another time.

17 to 23: Reflects a moderate commitment to weight management, but you still need to work on motivation.

24 or higher: Reflects high motivation. This could be the best time to begin losing weight.

---

keeping daily journals, and they keep close tabs on their weight, quickly jumping into action with well thought out strategies at the first sign of a three-to-five-pound weight gain. They make their health a priority, nurture support from themselves and others, and are good problem solvers. It's no surprise that they exercise a lot and permanently shave fat and calories from their diets. What is surprising is that the majority report they enjoy food, don't feel deprived or as if they're even on a diet. They don't spend extra time thinking about their weight or food, yet are happier and more self-confident as a result of the lifelong changes. They also consistently report that the weight-loss process gets easier the longer they stick with it.

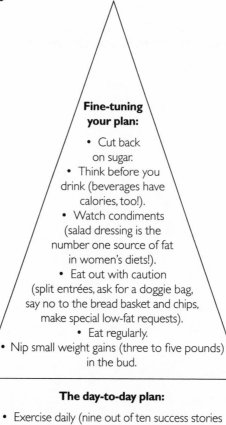

**Fine-tuning
your plan:**

- Cut back
on sugar.
- Think before you
drink (beverages have
calories, too!).
- Watch condiments
(salad dressing is the
number one source of fat
in women's diets!).
- Eat out with caution
(split entrées, ask for a doggie bag,
say no to the bread basket and chips,
make special low-fat requests).
- Eat regularly.
- Nip small weight gains (three to five pounds)
in the bud.

**The day-to-day plan:**

- Exercise daily (nine out of ten success stories
exercise regularly, even daily; they vary exercise
from day to day and season to season).
- Adopt a low-fat, fiber-rich diet. (Focus on vegetables,
fruit, whole grains, legumes, and nonfat milk products.
Use meat as a condiment.)
- Closely monitor your progress (i.e., preplan meals, cut portions,
have a shopping list, check calories, weigh yourself,
keep a food and exercise diary).
- Convert negative self-talk to positive self-talk.
- Stay motivated (list pros and cons, establish nonfood rewards).
- Encourage support. Seek people with similar health goals.

**The first steps to success:**

- Believe you can succeed.
- Take responsibility. Accept there are no quick fixes. This process is up to you and for you.
- Develop a plan you can live with for life (include favorite foods in moderation).
- Acknowledge it won't be easy.
- Create problem-solving strategies (don't solve emotional problems with food,
deal with high-risk situations, plan relapse tactics).
- Set realistic goals to lose weight gradually.

---

**GRAPH 7.1     The Healthy Woman's Weight-Loss Pyramid**

While every success story is unique, there are common themes, such as nine out of ten successes exercise daily and all follow low-fat/high-fiber diets. More important than diet and exercise is a change in attitude.

The Healthy Woman's Weight-Loss Pyramid reflects that. The three tiers are equally important, but are ordered in terms of what to do first, with the tips in the bottom tier representing steps you should take first, followed by day-to-day tips to follow in the middle tier, and finally fine-tuning tips at the top. All the tips within each tier are equally important and will vary from person to person. Select the tips from each tier, in order, that pertain to you. Focus on these in designing your personalized successful-change program.

---

"Those successful at weight loss have accomplished a powerful, yet simple task; they've learned that food isn't the issue; it's only the symptom," states Lauren Mellin, M.A., R.D., author of *The Solution* (Regan Books, 1997), a book regarding a program developed at the University of California, San Francisco, that has been very successful at ending the weight battle for thousands of chronic dieters. "Food stops serving the role of nurturer when people learn to nurture themselves and set realistic limits. As a result, their lives work better and they no longer need to overeat."

Thousands of people have proven that weight-loss success is possible. So, here are the ten no-fail steps guaranteed to stop the diet merry-go-round and help you negotiate permanent peace with your weight and health. You'll tame the shrew within you and feel the best you've ever felt. At least that's what the hoards of people who have crossed the dieting finish line tell us! Read on. You'll also find hints and tips on how to develop a weight-loss program that will make you a success, too.

## *Ten Steps to Losing Weight and Keeping It Off*

Permanent weight management is not just a matter of eating less. If you're serious about reaching and sustaining a realistic weight, then *commitment* must become your middle name. People who are successful at keeping weight off typically have histories of repeated failed dieting attempts. What made the difference the last time was their commitment to change, including decisions to permanently change the way they ate and thought, how much they moved and how well they organized their lives, solved problems, and strategized. It also means taking a hard look at the role food plays in your life, since what you weigh is a reflection of how you live. Those skills can be summarized in the following ten steps.

## Step 1: Plan Ahead

There's a saying that "failing to plan is planning to fail." Nowhere does that apply more than with weight management. Successful losers learn to set realistic expectations and limits on themselves. Continually ask yourself, "Is this reasonable for me at this time in my life?" Then, plan your meals, your daily exercise, and how you will handle personal high-risk situations from stress, parties, and travel to eating in restaurants and boredom. Anticipate problems and go into battle well armed with a plan. Even have a plan for when you slip off your plans. Leave little to chance. "Successful losers pay attention. They watch their weight, self-monitor their eating and exercise habits, and have backup plans for how they'll handle problem situations," says Dr. Klem.

Planning begins by setting realistic weight-loss goals of no more than one to two pounds a week. It also means time spent up-front keeping records, finding solutions to barriers (what's keeping you from eating right or exercising more?), and educating yourself on nutrition basics, from reading labels to eyeballing portions. Refer to chapter 8 for information on how to keep a food diary, set goals, develop a plan, and manage tough situations.

## Step 2: Pay Attention

Monitoring your progress is one of the most important habits you can develop. For the first few weeks of a weight-management program, keep a food journal and record what, how much, when, and where you eat, as well as your hunger level and mood before and after the meal. This boosts self-awareness, keeps you focused on your goals, provides invaluable feedback, and is the critical first step in designing strategies.

Most important, pay attention to your needs. "Develop the habit of checking your feelings at least five times during the day by asking yourself 'how do I feel' and 'what do I need,'" suggests Mellin. Weight maintainers also keep close track of their daily exercise and their weight. Some weigh and measure their food in the beginning, until they can accurately eyeball correct portions. Others find that jotting down how much time they spent sitting or lying down was the motivation they needed to start exercising.

## BOX 7.1    Take the Stairs

Being a fit chick means seriously pumping iron or running marathons, right? Not necessarily. According to studies from the University of Pennsylvania School of Medicine in Philadelphia and the Cooper Institute for Aerobic Research in Dallas, you benefit as much from increasing your daily activity—like taking the stairs instead of the elevator or walking instead of driving short distances—as you do from a structured exercise program. In the Pennsylvania study, overweight women either took aerobics classes for up to forty-five minutes three days a week (totaling about 1,500 calories/week of exercise) or they accumulated thirty minutes daily of moderate-intensity physical activity within their normal daily routines.

The results were astonishing! Women who increased their lifestyle activity lost about the same amount of weight compared to the women who followed a traditional aerobic exercise program. The more they moved during the day, the greater the benefits. "Compared to the exercisers, the women who increased their lifestyle activity had a greater tendency to maintain their weight loss because they continued to stay more active, while many of the exercisers dropped out of the aerobics class," says Thomas Wadden, Ph.D., one of the study's investigators and director of the Weight and Eating Disorders Program at the University of Pennsylvania.

How did the women boost their daily activity? According to Dr. Wadden, they stopped using their kids as servants, took miniwalks of one to five minutes several times during the day, and threw out the television remote control. Some answered the phone or went to the bathroom on a different floor at work or got up to talk to their coworkers rather than e-mailing them. "Ultimately, weight loss is about calories in and calories out, and you can package those calories out as either high-intensity workouts or moderate-intensity activity distributed throughout the day," says Wadden.

Be honest, specific, and complete in your record keeping. (Diet successes are consistently more accurate about portion size than are diet failures.) Record information at mealtime, since memory is highly inaccurate. Return to record keeping at the first sign of weight gain. Use "The Daily Food Record" on page 149 to stay on track.

## Step 3: Keep Moving

The most important predictor of whether or not you will succeed at permanent weight loss is physical activity. While some studies recommend burning at least 1,500 calories a week exercising, Dr. Klem says the NWCR shows many people need to move much more than that. "Successful losers are very active, expending about 2,800 calories a week in physical activity, which is the equivalent of walking four miles every day," says Dr. Klem. She cautions that they probably didn't start out at that level of exercise, but gradually increased their activity during weight loss so that by the time they were seasoned maintainers they were very active.

While most maintainers walk for exercise or combine activities such as aerobics or swimming, how you burn the calories doesn't seem to matter. In fact, recent evidence shows that even just taking the stairs or using a push lawnmower might do the trick.

## Step 4: Eat a Low-Fat, Low-Calorie Diet

Contrary to the latest diet craze to eat more protein and less carbohydrates, people who lose weight *and* keep the weight off make carbohydrate-rich foods, like whole grains and vegetables, the mainstay of their diets. They also watch their intakes of calories and fat. "Calories are the main focus, with fat being important only because it is a concentrated source of calories," says John Foreyt, Ph.D., a psychologist at Baylor College of Medicine in Houston who has extensively studied successful dieters. The success stories also eat regularly, dividing their food intakes evenly throughout the day. They create an individualized plan based on the same healthy foods they ate while dieting; they're just a little freer with their choices. How free can you be? Try adding 100 calories to your weight-loss diet every few days until your weight stabilizes.

## Step 5: Be a Problem Solver

People who succeed at weight loss are confronted with the same high-risk situations as their diet-challenged friends. The difference is that diet failures fall victim to the situation, while diet successes control these situations by creative problem solving. For example, the number one predictor of relapse is emotional issues, such as stress. "Successful weight managers have mapped out their trouble-prone situations along with effective solutions. They call ahead to ask if the restaurant will serve low-fat foods, they bring fruit platters to parties, and they pack their own lunches so they're not tempted by the doughnuts at work," says Dr. Foreyt.

From your diet records, you'll identify high-risk situations. Write them down on the left-hand side of a piece of paper and develop plans for handling these situations on the opposite right-hand side. Revise your plans as needed using the suggestions in chapter 8.

---

**TABLE 7.2    Time-Tested Strategies to Lose Weight and Keep It Off**

1. *Make exercise fun.* Listen to books on tape while you walk the dog, read a book on the exercise bicycle, vary your workouts with the season.

2. *Eat two fruits and/or vegetables at every meal and one at every snack.* You'll meet your daily quota of eight to ten servings, feel full, and automatically cut back on fat and calories.

3. *Take a little hike, every hour.* If you don't have time for an hour workout, set your watch alarm on the hour and take a five-minute brisk walk around the office. Over the course of an eight-hour shift, you'll accrue forty minutes of exercise.

4. *Turn off the tube.* Hours of television watching are directly proportional to weight gain. Go for an after-dinner walk, ride the exercise bike, do laundry, or paint the living room instead.

5. *Just say no.* Listen to your body and eat only when you're hungry, not because the food is there or because someone offers it.

6. *Drink first.* We often confuse thirst with hunger, diving for the ice cream when it's water our bodies need. Drink a glass of water and wait fifteen minutes before giving in to a craving. You may find that the hunger subsides.

7. *Challenge yourself.* If you're comfortable walking at a moderate pace, go up a short hill during your next walk or pick up the pace.

8. *Be a lark.* Exercise in the morning so you don't spend the rest of the day making up excuses why you can't exercise.

9. *Be an expert.* Learn to read labels and purchase mostly foods that contain no more than 3 grams of fat for every 100 calories (or approximately 30 percent fat calories).

10. *Doggie bag it.* Most restaurant servings are platters, not portions. Put half the serving in a doggie bag for tomorrow's lunch.

11. *Skip the fat-free desserts.* Ounce for ounce, most fat-free desserts are just as calorie-dense as the higher-fat versions. Even if they are low-calorie, you aren't doing yourself any favors by eating the whole box. Stick to the serving size on the label.

**12.** *Eat less.* Cut your typical portions of everything except vegetables and fruit by one quarter.

**13.** *Hang out with exercisers.*

**14.** *Remember, the calories in beverages count.* Especially those in gourmet coffee drinks, fruit juices, or smoothies.

**15.** *Watch out for extras.* A tablespoon of mayo on a turkey sandwich doesn't seem like a lot, but over the course of one year that daily mayo equals ten and a half pounds of excess body fat.

**16.** *Don't assume you can exercise away anything you eat.* A café mocha is the calorie equivalent of a one-hour jog.

**17.** *Get enough sleep.* You're more likely to overeat and choose all the wrong foods (candy, chocolate, sugar, and caffeine) when you're tired.

**18.** *Purchase a step counter.* This small device straps to your ankle and is a great incentive to boost the number of steps you take every day.

---

## Step 6: Healthy Self-Centeredness

Chuck the "Good Girl" syndrome. When you put other people's needs before your own—by cooking what they prefer or trading your exercise time to complete a project at work—your weight-management efforts are shoved to the back burner. Instead, develop a healthy sense of self-centeredness. When women learn to identify how they feel and what they need, they no longer turn to food to fulfill themselves. Instead they call a friend if they're lonely, cry if they're sad, and eat only when they're physically hungry. Generating the motivation to succeed also requires that you truly want to lose the weight for you and your health, not because your significant other makes a snide comment about your weight, your mother pressures you to do it, or because you want to look like a knockout at your sister's wedding or class reunion. In other words, take care of, even pamper, yourself every day, including making daily exercise a number one priority.

## Step 7: Think Positively

What's on your mind is just as important as what's on your plate. Listen to your self-talk, those thoughts that repeat over and over like a mantra. Successful dieters use positive self-talk, reinforcing their efforts with an internal dialogue of support and encouragement. They also have a firm conviction that they will succeed. "Somewhere along the way toward diet success, these people develop a strong belief in themselves. They stop seeing themselves as diet failures and start defining themselves as people who take control and are successful," says Fletcher.

To boost your self-efficacy, find successful role models, emulate them, and ask them how they made healthy choices, started and stayed with exercise, or bolstered their self-esteem. Replace negative internal messages ("I can't do this," "I'm no good") with positive, supportive ones ("I'm making great progress," "I can do anything I set my mind to do").

## Step 8: Team Work

It's tough to stay on the diet track when everyone is eating chocolate eclairs. You need to convert sabotage into support to keep you going through the tough times and to provide valuable feedback. Most successful weight managers have surrounded themselves with supportive family members and friends, or regularly attend a support group. They include their loved ones in their new eating and exercise plans.

Encouraging support takes two skills: asking for it and modeling it. Use assertive (not aggressive or passive) communication skills to ask specifically for the type of help and support you need from friends and family. If you lose weight through a clinic or program, stay in touch with fellow weight managers. (See chapter 8 for more tips on how to encourage support from friends and family.)

## Step 9: Revel in Imperfection

Never say never or always. Successful dieters give themselves permission to be imperfect. Successful weight managers often accept a weight heavier than their dream weight, one that is comfortable but doesn't require starvation regimens or fanatic exercise programs. They also realize that slips are normal and expected. They allow themselves treat foods that others label as forbidden. The secret is they don't let one day of missed exercise or one piece of chocolate cake undo all their efforts. If they go overboard, they pick themselves up and start over again at the next meal or the next day.

The trick here is to have an early-warning plan to prevent slips from progressing to relapse. Reinstate record keeping, cut portions, or exercise ten extra minutes a day when your weight moves out of a three-to-five-pound buffer zone.

Remember: There are no mistakes, only feedback. Chapter 8 has more information on how to handle slips and avoid relapse.

### Step 10: Pat Yourself on the Back

What will keep you motivated to stick with your weight-management efforts? What will sustain your determination? What are the benefits to finally saying so long to the diet roller coaster? Making sure your new habits are positively reinforced is the most powerful way to motivate yourself to stay on track. Use your creative problem-solving skills to develop an ongoing list of nonfood bonuses you give yourself for meeting certain goals or when you just need a boost. It could be clothing, a movie, stars on the calendar, or quarters in a jar for every day you exercise (use the money to buy yourself new exercise equipment), a manicure, or planting flowers. Use the "If . . . then" rule. *If* you reach your goal, *then,* and only then, do you get the bonus. Use lots of rewards at the start to keep you motivated to stick with it. Later on, as diet changes become habits, how good you feel and look will be reward enough.

## *Your Diet Game Plan*

While the research on weight and obesity is complex and sometimes confusing, the guidelines for managing weight are straightforward. The tried-and-true guidelines for losing weight and keeping the weight off include:

1. Combine a healthful mix of the energy nutrients, with 55 to 65 percent of calories from carbohydrates, 20 to 25 percent of calories from fat, and 10 to 20 percent of calories from protein.
2. Consume no less than 1,500 calories (with an additional 500 calories for taller or more active women) daily. If you can't lose weight on this calorie intake, then increase your daily exercise.
3. Choose nutrient-packed foods to ensure you meet your daily needs for all vitamins, minerals, fiber, protein, phytochemicals, and more (you'll still need to consider a multiple when intake falls below 2,000 calories).
4. Plan to lose weight gradually, or approximately one to two pounds a week. This ensures you lose fat, not muscle or water weight.

## What's a Desirable Weight?

Good question! The hidden message from viewing fashion models is "the thinner the better"; however, most of us know by now that striving for ultrathinness is harmful to our egos and our health. We're ready to aim for something a little healthier and more realistic. But the researchers can't even agree on the "ideal" weight for our health.

David Levitsky, Ph.D., professor of nutrition and psychology at Cornell University, reports that a few extra pounds won't hurt you and might be healthier in the long run than being underweight. "While there is no question that obesity is associated with all kinds of health risks, gaining twenty to thirty pounds over a lifetime does not pose a health risk and, actually might improve your health profile," says Dr. Levitsky. No one knows why heavier people live longer than their lean counterparts, but Dr. Levitsky speculates that while being underweight probably doesn't directly cause health problems, a slightly heavier person who becomes sick might have more "reserves" to fight the disease longer than would a skinny person.

The Cornell study is in stark contrast to other studies that found a strong link between even moderate weight gain and disease risk. According to researchers at Harvard Medical School, relying on the Metropolitan Life Tables could give us a false sense of security. In reviewing weights and disease rates in more than 115,000 women, the Harvard researchers found that modest weight gain (eleven to eighteen pounds) in the middle years, even though the women's weights were considered normal, raised their risks for developing heart disease by 25 percent. A gain of more than eighteen pounds raised disease risks even higher. The lowest disease rate from all causes was observed among women who weighed at least 15 percent less than the average for women of similar age and in women who maintained a stable weight throughout life.

The Cornell and Harvard findings are not as contradictory as they appear and might distill down to who is losing weight and why. The Cornell study pooled data from nineteen studies that included men and women. "The link between underweight and mortality is strongest in men, while lower weights have less of an effect on mortality in women," says Dr. Levitsky. Then there is the issue of confounding factors, such as cigarette smoking and undiagnosed disease such as cancer. "Most studies that have looked at mortality risks and weight have not controlled carefully for these confounding factors," says Walter Willett, M.D., Dr.P.H., at the Harvard School of Public Health in Boston, and head researcher of the Nurses' Health Study.

Other studies bear this out. In a study conducted at the National Center for Chronic Disease Prevention and Health Promotion in Atlanta, researchers found that *intentional* weight loss, that is healthy people dieting to lose weight, reduces disease risks, while a study from the National Institute of Aging in Bethesda concluded that *involuntary* weight loss that results from illness or cigarette smoking was a major contributor to disease and death.

The bottom line? There isn't one that is agreeable to everyone. Obviously, being too thin is harmful if it results from unhealthy habits or disease. On the other hand, being very overweight or obese is definitely a serious health hazard for everyone, especially women. The middle ground of weight gain, where love handles and soft curves reside, is the hot seat of controversy. A few extra pounds on a woman who exercises and is otherwise fit, is not a problem. However, love handles combined with a couch-potato lifestyle might well cut short your healthy years.

Everyone agrees on one issue: prevention is the best medicine when it comes to health and weight. If you are gaining a few pounds every year and those extra pounds are fat not muscle, take it as a sign you should nip future weight problems in the bud by starting and sticking with a daily exercise routine and low-fat diet. And while body fat is the weight you want to monitor, the bathroom scale is still a reasonable way to track your gains and losses. "Body weight is a more sensitive indicator than body fat, if for no other reason than the scale will detect a five-pound weight loss long before body-fat calipers measure a small shift in body fat," says Dr. Willett. The good news—it's never too late to start!

## What about Yo-Yo Dieting?

For years, we were told that repeatedly losing and regaining the same ten pounds was harmful to our health and made future weight loss that much harder. However, a panel of experts from the National Institutes of Health reviewed more than forty scientific studies on yo-yo dieting and concluded that there is "no compelling evidence that weight cycling has adverse effects on the body . . . or future efforts at weight loss."

While yo-yo dieting might not be as harmful as once thought, it is by no means considered safe for long-term health and emotional well-being. In contrast, even modest weight loss in overweight people improves health and avoids the weight cycling posed by repeated attempts to get thin.

## Time-Proven Diet Skills

While the weight war is waged in the laboratory and on the streets, the common soldier who wants to keep her health and her waistline intact must rely on the only sound, time-proven skills for permanent weight management.

1. Maximize nutrients.
2. Cut back on fat, sugar, and refined grains . . . in that order.
3. Take daily exercise seriously.

*Focus on Plants:* The basis of a successful weight-management eating plan is to emphasize fruits, vegetables, and whole grains, with moderate amounts of calcium-rich (nonfat milk) and iron-rich (extra-lean meats, chicken, fish, or legumes) foods. Plan your meals and snacks around fruits, vegetables, whole grains, and legumes so that they constitute at least three-quarters of the foods in your eating plan. By doing this, you will automatically cut back on fat, sugar, and unnecessary calories. However, even the best diet can't guarantee optimal intake of all nutrients when it drops below 2,000 calories. So, consider taking a moderate-dose, well-balanced vitamin and mineral supplement.

*Lose Weight Gradually:* You want an eating plan you can live with for life and one that will allow a gradual weight loss of no more than two pounds a week. Strive for no less than 1,500 calories if you are short or relatively inactive (add an additional 500 calories if you are tall and/or active). You should increase exercise, not cut calories further, if you can't lose weight on this low-calorie plan.

*Eat Regularly:* When you eat those calories also is important. Large, infrequent meals might set up a feast-or-famine scenario where the body stores more calories as fat as a safeguard against what it perceives as a famine. In contrast, dividing the same amount of calories into five or more little meals and snacks encourages the body to burn the food for immediate energy rather than store it in the hips and thighs. Space your meals, starting with breakfast, so that no more than four hours goes by between a light meal or snack.

*Commit to Health:* Keep in mind that your ultimate goal is not just a certain figure or a number on the bathroom scale, it is a lifelong commitment to be the best and healthiest you. This plan requires a lifetime commitment, not to lose weight and keep it off, but to modify habits so they support health and, ultimately, maintain the best weight for you.

## *Fifteen Diet Tricks That Work*

The road to successful weight loss is as varied as the people who reach their goals. Sometimes even small changes in what, when, or how you eat can produce dramatic results on your weight. Here are a few quick tips to help you on your way to success.

1. Eat breakfast. People who eat breakfast are much less likely to overeat later in the day. A healthful breakfast takes only five minutes and is as simple as juice, fruit, and cereal.
2. Bring foods with you. Pack one snack for each four hours you'll be gone. Pack your briefcase, glove compartment, or desk drawer at work with oranges, apples, yogurt, bread sticks, string cheese, and other quick-fix healthful snacks.
3. Eyeball portions. A half-cup serving of rice is the size of your fist, an ounce of cheese is the size of a large marble, a three-ounce serving of meat is the size of a cassette case, and two tablespoons of salad dressing is the size of a Ping-Pong ball.
4. Include your favorite foods. If you love a glass of wine in the evening or a cookie at the midmorning break, then drop something else during the day or walk an extra mile at lunch. If cheddar cheese is your downfall, use the sharpest type and slice it thin, then cut fat calories elsewhere.
5. Drink water. Meet your daily quota of six to eight glasses, curb appetite, and possibly avoid late-night cravings by keeping bottled water in the refrigerator or filling a container with eight glasses of water and drinking one glass every one to two hours.
6. Eat slowly. It takes up to twenty minutes for signals from the stomach to reach the brain; if you are wolfing down food, you could be stuffed before those signals hit. Instead, put the fork down between bites, focus more on the conversation, take small bites, or wait fifteen minutes before going back for seconds.
7. Cut one hundred calories each day. Lose one pound a month by simply replacing that candy bar with an orange and banana, the half cup granola with two cups of Cheerios, or half cup of frozen broccoli in cheese sauce with half cup steamed fresh broccoli.
8. Lose weight gradually. You are more likely to lose fat weight and maintain the loss if you take it slow—no more than two pounds a week. Bet-

ter yet, forget the scale and monitor your weight by how your clothes fit or by the notch on your belt.

9. Eat consciously. Don't nibble while cleaning up the kitchen, taste while cooking, eat from the serving bowl, or graze from someone else's plate.

10. Cut out or limit alcohol. Alcohol stimulates appetite and erases your willpower. Limit wine, beer, or other alcoholic beverages to special occasions. Serve these beverages in small glasses and intersperse alcohol with calorie-free beverages.

11. Throw it out. If those brownies or homemade cookies beckon to you, get rid of them . . . now! Drown them in water, dump them down the disposal, feed them to the dog, or bury them under garbage in the trash.

12. Brush your teeth. This can stop the cravings or uncontrollable grazing from the refrigerator by eliminating the taste of food from the mouth and signaling the body that eating is over.

13. If you can't live with it, don't buy it. Just say no to tempting foods at the grocery store if they are likely to beckon you to indulge at home. Also, store tempting foods out of sight.

14. Go spicy. Overeating and food cravings can be an underlying search for flavor. Add chilies to chicken sandwiches, salsa to scrambled eggs, or curry to sauces. Try hot cuisines, such as Thai, Szechuan, or Indian.

15. Stay busy. Keep your hands busy by sewing, manicuring your nails, addressing envelopes, or exercising during your craving-prone time of day, such as watching TV or reading.

# CHAPTER 8

# *Changing Habits*

**H**abits develop slowly. Day in and day out, year in and year out, each of us repeats the same patterns and routines until they are well-worn habits. Changing these habits also takes time. Telling yourself to eat right or exercise more won't make lifelong habits go away. If you try to force yourself to do something, such as stop snacking or begin a strenuous exercise program after years of inactivity, you are likely to fail. Repeated failures convince you that you didn't have what it takes to make a healthful change. Nothing could be farther from the truth!

The nice thing about habits is that we developed them ourselves. That means we can relearn or replace any habit with a new one. It is not a matter of willpower. It is a matter of really wanting and being ready to make the change, then following a few simple steps and practicing new behaviors until they become second nature. Identifying lifelong habits that need to be changed, setting realistic goals, practicing effective strategies for developing new habits, and sticking with it are the foundations for success, whether your goal is to eat better, lose weight, exercise more, or create more happiness in your life. Make changes gradually—they are more likely to stick with you that way. The good news is the process gets easier with each step!

## *Step 1: Set Realistic Goals*

Goals are your road map for making changes. Without them you won't know where you are going or even if you got there. If you set unrealistic or perfectionist goals, you will feel like a failure even when you make tremendous progress. In fact, an unrealistic goal, not lack of willpower, often is the cause of many failed attempts to successfully lose weight or stick with an exercise plan. On the other hand, when you set realistic goals, you feel successful each step of the way. For a goal to be useful, it must be specific, realistic, and flexible.

## Specific Goals

Goals must be measurable and precise. You should know exactly when you've reached a goal. Always include *what, when, where,* and *how* in each goal. For example, goals to "exercise more" or "reduce fat intake" are too vague, but goals such as "I will jog for thirty minutes during my lunch hour, five days a week, for the next six months," or "To reduce my fat intake, I will spread apple butter instead of butter on my toast in the morning" are specific. They let you know when you are successful and how much progress you've made along the way.

## Realistic Goals

Goals should take into account where you are today and what you are likely to accomplish with reasonable effort. Unrealistic goals are a setup for failure, so avoid perfectionist goals that use words such as "always," "never," or "every day." The more realistic your expectations, the more successful and motivated you will be. One way to test a goal is to ask yourself "Would I want a friend to meet these expectations?"

## Flexible Goals

Remember to stay flexible. Modify your goals if you find they are too easy or too difficult. Routinely evaluate your progress. Ask yourself each week, "How am I doing? Am I meeting my goals? Are my goals still realistic?" If you are not meeting your goals, that doesn't mean you are bad or lack willpower; it merely provides feedback on how to adjust your goals or strategies to achieve success. Goals should be challenging, not overwhelming. Also, pick goals you want, not goals someone else wants for you.

**WORKSHEET 8.1    My Roadmap to Success**

Complete the following worksheet each week. Use the checklist to monitor your success by summarizing your ministeps in the lefthand column. Then give yourself credit by making a tally mark under the appropriate day each time you accomplish a ministep. There can be more than one tally mark per day. Use this sheet as a master copy.

Date/Week: _____

Long-Term Goal: _____

This Week's Short-Term Goal: _____

Each day's Ministeps (include details such as when, where, how often, with whom)

1. _____
2. _____
3. _____

| | MON | TUES | WED | THURS | FRI | SAT | SUN |
|---|---|---|---|---|---|---|---|
| Ministep 1: | | | | | | | |
| Ministep 2: | | | | | | | |
| Ministep 3: | | | | | | | |

## Minigoals: One Step at a Time

For a goal to be realistic, it should be broken into ministeps. The path to long-term success is lined with hundreds of small accomplishments. For example, a long-term goal to lose twenty pounds can be divided into short-term minigoals to lose one to two pounds a week for the next ten to twenty weeks. The steps you use to reach that short-term goal might include walking an additional two miles a day, replacing negative thoughts with supportive thoughts, and substituting baby carrots for potato chips at the midafternoon snack.

## *Step 2: Keep a Journal*

No matter how determined you are to eat better, exercise more, or lose weight, you will waste a lot of time with one quick trick after another if you don't first stop and evaluate what you need to change to reach your goals. Most successful dieters keep a journal. A diet and exercise journal helps you accurately identify what eating or exercise patterns are interfering with reaching your health goals. When you take the time to write down when, what, and why you eat; how you feel when eating; and how other people influence what and how much you eat, you obtain valuable feedback on what habits need modifying to reach health goals.

You should keep detailed records for at least two weeks at the start of any habit change. The records should contain lots of information related to eating, such as thoughts, events, or circumstances that trigger eating. After a week or two, you should notice patterns. Do you find that you are more likely to grab a candy bar midafternoon on days when you skip breakfast? Do you eat more food when you eat with friends, or do you tend to eat the wrong foods when you are angry? Some eating patterns are useful or at least not harmful. Other patterns, such as snacking on doughnuts at the midmorning break, will interfere with health goals and are targets for change. From the information you gather on your records, you can develop strategies tailored to your individual needs, lifestyle, and time demands.

### Write It Down While It's Fresh in Your Mind

Keeping records is not a test. There are no right or wrong answers, only feedback for making changes. The more honest and thorough you are in journal keeping, the more you will learn about your habits.

Record information immediately following or while you eat. If you wait until the end of the day or the next day to write down your food intake, you're likely to forget what you ate and how much. Studies repeatedly show that people who estimate their food intake inevitably underreport their food intake by up to 700 calories a day, while they overestimate how much they exercise. This sloppy record keeping will do you no good. You must be accurate, and to be accurate you must write it down immediately.

You might find that keeping a journal changes what you choose to eat. You don't want to write down a candy bar, so you skip this favorite midafternoon snack. But your journal is supposed to give you feedback and it can do that only if the information truly reflects your typical eating habits. So, use a different color pen to mark foods that you normally would have eaten if you hadn't been keeping a diary.

Keep records whenever you need feedback on why you are gaining weight, have fallen off the healthy-eating wagon, or stopped exercising. Although keeping records takes time and commitment, it is one of the most important lifestyle-management skills you will learn!

## *Step 3: Analyze Your Records*

After recording your eating behaviors for two weeks, the next step is to analyze those records and look for patterns that might interfere with following the Healthy Woman's Diet.

Behavior doesn't just happen. You don't find yourself sitting on the couch eating a bag of cookies for no reason. Everything you do is always preceded or triggered by something—a person, an emotion, an event. In addition, everything you do is followed by a consequence or reward. For example, the reward for watching a TV show, having lunch with a friend, or going to a movie is that it is fun. You might nibble on chips while reading the newspaper as a way to relax. That extra serving of dessert might be triggered by an argument with your boss; the reward is the dessert, which helps you cope with anxiety or anger. Eating a high-fat lunch at a fast-food restaurant might meet your need to socialize with friends.

Keeping a journal helps you identify the triggers that cause you to choose the wrong foods. Sometimes the trigger is external—you have the urge to eat after you smell the food cooking, see or hear someone eating, watch a commercial on TV, notice the time of day, see an ice cream store, or attend a football game. Sometimes the trigger is internal. Thoughts such as "Everyone else eats this way, why can't I?" or "One bite won't hurt" are triggers that lead you to eat all the wrong stuff. Other internal triggers include feeling relaxed, happy, angry, anxious, fatigued, or bored. Try to identify from your food journal what external and internal triggers interfere with reaching your nutrition, weight, or exercise goals.

**WORKSHEET 8.2**    **The Daily Food Record**     **DATE:**

After each meal and snack, fill in the time and complete each column of the Food Record. Use the following scale for the "Hunger" category: 0=not hungry, 5=starving. Use this sheet to make additional copies.

| Time | Food/ Beverage | Amount | Hunger | Where? | With Whom? | Doing What Else? | Feelings Before/After |
|------|------|------|------|------|------|------|------|
|  |  |  |  |  |  |  |  |
|  |  |  |  |  |  |  |  |
|  |  |  |  |  |  |  |  |
|  |  |  |  |  |  |  |  |

## Consequences: The Whys of What You Do

When consequences of an action are positive, you are likely to repeat the action again. If grabbing a Big Mac saves time during a busy workday, you are likely to pull into the drive-up window again. If you are praised for your homemade cheesecake, you probably will make it (and eat it) again. The secret is to identify what happened before and what resulted from your inappropriate eating. Once you know this, you can develop new strategies for getting your emotional, social, or other needs met and still stick with your nutrition goals.

The following questions can help you glean the most out of your records:

1. How do other people influence how, what, when, and where I eat or exercise?
2. Are specific thoughts, emotions, or attitudes associated with eating? Do loneliness, boredom, or unpleasant feelings influence my eating?
3. What happens just before I eat?
4. Did alcohol influence my food choices?
5. Am I likely to eat based on the time of day? The sight of food? The smell of food? After a glass of wine? At a party?
6. What prompts me to eat high-fat or high-calorie foods?
7. How much caffeine do I consume? Do caffeinated beverages influence my eating habits?
8. What times of day do I usually eat? Do I skip meals? How is my total day's food intake distributed throughout the day?
9. How hungry am I when I eat? What am I doing while I eat?
10. What excuses do I use to eat?
11. Are specific thoughts, beliefs, or attitudes associated with problem eating?
12. What precedes inappropriate eating or snacking?
13. What foods are difficult to resist?
14. How fast do I eat? How often do I eat too fast?
15. What is the effect of exercise on my eating habits? Do I eat more, less, or differently?

## *Step 4: Develop a Plan*

After you set realistic goals, identify the behaviors you want to change, and recognize what triggers these habits, the next step is to develop new habits that will help you reach your goals.

Strategies for counteracting bad habits come in three forms.

- Avoid or eliminate whatever triggers the eating. For example, Gail couldn't resist the ice cream store on her way home from work, so she now drives a different route.
- Learn a new habit for an old situation. For example, if you snack on cookies when watching television, take this time instead to polish your nails, ride an exercise bicycle, or mend clothes. You also could replace fatty snacks with more healthful ones.
- Create a new situation for a new behavior. For example, Margaret headed for the coffeepot when she woke up in the morning. She chose instead to place her walking shoes on top of the alarm clock and, when she reaches over to shut off the clock she also reaches for her shoes, puts them on, and sets out for a quick morning walk to wake herself up. Developing friendships with fellow exercisers, taking a low-fat cooking class in the evening when you normally would be snacking on the couch, or bringing a nutritious lunch to work rather than going out to lunch are other examples of establishing new situations for developing new habits.

## *Step 5: Manage Tough Situations*

Tough situations are ones where you are most likely to revert back to old habits. Without a plan, it is difficult to stay on track. Say your goal for the week is to avoid all fried foods, but here you are at a party nibbling on fried appetizers. You can either stop as soon as you realize what is happening and find something else to do until a better choice comes to mind, or you can eat the appetizers and take time later to learn from your mistake by planning how you will handle the situation in the future.

Your records will come in handy for identifying tough situations, where you are likely to overeat, eat high-fat or high-sugar foods, skip exercise, or skip meals. Whether it is a party, a vacation, a person, or a mood, if you plan ahead, you avoid caving in during tough situations.

## *Step 6: Develop Support*

The people who are most successful at making changes in their eating and exercise habits are those who have strong social support from family, friends, coworkers, or other people. These people help you through slip-prone times, encourage you and build your self-confidence, and even join in the healthful changes you are making in your life. Most people will be supportive of your desires to eat more healthfully or exercise. However, any change in life can trigger changes in interpersonal relationships that can be both good and stressful.

### TABLE 8.1    Tips for Developing New Habits

- Shop from a list and do not shop when hungry.
- Do not bring tempting food into the house.
- Store food out of sight and immediately put away leftovers.
- Enter the house through a door away from food.
- Do not put bowls of food on the table at meals.
- Arrange business meetings at times other than lunch.
- Eat slowly. Put the fork down between bites.
- Monitor portion size.
- Sit down to eat.
- Leave food on your plate.
- Schedule tempting foods into your food plan.
- Redefine "problem" foods as "foods I eat occasionally." Then define "occasionally."
- Plan social events around exercise, rather than eating.
- Eat only at a designated eating spot.
- Eat at regular intervals of four to five hours.
- Plan ahead what and when you will eat before attending a party.
- Replace negative thoughts with encouraging ones.
- Ask for support, help, and encouragement from friends and family.

Sometimes support must be nurtured and encouraged. The more you encourage support from others by openly and honestly asking for help or encouragement and by modeling supportive behavior (i.e., treating other people as you want to be treated), the more likely you will receive the type of support you need.

## Step 7: Practice Makes Habits

Realistic goals, accurate record keeping, creative strategies, and a strong social support set the stage for making changes in how you eat and exercise. But the standing ovation only comes from practice. Including the new habit in your routine every day, day in and day out, is the way old habits are replaced with new ones. The key is to practice, practice, practice.

Fortunately, the process gets easier with each step and soon you automatically choose healthy foods. You even lose the taste for fattier foods. Many food habits are only conditioned reflexes; you eat just before going to bed every night and soon your body craves a before-bed snack. By practicing a new habit, such as drinking a glass of water, riding your exercise bike for fifteen minutes, or giving yourself a facial just before bed, the body soon unlearns the food craving.

Slowly converting your diet to the nutritious Healthy Woman's Diet is much like learning to ride a bike. Practice, determination, patience, and encouragement are essential for success. Sometimes you fall off. That's all right as long as you get back on the bike and keep trying. Sometimes the process isn't fun. So what! Lots of things in life are not always fun. Do it anyway. The fun, health rewards, energy, new looks, and feelings of confidence will come as long as you keep at it.

## Step 8: Reward Your Efforts

Motivation is the fuel that drives you toward your goals. It is the basis for all habits and especially habit change. Regardless of your health goals, motivation is the key to sticking with it.

Willpower is only a small fraction of what keeps a person on track. Gritting your teeth during high-risk situations inevitably leads to failure, which is probably why many women feel that motivation is a gift—you either have what it takes to stick with it, or you don't. Nothing could be farther from the truth. Anyone can stay motivated and everyone can reach their goals, while enjoying the process; all it takes is a motivation plan.

## What Is a Reward?

Rewards are things that happen during or immediately following a new behavior that increase the likelihood of your wanting to do the behavior again. Going to a movie tonight if you follow your eating plan today might be just what you need to motivate yourself to stick with it, whereas planning a trip to Mexico when you have lost twenty-five pounds is too far in the future to help you out today.

An effective reward must increase the likelihood of your doing the new habit. What works for one person might not work for someone else. If putting a quarter in a jar toward the purchase of a new set of wineglasses every time you use low-fat cooking methods doesn't motivate you to follow your plan, then it is not a reward for you. When people say "Rewards don't work," what they really are saying is "I haven't found a reward that works for me."

Rewards are as varied and unique as the people who use them. You can celebrate accomplishments with money, tally marks on a graph, tokens in a jar, or stars on the calendar that can be exchanged for other rewards such as going to a movie or buying a book. Rewards can be activities, such as gardening or fishing. Rewards can be praise from friends or positive thoughts. However, never use food as a reward.

There are a few rules to using rewards.

- Plan daily how, when, and for what you will reward yourself.
- A reward is only effective if you follow the "if . . . then" rule. In other words, "if" you eat a low-fat lunch, "then" (and only then) do you get to watch your favorite TV show. No low-fat lunch, no show.
- Use more or multiple rewards at the start of a new behavior. For example, following the Healthy Woman's Diet might require using several rewards daily in the beginning. Later on, how you feel and the taste of the food might be rewards in themselves and fewer rewards will be needed.
- Finally, just as strategies must be updated frequently, a motivation plan also must be reviewed and updated. A reward that works today might not work once a health goal has been reached. In addition, a

reward that works for changing one habit might not work when you tackle a new habit change.

## Step 9: Handle Slips to Avoid Relapse

Everyone trying to change eating or exercise habits occasionally slips off their plans. Giving in to the taste of a favorite high-fat food, a lack of time leading you to grab a bag of potato chips because they are convenient, or believing it takes longer to cook healthy foods are some of the most common excuses for slips and relapses. The secret is not allowing the slip to progress to a relapse. People in the National Weight Control Registry (see chapter 7) who have successfully lost weight and kept it off typically have learned to identify a slip and handle it before it progresses to a relapse. The sooner you recognize that you are reverting to old habits and use that experience to learn more about yourself, the easier it is to prevent that slip from progressing and to avoid it in the future.

Self-talk is important in handling slips. Negative thoughts and attitudes reinforce that you are bad, a failure, deprived, or lack willpower and will encourage a

---

**TABLE 8.2    Learning from Your Mistakes**

If you are struggling with slips and relapses, ask yourself some or all of the following questions:

1. What are the emotional states that challenge me the most? Am I likely to eat inappropriately when I am bored, happy, tense, relaxed?
2. How have I prevented slips from progressing into a relapse in the past?
3. How do worries about my willpower interfere with my health and fitness goals?
4. What type of positive thoughts help me counteract self-defeating thoughts? What self-talk can I use to stay on track?
5. What is the most consistent and strongest reward for my efforts to change health-related behaviors?
6. What do I foresee to be my biggest challenge to long-term health and fitness management? What can I do to minimize this challenge in the future?

---

slip to progress. On the other hand, positive self-talk lets you use the slip to re-evaluate and revise health and fitness plans and encourages long-term success. Monitor your self-talk and replace negative thoughts with positive ones.

When you realize you have slipped from your eating or exercise plans, review your goals, records, strategies, and motivation plan. Identify the troublesome situation and plan how you will cope with it in the future. Focus on the long-term benefits of feeling your best, rather than the short-term payoffs of overeating, eating unhealthful foods, or skipping exercise. A piece of cake might taste good now, but the long-term effects might lower self-esteem, cause weight gain and frustration, interfere with optimal health, or prevent you from wearing that "little black dress."

---

**TABLE 8.3     The Maintainer's Questionnaire**

Ask yourself the following questions when analyzing your food records:

1. What do I want to improve in my maintenance habits?
2. What do I need to continue doing or thinking?
3. What do I need to do more frequently?
4. What characteristics of a healthy person do I currently exhibit?
5. What do I want to be doing or thinking three, six, or twelve months from now?
6. How much progress toward my goals do I want to have made in three months?

The answers to these questions provide you with information to update goals, develop minigoals, and practice new strategies.

---

## *Step 10: Keep It Up*

Learning to choose healthy meals, losing weight, or beginning any new health habit is the first step. The bigger challenge is maintaining the change. The work is not over when you reach your goals. Maintaining those goals requires that you continue practicing the same key steps that helped you get there.

First, never assume you've made it. Overconfidence is your worst enemy. Breaking an old habit—from nail biting to eating high-fat foods—is a lifetime process that requires careful attention, so don't be fooled into thinking that you have overcome your old habits forever!

Second, no one is powerless, helpless, or hopeless when it comes to food. Just the opposite—women who believe they can make a difference in their lives show increased power and ability to do so. Women who believe they can't make a difference are riddled with feelings of self-doubt, helplessness, and hopelessness, which undermine success. Remind yourself that it is not how many or how big your obstacles, but how you handle and think about them that determine success or failure. You are limited only by your own expectations, aspirations, and beliefs. In short, you get what you think you deserve.

Finally, surround yourself with people who also take their health seriously and who support your efforts. Strengthen your skills by repeating situations that you have handled successfully. Frequently monitor your thoughts and attitudes and act immediately at the first sign of a slip. Pay attention to your successes, be patient, and stick with it!

# PART II

# *Life Events*

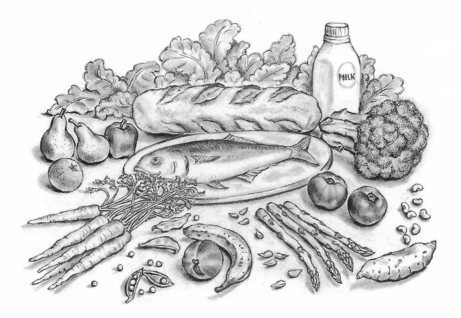

# CHAPTER 9

# Nutrition, Exercise, and Sports

Fitness has become a way of life for many women. Some women exercise for health or weight reasons. For other women, the love of exercise has grown beyond recreational or weekend sports; they work out intensely for personal enjoyment and occasional competition. Then there is the female athlete, someone who trains every day for a specific event and whose life revolves around training and competition.

The study of physical activity is broad, ranging from the health benefits of moderate exercise for the average woman to optimal sports performance for the competition athlete. Although the issues pertinent to these two ends of the spectrum might appear unrelated, in reality, many physiological and nutritional factors are common for all women engaged in physical activity.

## Why Exercise?

If you exercise regularly, you've probably noticed a few differences between how you feel and manage your life and how your sedentary sisters, friends, and coworkers get by. Women who exercise regularly

- have more energy and are healthier than women who are sedentary.
- are less likely to develop hypertension, heart disease, cancer, memory loss, depression, premenstrual syndrome (PMS), serious side effects of menopause, or diabetes.

- are less likely to die from age-related diseases, such as heart disease or diabetes.
- live longer than their couch-potato counterparts.
- have an easier time managing their weights, maintain weight losses after dieting, and have less abdominal fat, which lowers their risk for age-related diseases.
- are stronger and more independent as they age.
- feel better, more satisfied and happier with their lives, and younger throughout life.
- look younger, as much as twenty years younger, than their sedentary friends.
- maintain their independence longer than do women who don't exercise.

It doesn't matter whether you are a recreational walker or an Olympic athlete, you experience similar health benefits from physical activity.

## What Do Athletes and Exercisers Eat?

Running your fastest race, playing your best game of tennis, or lifting the most weight is a satisfying accomplishment. It is also the outer reflection of an inner symphony of complex metabolic and physiological adaptations to the stress of exercise training. This response to exercise results from progressive increases in how long, how hard, and how often you exercise. Performing at your best happens only if all the nutrients needed for the growth and maintenance of body tissues are present during training, competition, and recovery from exercise.

Women athletes continually search for the perfect diet or the right combination of nutrients to maximize exercise performance. Even recreational exercisers want to enhance their health and exercise programs by eating the right foods in the right combination. Ironically, several studies report that women athletes and exercisers do not always eat right. For example, their diets are often low in calories and carbohydrates, as well as several nutrients, including vitamins C, $B_1$, $B_6$, and E, and minerals, such as calcium, copper, iron, magnesium, and zinc.

The common belief that you'll eat more if you exercise is incorrect. Most studies show that women who exercise don't compensate by eating more and, in many cases, eat fewer calories than it takes to maintain their weight, causing them to lose weight. If you have a few pounds to lose, then exercise is a must for any weight-loss plan. However, many competition athletes don't need to lose weight. For them, poor diet at a time when nutrient needs are at an all-time high can jeopardize exercise performance and general health.

## How Much Should an Athlete Weigh?

Women who exercise have more muscle and less body fat than women who do not exercise. The more intense and frequent the exercise, the more the ratio shifts toward muscle and away from body fat, regardless of age. Don't worry about bulking up. Even with strenuous strength training, a woman won't build the muscle mass that men do because she doesn't have the male hormones—called androgens—required for building massive muscles. Compared to men, women have about two-thirds the strength, but are more flexible. Lean women also have approximately 10 percent more body fat than do men of the same age, weight, and fitness.

Because body fat does not contribute to athletic performance, many women athletes want to lower their percentage of body fat. There is no general agreement on optimal body fat for athletes in any sport, and body fat percentages range from 6 to 20 percent in elite women athletes, such as runners. However, researchers do agree that reducing body fat below 12 to 15 percent jeopardizes health. In addition, the dietary practices used to severely reduce body fat, such as fad dieting, are always harmful to health and often undermine exercise performance. In fact, these diets backfire. According to a study from Georgia State University in Atlanta, athletes who severely cut calories end up with higher body fat percentages than athletes who don't diet, probably because energy deficits lower resting energy expenditure, resulting in increased fat deposition.

*Eating Disorders:* Eating disorders are more common in women athletes than in the general public. Estimates are as high as 72 percent of women athletes battle eating disorders. One study from Kent State University found that one in every four women who ran more than thirty miles a week had signs of an eating disorder. Red flags that you might be bordering on an eating disorder include:

- Prolonged dieting.
- Frequent weight fluctuations.
- Sudden and dramatic increases in exercise training.
- Preoccupation with food and body weight.

Amenorrhea, or cessation of the menstrual period, is a major symptom that you're not eating enough or you are exercising too much. Women exercisers who have stopped having monthly periods are at high risk for bone loss today, are four times more likely to develop stress fractures, and are at risk for osteoporosis later in life. If you are an avid exerciser or athlete whose period has stopped or is erratic, consult your physician.

---

**TABLE 9.1    What Is Your Risk for Disordered Eating?**

Answer the following questions to assess your risk for disordered eating.

| **Question** | **Frequently** | **Sometimes** | **Never** |
|---|---|---|---|
| **1.** I skip at least two meals a day. | | | |
| **2.** I eat big meals or feel out of control with my eating. | | | |
| **3.** I eat when I'm not hungry. | | | |
| **4.** I use laxatives, diuretics, vomiting, or stimulants to lose weight. | | | |
| **5.** I have had stress fractures. | | | |
| **6.** I exercise more than other people and hide extra workouts from my friends and family. | | | |
| **7.** I am disgusted with, and often feel guilty or depressed about, my eating. | | | |
| **8.** I hide the food I eat from other people. | | | |
| **9.** I have fewer than 10 to 13 periods every year. | | | |
| **10.** I lie about how much food I eat. | | | |

The more "frequently" and "sometimes" you answered the question above, the more likely you are to be battling disordered eating.

Adapted from Wiggins D, Wiggins M: The female athlete. *Clin Sp Med* 1997;16:593–612.

---

# *Do Athletes Need More Protein?*

Your body needs protein for growth, repair, and maintenance of muscle and other lean tissues. Women who are building muscle during the beginning stages of weight training need more protein to supply the building blocks for muscle. Other sports that build endurance, not muscle, such as running or bicycling, don't place a demand for more protein on the body, so protein needs are not much higher than the general public. Even with weight training, the increased need is slight and levels off when you stop increasing the amount of weight you lift. Most women are consuming more than enough protein already without needing to add additional sources.

*How Much Do You Need?* According to researchers at the University of Western Ontario, physically active women might need up to twice the protein of sedentary folks, or about 1.8 grams per kilogram of body weight (123 grams a day for a 150-pound person). Even this increased amount is easy to meet, since a bowl of whole-grain cereal with soy milk for breakfast and a turkey sandwich and glass of nonfat milk at lunch supply more than half the requirement. Add a serving of fish, a baked potato, and another glass of nonfat milk for dinner and you've more than met your protein requirement. The only active people who might need a protein boost are vegetarians and seniors, since they are the ones least likely to reach their protein quota.

*Amino Acid Supplements:* While most amino acid supplements aren't worth the extra cost, branch-chain amino acids (BCAA), such as leucine, isoleucine, and valine, might improve athletic performance, according to a study from Rutgers University. In this study, athletes participated in two events in the heat followed by cycling to exhaustion. Those who consumed a BCAA-fortified drink exercised longer than did other athletes. Muscles use BCAAs for fuel during intense exercise. When glycogen stores are low, more BCAAs are used for energy, suggesting that intense exercise breaks down muscle tissue when glycogen is depleted. Athletes who supplement their diets with BCAAs sometimes prevent this exercise-induced muscle loss and, in some cases, might improve muscle mass.

*Creatine:* Creatine is a natural dietary nutrient and is made in the body from other amino acids. It is a component of phosphocreatine, which is the high-octane fuel in muscles during short bursts of high-intensity exercise. It also stimulates mitochondria, the cells' energy powerhouses, and reduces lactic acid that otherwise accumulates in muscles during intense exercise (lactic acid is what causes that burning sensation and limits the amount of intense exercise an athlete can do). Taking creatine supplements boosts levels of phosphocreatine in muscles by 20 to 30 percent. As a result, more energy is formed, an athlete doesn't tire as easily, and recovery is quicker from intense exercise.

Several studies show that taking creatine supplements improves short-term muscle strength and the body's ability to perform intense athletic events, such as competitive basketball, soccer, sprint swimming, weight lifting, and hockey, as well as short events in track and field. Competition cyclists pedal more intensely for short bursts, people lift greater weights and can complete more repetitions, and sprinters jump higher when supplementing with creatine. Even 1.5 grams of supplemental creatine daily was enough to produce a 46 percent increase in muscle size in one study. Creatine appears to be effective for both elite or highly trained athletes and nonathletes. However, it won't improve aerobic or endurance performance, such as walking, swimming, jogging, or bicycling.

What dose is best? Most people consume about one to two grams daily from meat, fish, and other animal products, and excrete about two grams in the urine as creatinine. Most studies have used 20 to 30 grams of supplemental creatine a day during the first five to six days to "load" the muscles, then drop that dose to two to five grams a day as maintenance. No one really understands exactly how creatine works or at what doses it is safe, and the research supporting its use has been small (9 to 14 subjects) and short (three days to a few weeks).

**TABLE 9.2    Creatine Content of Selected Foods**

| FOOD | CREATINE CONTENT (GRAMS/KG) |
|---|---|
| Herring | 6.5 |
| Beef | 5.5 |
| Pork | 5.0 |
| Salmon | 4.5 |
| Cod | 3.0 |
| Milk | 0.1 |

Creatine supplementation for up to eight weeks has not shown any major health risks, but few safety data are available. Theoretically, creatine supplements could suppress the body's natural ability to manufacture this compound or could lead to kidney damage. But these concerns are unsubstantiated at this time. Another concern is that there is no guarantee that a creatine supplement is pure, since there's little or no government regulation. Because the dose is so high for creatine, impurities could theoretically produce a host of harmful effects. At this time, it's an individual decision whether you want to take the risk to reap the benefits of creatine.

## *Carbohydrates: First Fuel for Exercisers*

Whether you exercise for fun or competition, carbohydrates are your main fuel. Your body will need this quick fuel for all stop-and-start anaerobic sports, from tennis and volleyball to sprinting. Carbs also are the kindling fuel necessary for burning fat during endurance sports, such as race walking, running, swimming, cross-country skiing, and cycling.

Your body stores carbohydrates as glycogen in muscle and the liver. Daily high-intensity training and/or endurance events lasting more than one hour deplete these stores and jeopardize performance. Stockpiling ample glycogen stores by eating lots of carbohydrate-rich foods boosts your tolerance for repeated days of heavy training or prolonged exertion. This is the underlying reason for the diet practice of "carbohydrate loading" or consuming carbohydrate-fortified drinks during heavy endurance training and competition events.

Most physically active women don't need to carbohydrate load. They just need to fuel their bodies regularly with a reasonable amount of high-quality carbohydrates. If you exercise for less than an hour, four times a week or less, then the Healthy Woman's Diet provides all the carbohydrates you need to meet your exercise needs. If you engage in vigorous physical activity more than four hours a week, you should boost your carbohydrate intake to about 60 percent of calories by adding a few more servings of fruits, vegetables, whole-grain breads and cereals, and cooked dried beans and peas to your daily diet.

*Low-Carbohydrate Diets:* The latest popular low-carbohydrate diets are a big mistake for everyone who exercises—especially women. Depriving your body and brain of its primary fuel results in lowered glycogen stores, reduced athletic performance, and altered mood, including increased tension, depression, fatigue, anger, mental confusion, and reduced vigor.

*Before Competition:* How the body uses carbohydrate before, during, and after exercise is influenced by the amount of carbohydrate consumed on the days prior to and the hours after exercise. A high-carbohydrate diet consumed during the week prior to an endurance event will have a greater impact on stocking the body's glycogen stores than will a big "preevent meal" the night before the event. In addition, athletes who consume carbohydrate-rich snacks with or without branched-chain amino acid supplements before and during exercise suffer less fatigue than do athletes who don't snack, state researchers at the University of South Carolina in Columbia. Eating a high-carbohydrate snack after exercise also increases muscle glycogen stores by 100 percent.

*During an Event:* Drinking or eating easily digested forms of simple carbohydrates during lengthy aerobic exercise (i.e., one hour or more of running, brisk walking, cycling, swimming, or aerobic dance sessions) helps slow the rate of muscle glycogen depletion, maintain blood sugar concentrations, and prevent fatigue. However, the best proportion of glucose to water remains somewhat controversial.

Sports drinks and fruit juice that contain too much carbohydrate slow the rate of emptying from the stomach and limit the delivery of fluids to the body during exercise. Dilute fruit juice to help speed absorption of fluids. Beverages containing glucose polymers, such as maltodextrin, also help maintain a high blood sugar level when consumed during endurance events and do not affect fluid replacement any more than does water ingestion. Isotonic beverages are the best.

## Drink It Up

When you're not performing up to par, look first to your water bottle. Dehydration is the most common cause of reduced athletic performance. A dancer might lose two to three pounds of water during a practice, while a runner can lose five pounds or more of water during a race. In fact, you lose body water every time you work out. The first sign of dehydration is fatigue, which is accompanied by increased risk for injuries. Water is the best fluid replacement, while soda pop, tea, and coffee have mild diuretic effects, so are not as effective in replacing fluid losses.

Thirst is a poor indicator of fluid needs. If a glass of water quenches your thirst, you probably need two or more glasses to rehydrate. A general rule for exercisers is—drink twice as much water as is needed to quench thirst, or at least ten eight-ounce glasses every day. Drink even more if you perspire heavily or work out in hot or humid climates. Athletes and exercisers alike should drink water prior to, during, and following all training and sports events, as well as regularly throughout the day.

Fluid loss during exercise is well documented. However, electrolyte losses—potassium, sodium, and chloride—and their effects on performance remain controversial. Your body does lose more water than electrolytes during exercise. This is especially true in the well-trained, acclimatized athlete who perspires more, but loses less electrolytes than does the untrained exerciser. Replacing electrolytes prior to fluid replacement only aggravates the dehydrated body, since this super-concentrates electrolyte levels in the blood. Always drink water first, then worry about replacing electrolytes.

Drinking potassium-containing beverages during intense exercise has no additional benefits than drinking plain water. Athletes consuming electrolyte-replacement drinks show no differences in body temperature, blood volume, or blood levels of potassium, chloride, calcium, or sodium compared to athletes consuming nonelectrolyte-containing drinks. In addition, any potassium lost during exercise can be replaced by eating a few servings of fruits or vegetables later in the day. Of course, you're likely to drink more if you like the taste. So, if you won't drink water, but you will drink a sports drink, then choose the sports drink.

## Vitamins and Exercise

Exercise revs up your metabolism. Millions of enzymes are recruited to meet the increased demands. Every cell, every tissue, every organ comes into play. Circulation increases, as does respiration. The kidneys and liver and other filtering organs work overtime, not to mention the nerves, muscles, and brain. All of this activity requires vitamins.

*The B Vitamins:* B vitamins are important for converting calories into energy for the muscles to use during exercise. Theoretically, requirements for many of the B vitamins, including vitamins $B_1$, $B_2$, $B_6$, niacin, pantothenic acid, and biotin, should increase when calorie intake increases. As long as quality carbohydrate-rich foods, such as whole grains and starchy vegetables, are consumed, then the intake of B vitamins also will increase. Limited research shows that exercise might alter vitamin $B_6$ metabolism and slightly increase the need for vitamin $B_2$, but there is little evidence that intakes of any of the B vitamins or the B complex in amounts greater than recommended levels improve exercise performance.

*The Antioxidants:* Athletes and recreational exercisers breathe in more oxygen than do sedentary women. Consequently, they are exposed to greater quantities of oxygen fragments called free radicals. (See pages 237 to 240 for more information on free radicals.) Repeated or long-term exposure to free radicals impairs athletic performance, while consuming an antioxidant-rich daily diet helps prevent free radical–induced tissue damage, decrease muscle fatigue, and improve endurance performance and high-altitude training. Research shows that some exercisers might benefit from the combination of an excellent diet and moderate-dose supplementation with the antioxidants. For example,

- Vitamin E supplementation might prevent exercise-induced free radical damage to tissues in athletes, state researchers at Tokyo Medical University in Japan.
- Muscle damage and inflammation following strenuous exercise is at least partially caused by free radicals. Antioxidant supplementation helps counter this generation of free radicals and prevent exercise-induced muscle damage, state researchers from Vrije University in Amsterdam.
- Researchers at the University of North Carolina found that supplementing athletes' diets with vitamin C reduced free radical levels in the blood following exercise.
- In a study from Arizona State University, subjects exercised more efficiently and with less fatigue when they supplemented with vitamin C.

The antioxidants also might help protect exercisers from the damaging effects of air pollution. Ozone is a component of air pollution that reacts with cell membranes to form free radicals. It also impairs immune function. Vitamin E and other antioxidants protect tissues from this damage, thus potentially increasing resistance to infectious diseases and cancer.

# Minerals and Exercise

Exercise might increase urinary and sweat losses of certain minerals, including iron, magnesium, and some trace minerals. Unless these minerals are replaced, these losses could affect exercise performance and general health today, and disease risk in the future.

*Calcium:* Women typically consume too little calcium, and women exercisers are no exception. Low calcium intake increases your risk for stress fractures, shin splints, strains, and poor ability to heal bone fractures. In later years, you'll be at increased risk for osteoporosis. Women exercisers also lose calcium from bone during periods of inactivity such as recovery from sports injury, stress, low vitamin D intake or exposure to sunshine, or when they consume high-protein diets.

As mentioned above, many competition athletes cut calories or exercise so intensely that they stop menstruating, a condition called amenorrhea. These athletes often have the bone density of women ten years older and many women with long-standing amenorrhea have the bones of women twice their age. A primary treatment is reduction in exercise training and increased weight gain and/or calorie consumption. Researchers at Brown University School of Medicine recommend that all women athletes with irregular periods should take 1,500 mg of calcium and 400 IU to 800 IU of vitamin D to reduce the risk for osteoporosis.

*Chromium:* Limited research shows that moderate increases in chromium, in the form of chromium picolinate, might maintain or even increase muscle mass while fat is lost. Although chromium is essential in protein and carbohydrate metabolism and, thus, may participate in muscle growth and function, there is no evidence that these "anabolic" effects are significant. Since nine out of ten people do not consume adequate amounts of chromium, increasing dietary intake to the recommended levels of 50 mcg to 200 mcg daily is beneficial.

*Iron:* As many as 80 percent of exercising women consume inadequate amounts of iron and the increased metabolic demands of even moderate exercise aggravate an otherwise borderline condition. If your exercise performance doesn't improve with time, or if you find yourself increasingly more tired than usual after a workout, you might be iron deficient. Other symptoms of iron deficiency include lethargy, irritability, poor concentration, and headaches. Iron deficiency in athletes can result from poor dietary intake, increased metabolic requirements, increased breakdown of red blood cells caused by training (called footstrike hemolysis), and/or increased iron losses in sweat.

You don't have to be anemic to feel the effects of iron deficiency, especially if you're an avid exerciser, according to a study from Cornell University. Young women who are physically active are at high risk for iron deficiency, yet this condition can progress undetected, since it does not show up on a routine test for iron-deficiency anemia. Whether you have symptoms of poor iron status, sports anemia, or iron-deficiency anemia, it is best to have additional blood tests beyond just the hemoglobin and hematocrit test. The serum ferritin, total iron binding capacity (TIBC), and transferrin tests are sensitive indicators of preanemia. If any or all of these tests conclude that you are iron deficient, your physician will recommend you take an iron supplement.

*Magnesium:* This mineral helps maintain muscle tissue. It helps convert glycogen to energy, regulate muscle building and relaxation, coordinate muscle and nerve communication, and regulate the heartbeat and blood pressure. One study reported improved muscle strength when magnesium intake was increased to 490 mg daily for a 135-pound woman.

Strenuous exercise alters magnesium concentrations in muscle and blood, which might affect performance and general health. Blood levels of magnesium are low after endurance exercise, such as marathon running or cross-country skiing, and remain below preexercise values for as long as several months after the strenuous training session or competition event. Stressful conditions, including intense exercise, elevate the stress hormones, which increase urinary loss of magnesium. Making sure you get enough of this mineral becomes even more important if you are an avid exerciser or competition athlete. To add to the risk, dietary surveys show that many women often choose diets that contain too little of this mineral.

While 350 mg of magnesium might be adequate for the recreational exerciser, higher amounts of 400 mg to 450 mg might be necessary for women engaged in strenuous activity. Make sure you include in your daily diet several servings of magnesium-rich whole grains, soy products, nuts, dark green leafy vegetables, and legumes. If you choose to supplement, don't go overboard with this mineral, since amounts greater than 500 mg have a laxative effect.

*Zinc:* Women who tire after a workout or have trouble improving in their exercise performance should look beyond just iron. Marginal zinc intake is common in women unless they regularly consume red meat. In fact, even menus designed by dietitians and based on the U.S. Dietary Guidelines are frequently low in both iron and zinc. Strenuous exercise increases urinary and sweat losses of zinc, which would compound the problem unless dietary or supplemental intake is increased. According to a study from Kumamoto University School of Medicine in Japan, women distance runners with marginal zinc status had reduced red blood cells, lowered hemoglobin levels, and reduced blood levels of iron and total protein, compared to runners with adequate zinc levels. All of these changes in blood values are indicative of reduced oxygen-carrying capacity of the blood, which would affect exercise performance and general health. Boost intake of zinc by eating whole grains, extra-lean red meats, legumes, or seafood and/or taking a supplement that contains 12 mg to 25 mg of zinc.

## Caffeine and Exercise

Will a cup of coffee improve your morning workout or running time? Maybe, but only if you're planning to exercise for a long time. Caffeine improves fat burning for aerobic activity. Since the primary cause of fatigue in endurance events is glycogen depletion, increasing levels of special fats called free fatty acids helps spare glycogen and so might improve performance. However, if caffeine is effective, it would only help if you're exercising to exhaustion, such as running a marathon or cycling for hours. On the other hand, some studies show no benefits from caffeine.

## Should Exercisers Supplement?

Do you benefit from supplements? It depends on what you expect from the supplements. All the research so far has been conducted on competition male athletes; there is virtually no research on recreational exercisers or active older adults, and very little research on women athletes.

When it comes to athletes, vitamin and mineral deficiencies will compromise exercise performance, while correcting these deficiencies improves performance. For example, marginal deficiencies of vitamins $B_1$, $B_2$, $B_6$, or C reduces endurance performance. Deficiencies in athletes are rare and, except for cases where overt deficiencies are corrected, seldom has the research shown that supplements actually improved athletic ability, such as enhanced oxygen uptake, endurance capacity, or strength. However, nutrient imbalances have been noted, which could have secondary effects on athletic performance by compromising general health. In addition, while nutrient requirements are only slightly raised in all but the most strenuous training programs, many athletes have difficultly eating perfectly to ensure optimal nutrition.

Beyond athletic performance, vitamin and mineral supplements show promise in enhancing immune function, speeding recovery from illness and injury, and preventing disease and infection. Researchers at the University of Connecticut state, "Vitamins must be viewed beyond their classical roles; they also have many nonenzymatic functions, such as antioxidants, hormonelike, and regulatory activities." For example, exercise generates an additional oxidative stress on the body through increased oxygen consumption, metabolism, and mechanical processes such as joint compression and trauma. This oxidative stress is held in check by the antioxidant nutrients.

Other studies have looked at the impact of exercise on mineral status. Chromium deficiency is possible in athletes who train strenuously, especially since typical chromium intakes are already low. Profuse sweating increases losses of iodine, iron, zinc, and other trace minerals, while magnesium supplements might enhance exercise performance. Calcium intakes also are typically low in athletes' diets, and supplements may be necessary to achieve a consistent intake. On the other hand, excessive intake of one mineral, such as zinc, can produce secondary deficiencies of other minerals, such as copper or iron. Vitamin and mineral supplements, just like the diet, should be balanced and doses should be moderate.

If you are a weekend athlete or you exercise four hours or less each week, then the Healthy Woman's Diet is all you need, since it provides recommended levels of all vitamins, minerals, phytochemicals, fiber, and other nutrients. A moderate-dose multiple vitamin and mineral supplement would provide nutritional insurance only when dietary habits are not optimal or consistent.

The athlete engaged in frequent strenuous training and competition would benefit from both a nutritious diet plus a moderate-dose vitamin-mineral supplement to ensure adequate intake of all nutrients. Also consider taking extra antioxidants, such as vitamin E. There is no reason to take megadose levels (i.e., more than ten times the recommended amounts) of most nutrients and there is no need for protein powders or other fabricated nutritional products. Also steer clear of gimmicky supplements. They typically do much less than they promise. For example, ginseng supplements did not improve athletic performance in men and women who took 200 mg of 7 percent ginseng for three weeks, according to a study from Louisiana State University. (See chapter 6 for additional guidelines on choosing a supplement.)

## *Special Dietary Concerns*

Several problems experienced by athletes and exercisers are related to, or can be improved with, diet.

*Diarrhea:* If you experience diarrhea during training or competitions, try training at different times of the day. In addition, examine the fiber or magnesium content of your diet, since excessive intake of either could result in diarrhea. Cut back on coffee, since it increases gastrointestinal motility and, in combination with exercise, could cause diarrhea.

*PMS:* Athletic performance is not necessarily compromised by premenstrual syndrome (PMS). Female athletes have won medals while performing during menstruation and there is no evidence that menstruation limits athletic performance. The nutritional guidelines for helping limit or prevent PMS symptoms are outlined on pages 362 to 366.

*Pregnancy:* If you are pregnant and continue to train and exercise, you must consume a diet that meets the increased calorie needs for training, plus the calorie and nutritional needs of pregnancy. Any nutritional deficit is harmful to the developing baby, so optimal nutrient and calorie intake must be guaranteed prior to, during, and following pregnancy. In addition, a physician should be consulted before strenuous or new forms of exercise are practiced.

*Oral Contraceptives:* Women exercisers and athletes who take oral contraceptives might be at risk for several marginal vitamin deficiencies. For example, some oral contraceptive users have lower blood levels of folic acid, vitamin $B_{12}$, vitamin $B_6$, vitamin C, and vitamin $B_2$. The added demands of exercise might aggravate these lowered levels, unless dietary intake is increased.

## *One Last Word*

Perhaps you exercise for the pure enjoyment of the sport. Or maybe because you are concerned about your health. You might push your limits because you want to be even more fit or because you enjoy the challenge and competition. Whatever the reason, total health—physical, emotional, and spiritual—should be considered, as well as exercise performance, when choosing a nutritional plan.

Any dietary practice, fad, or gimmick that promises improved strength, endurance, or performance at the cost of your health is a red flag for disaster. What you want is a diet that maximizes exercise performance, since this is also the diet that ensures optimal health and fitness throughout life. The foundation of that diet is a wide variety of minimally processed, real foods, like those you'll find in the Healthy Woman's Diet.

# CHAPTER 10

# *Pregnancy and Breast-Feeding*

What you eat prior to, during, and immediately following pregnancy is more important than at any other time in your life. Every bite you take, every sip of water, every milligram of iron in a forkful of meat, every microgram of folic acid in a spinach salad, every smidgen of vitamin C in a gulp of orange juice is fueling your baby's future health. In fact, a wealth of new research shows that what you eat while pregnant will not only have a major impact on the outcome of your pregnancy, the weight and health of your newborn, and whether or not you develop complications during pregnancy and delivery, but in large part also will determine whether or not your baby will some day be at risk for heart disease, cancer, diabetes, obesity, hypertension, and more. What you eat might even affect how much you enjoy being a mom.

Don't worry. You don't have to live on brewer's yeast and sprouts to have a healthy baby. You can still eat foods that come in a box or a bag, eat out several times a week, and order pizza to go as long as you also follow a few simple eating-for-two dietary guidelines.

## *Gearing Up for and Getting Pregnant*

In the old days, a baby was thought to be the "perfect parasite." Regardless of the mother's nutritional status, the baby would draw all necessary nutrients from the mother's nutrient stores. For example, the mother should, but didn't have to, drink milk because the baby would siphon calcium from the mother's bones and teeth (thus, the old wives' tale that you lose a tooth for each child).

---

**TABLE 10.1    Preparing for Pregnancy**

Answer yes or no to the following statements:

_____ **1.** I don't drink alcoholic beverages.

_____ **2.** I don't smoke cigarettes, and I avoid other people's smoke.

_____ **3.** I don't drink caffeinated beverages (coffee, tea, cola) and limit my intake of decaffeinated coffee to two cups or less each day.

_____ **4.** I don't take medications, except those that are monitored by a physician.

_____ **5.** My weight is desirable for my height.

_____ **6.** I eat a low-fat, low-sugar diet based on fresh fruits and vegetables, whole grains, legumes, nonfat or low-fat milk products, extra-lean meats, and fish.

_____ **7.** I consume at least 2,000 calories daily or, if not, I take a moderate-dose multiple vitamin/mineral supplement.

_____ **8.** I take extra supplemental iron and folic acid.

_____ **9.** I include relaxation time and effective coping skills in my daily routine.

_____ **10.** I exercise at least five days a week for at least thirty minutes each day.

_____ **11.** I have an obstetrician/gynecologist that will monitor my pregnancy on a regular basis.

You should answer yes to all of the above to ensure the best environment for your baby's growth.

---

Today, experts recognize that a baby is more of a passenger than a parasite, competing with the mother for nutrients. Therefore, every choice you make, from the cereal you select to the supplements you take, directly affects your baby. Some essential nutrients come from the limited tissue stores you stockpiled prior to pregnancy if your diet was optimal. Other nutrients are not stored in the body or are stored in such limited amounts that the diet is virtually the only place your baby can get what is needed.

Consequently, nourishing a baby begins before conception. You don't want to enter pregnancy nutritionally compromised if you can help it, since it is difficult to catch up once the pregnancy process begins. In addition, your baby will have accomplished much of its critical growth in the first four weeks before you even know you're pregnant. Nutrient deficiencies during this critical period can have lifelong consequences for your baby's health and development. Since one in every two pregnancies is unplanned, it is important to eat well throughout the childbearing years—from puberty to menopause—to ensure a healthy baby.

## Diet and Fertility

Your ability to maintain a regular menstrual cycle, become pregnant, and carry a healthy baby to term is directly and indirectly related to your nutritional status. Weight is a perfect example.

Overnutrition—that is, eating too much—results in obesity, which interferes with ovulation and menstruation and reduces your chances of pregnancy. Even moderate weight loss for an overweight woman often restores ovulation and fertility.

On the other hand, being too thin also jeopardizes your ability to conceive. The onset and maintenance of menstruation depends on maintaining both a desirable weight for your height and a certain amount of essential body fat. Overconcern with being too thin, fit, and lean that results in severe calorie restriction and abnormal eating habits also interferes with normal menstruation and fertility. Even if a poorly nourished woman becomes pregnant, she has a high risk of miscarriage or stillbirth. While the pencil-shaped body of a model might be attractive for a fashion magazine, being too thin is dangerous for the woman who wishes to maintain her health and fertility or desires a healthy, well-developed baby and a low-risk pregnancy.

All aspects of nutrition relate to fertility, since optimal health is essential for reproductive function. Poor intake of any of the major nutrients, including protein and fat, contributes to infertility. For example,

- Inadequate intake of the essential fatty acid, linoleic acid, found in safflower oil and other vegetable oils results in infertility, while optimal intake of vitamin C helps boost your chances of conceiving.
- Vitamin A maintains healthy epithelial tissue that lines all the external and internal surfaces of the body, including the lining of the vagina and uterus. In contrast, vitamin A toxicity from high-dose supplementation results in amenorrhea.
- Vitamin D performs an indirect role in fertility by aiding in the formation of a woman's pelvic bone. In fact, the misconception that

women should restrict weight gain during pregnancy originated from the days when vitamin D–deficient women with poorly formed pelvises often died giving birth to full-sized babies. In the old days, women were told to limit weight gain so their babies would be small enough to deliver successfully. (We now know it is much safer and healthier for women to eat better and develop a normal-sized pelvis that can tolerate delivering healthy-weight babies!)

- Although vitamin E improves fertility in some animals, it has no direct effect on fertility in humans. However, this antioxidant vitamin does affect the production and activity of hormonelike substances in the body called prostaglandins that influence reproduction.
- Deficiencies of any of the B vitamins result in lethargy, loss of appetite, and altered hormone metabolism that indirectly might affect reproductive function. For example, folic acid deficiency might result in infertility. In several studies, women who consumed folic acid–poor diets and who had been unable to get pregnant became pregnant within months of increasing folic acid intake. Supplementation with folic acid prior to conception also reduces the risk for birth defects, including neural tube defects such as spina bifida.

Several minerals are important in fertility. Optimal intake of manganese-rich foods, such as spinach, whole-grain breads and cereals, and cooked dried beans and peas, improves fertility, as do potassium-rich foods, such as fruits and vegetables. Zinc-rich foods, such as oysters, turkey breast, and wheat germ, reduce the risk of sterility, birth defects, delayed sexual maturation, and other reproductive disorders.

Your best bet for optimizing your chances of getting pregnant is to follow the Healthy Woman's Diet as outlined on pages 44 to 53. Maintain a desirable weight within 10 to 15 percent of your ideal. Obese women who are infertile or are experiencing amenorrhea (no menstrual periods) should consult their physicians or dietitians about safe, gradual weight loss before considering getting pregnant. (See chapters 7 and 8 for weight-management guidelines.)

The diet should contain at least 100 percent, but no more than 200 percent, of the recommended intake for all vitamins and minerals and reliable sources of linoleic acid, such as one to two tablespoons daily of safflower oil, and omega-3 fatty acids, such as fish. Well-balanced vegetarian diets can provide adequate nutrients and calories, but if poorly planned they can alter female hormone levels and might cause decreased ovulation and infertility. See chapter 2 for more information on designing well-balanced vegetarian diets.

While moderate exercise is a must, avoid excessive exercise that places extreme physical stress on the body and reduces body fat below levels needed to maintain normal menstrual function. Menstrual disorders are frequently reported in women who engage in strenuous physical activity.

---

**TABLE 10.2     Exercise Guidelines for Pregnancy**

The following guidelines are proposed by the American College of Obstetrics and Gynecology (ACOG) and are intended for women who do not have any additional risk factors for adverse maternal or perinatal outcomes.

1. Women can continue to exercise during pregnancy and will experience health benefits even from mild to moderate activity. Regular activity—at least three times a week—is preferable to sporadic activity.

2. After the first trimester, a woman should avoid any exercise that requires lying down in the supine position (on the back). This position reduces cardiac output (blood flow from the heart). Long periods of motionless standing also should be avoided.

3. Because oxygen available for aerobic activity decreases during pregnancy, a woman should adapt all exercise to accommodate this shift in oxygen supply. She should stop exercising if she feels fatigued and should not exercise to exhaustion. Non-weight-bearing activities, such as swimming or cycling, help minimize the risk of injury; however, even weight-bearing activity, such as jogging, can be continued with modification under many circumstances and with physician approval.

4. Any activity that poses a threat of abdominal trauma or the loss of balance and risk to the mother or infant's well-being should be avoided.

5. Women who exercise will require up to 300 additional calories to sustain normal body functioning and a gradual weight gain.

6. To counter any increase in body temperature, a pregnant woman should drink plenty of fluids, wear appropriate clothing, and avoid exercising in hot climates.

7. Many of the physical changes of pregnancy persist six to eight weeks after delivery, so exercise routines should be resumed gradually based on a woman's physical capability.

**Nutrition Basics**

The guidelines for eating well for a healthy pregnancy are simple and easy to follow. A woman who wants to get pregnant should include in her daily diet:

1. Eight to ten servings of fresh fruits and vegetables (including at least one serving of a dark orange vegetable, two servings of dark green leafy vegetables, and one serving of citrus fruit).
2. Six servings or more of 100 percent whole-grain breads and cereals.
3. Three servings of nonfat or low-fat milk, milk products, or calcium- and vitamin D–fortified soy milk.
4. Two to three servings of extra-lean meats, chicken without the skin, fish, or cooked dried beans and peas.
5. Six to eight glasses of water.

When and where you eat these foods is flexible, and often governed by necessity. You can choose a small snack for breakfast and a larger meal later in the morning if you don't like to eat right after getting up. You can eat four, five, or more minimeals and snacks, whatever fits into your routine and schedule. Plan at least two fruits and/or vegetables at every meal and at least one at every snack to ensure you meet the quota of eight to ten servings into your daily routine. Once you are pregnant, you also will need to adapt these guidelines to fit the roller-coaster ride of hormones, morning sickness, or heartburn. For example, morning sickness in the first trimester might mean you eat light meals in the early part of the day and larger meals in the evening, while a woman in her third trimester might select a large breakfast and a light evening meal in the last trimester when heartburn is a likely problem.

Avoid or limit caffeine (such as coffee, tea, and colas) and avoid alcohol, tobacco, and medications (unless recommended and supervised by a physician) while trying to conceive. Limited evidence shows that caffeine might increase the risk of stillbirths or birth defects, while alcohol can cause permanent physical and mental birth defects. No safe limit has been established for alcohol, so abstinence is a woman's best choice.

## The Weight-Gain Issue

One of the biggest issues for the pregnant woman is figuring out how much weight she should gain. If you don't gain enough weight, your baby also won't gain enough weight. These low-birth-weight infants are at high risk for disease, learning disabilities, and death. Complications during delivery also are common when the baby weighs less than 6½ pounds. (It is normal, however, for a short, healthy woman to give birth to a small, healthy baby.)

Optimal weight gain of twenty-five to thirty-five pounds in a slender woman helps ensure a healthy-sized baby. Underweight women should gain more weight, or approximately twenty-eight to forty pounds. Overweight women should not attempt to use pregnancy as a way to use up extra body fat, since stored body fat is not the stuff from which babies are made. A modest weight gain of no more than twenty-five pounds is recommended for these women.

Don't get carried away. Further weight gain beyond recommended amounts will not make bigger or healthier babies. It will make regaining a desirable figure more difficult after delivery. It is also not just total weight gain but the pattern of weight gain that is important—with a slow gain in the first trimester of about two to five pounds total (more if you are thin, very active, or tall and less if you are overweight, sedentary, or short), followed by a steady increase to approximately three-quarters to one pound a week in the last two trimesters.

## Nourishing the "We of Me"

You won't see many changes in your body in the first few weeks of pregnancy, but an enormous amount of growth is going on inside you. Two cells have divided and changed into millions of different cells that form rudimentary organs and tissues within the first few weeks. This rapid growth and differentiation demands a constant supply of all the forty-plus nutritional building blocks.

Your body also is changing. A new organ called the placenta develops inside the uterus and serves as the junction between your body and your baby's body, supplying twenty-four hours a day, seven days a week, the nutrients and oxygen needed to make a baby. The muscles supporting the growing uterus increase in size, as does the blood volume and the volume of other body fluids, the breast tissue increases in preparation for lactation, and there is an increase in the fat or energy stores. The overall gain in weight from increased maternal body tissues and the growing baby is dependent on a constant supply of nutrients and calories.

## Your Vitamin and Mineral Needs

All nutrition experts agree that the best place for the mother-to-be to get all the essential nutrients, including ample amounts of vitamins and minerals, is from her diet. The trick is getting enough.

Numerous studies report that women often fall short of optimal when it comes to nutrition during the childbearing years. In a study conducted by the U.S. Department of Agriculture, only 6 percent of women consumed recommended levels of vitamin $B_6$ before and during pregnancy. Babies born of mothers who did not eat well during pregnancy are found low in many nutrients, including vitamins A, E, K, and $B_2$; folic acid; and the minerals iron, copper, calcium, and zinc. This poor nutritional status in turn increases the baby's risk for a variety of illness from tumors, anemia, and poor digestive function to impaired brain function, suppressed immunity, and poor bone formation. In contrast, women who eat well and supplement responsibly before and throughout their pregnancies are most likely to have few complications during the pregnancies and delivery, give birth to healthy babies, and return to prepregnancy energy levels and body weights.

*Folic Acid:* The stakes are high when it comes to folic acid. This B vitamin is essential in normal cell differentiation throughout pregnancy, but especially in the first few weeks before a woman even knows she is pregnant. Ample folic acid allows cells to divide and change into the different organs and tissues. Less-than-optimal amounts of folic acid mean cells might not change in a normal fashion, increasing the risk for neural tube defects (NTD), such as spina bifida. NTDs are the second leading cause of death among infants who die from birth defects. Folic acid supplementation around the time of conception and during pregnancy reduces the risk of NTD, a condition where the embryonic neural tube that forms the future brain and spinal column fails to close properly. Even mild folic acid deficiency during pregnancy increases the risk for spontaneous abortion, low birth weight, and poor growth, while folic acid supplementation improves pregnancy outcome and increases birth weight, while lowering the risk for delayed growth.

A review from the University of California, Berkeley, of women's eating habits found that on any four days as few as 7 percent of women consumed even one folic acid–rich dark green leafy vegetable. It's no surprise that intakes for this

B vitamin typically are below recommended levels, placing many women at risk of having babies with NTD. To avoid this tragedy, women should consume at least 400 mcg to 800 mcg folic acid daily, from both food and supplements. (Folic acid is better absorbed from supplements than from food, so a combination of sources is the best.)

*Iron:* Iron needs increase considerably during pregnancy because of an increase in the mother's blood volume and the demands of the developing infant. The number of red blood cells in the mother's blood increases 20 to 30 percent, depending on the available supply of iron. The increased daily food intake during pregnancy usually provides only 1 mg to 2 mg. This inadequate consumption, coupled with low iron stores and inadequate dietary intake of iron prior to conception, makes iron deficiency a common occurrence in pregnant women. Daily supplementation of 30 mg to 60 mg of elemental iron is usually recommended to prevent anemia or marginal iron deficiency.

The consequences of iron deficiency are greater than anemia alone. The iron-deficient woman is less able to tolerate blood loss during delivery and is more susceptible to infection following delivery. Mild to severe iron deficiency increases the risk for spontaneous abortion, premature delivery, low-birth-weight infants, stillbirth, and infant death. Infants born of anemic mothers are at greater risk for developing anemia during the first year of life. All of these complications are avoided if iron intake from food and supplements is optimal prior to and during pregnancy.

*Calcium:* What are the consequences of not consuming enough of a nutrient? While clinical deficiencies are rare in most developed countries, marginal intake of nutrients is relatively common and can have long-lasting effects on the mother and the developing baby. For example, calcium intake remains a primary concern for pregnant, nursing, and postnursing mothers. Three out of every four women enter pregnancy marginally nourished in the mineral (i.e., the average calcium intake for women is less than 600 mg compared to the recommended 1,000 mg daily). Pregnancy and nursing increase the daily requirement by an additional 33 percent. Consequently, the majority of women are at risk for deficiency, despite their bodies' best intentions. Low calcium intake increases a woman's risk for preeclampsia (women at high risk for preeclampsia might need up to 2 grams of calcium daily), lead toxicity, high-blood pressure in the infant, loss of bone in the mother, and poor skeletal formation in the infant. Why play Russian roulette with your diet when the benefits are so great and the potential consequences of poor intake are so serious?

## Should You Supplement?

Studies repeatedly show that women who eat lots of nutrient-packed, low-fat foods and supplement sensibly have a better chance of maintaining optimal nutritional status and giving birth to healthy babies. Some studies conclude women must supplement in moderation to maintain optimal blood and tissue levels of nutrients. From early studies showing that iodine supplementation virtually eradicated the mental and physical retardation of cretinism to the more recent findings that folic acid taken prior to and following conception can dramatically reduce the risk of NTD, responsible supplementation has proven worth its weight in gold. Research is uncovering many reasons to supplement responsibly. For example,

- Women who supplement tend to have fewer low-birth-weight infants than do women who don't supplement.
- Magnesium supplementation decreases pregnancy complications and improves infant development.
- Calcium supplementation reduces the incidence of high blood pressure and might improve skeletal development in the baby.
- Mothers who supplement with fluoride or drink fluoridated water have children who are resistant to dental caries throughout life.
- Folic acid supplements taken prior to and following conception can greatly reduce the risk for having a baby with a neural tube defect.
- Taking a multiple during pregnancy lowers your baby's risk for developing cancer later in life.
- Zinc in a multiple improves birth weight and head circumference, as well as nerve development and behavior in babies.
- Studies on animals show that vitamin E supplements help prevent birth defects, while pregnant women who maintain optimal antioxidant status are less prone to DNA damage.

Supplementation is especially important for some women—strict vegetarians (especially with vitamin $B_{12}$, calcium, vitamin D, zinc, and iron) and women who are lactose intolerant (especially with vitamin D, calcium, and vitamin $B_2$), who are carrying more than one baby, or who smoke, or adolescent girls who are pregnant. However, most women before, during, and following pregnancy probably would benefit from a well-balanced multiple vitamin and mineral.

*A Moderate-Dose Multiple:* The secret to supplementation is to do it sensibly. For healthy women, a multiple vitamin and mineral is best. A multiple is a convenient, cost-efficient way to supply a balance of nutrients, while avoiding secondary deficiencies that result when a woman takes too much of one nutrient and crowds out another. In general, 100 to 200 percent of the Daily Value as listed on the label is sufficient, with the exception of iron, folic acid, and possibly the antioxidants, which may be taken safely in greater than Daily Value amounts.

*Calcium and Magnesium:* Most multiples do not contain enough calcium and magnesium, so consider supplementing your supplement with a calcium-magnesium tablet if you don't consume ample amounts of calcium-rich milk or fortified soy milk and magnesium-rich whole grains, soybeans, and dark green leafies. A supplement that contains 500 mg of calcium and 250 mg of magnesium will fill in the gaps of a not-so-perfect diet.

*Multiple Doses:* Supplements that provide nutrients in multiple daily doses allow a woman to take smaller doses several times a day for maximum absorption. They also provide flexibility. A woman can decrease the dose on "gold star" days and increase the dose on the days she doesn't have the time to eat a nutritious diet.

---

**TABLE 10.3    Calcium Tricks**

Tired of drinking four glasses of milk every day? Does the thought of another cup of yogurt put a damper on your already maxed-out appetite? You can obtain ample amounts of calcium without even knowing it. Try the following tricks for adding calcium to your diet:

1. Make creamed soups and cream sauces with evaporated nonfat milk instead of cream.
2. Cook your brown rice, oatmeal, or noodles in nonfat milk or fortified soy milk instead of chicken stock or water.
3. Add nonfat dry milk powder to recipes, such as muffins, breads, pancake batter, milk shakes, or even meat loaf.
4. Drink calcium-fortified orange juice or use calcium-fortified bread.
5. Substitute low-fat cheese for meat in lasagna, ravioli, or stuffed shells.
6. Use undiluted evaporated nonfat milk in mashed potatoes.
7. Use canned salmon with the bones in recipes.
8. Blend nonfat milk or fortified soy milk with fresh fruit to make a fruit shake.

---

*Extra Iron:* Iron supplements can cause constipation or diarrhea in some women; however, taking iron supplements in small doses throughout the day or starting the supplement program by taking a small dose and gradually increasing the amount can help offset these side effects.

*Stick to the Basics:* Pregnancy is not the time to experiment with supplements, since excessive intake of some nutrients can be dangerous. For example, megadoses of some nutrients, such as vitamin A, selenium, or fluoride, can produce numerous side effects ranging in severity from mottled teeth to birth defects.

Opponents of supplementation state that a supplement will provide a false sense of security, reducing a woman's concern about her dietary practices, which could result in poor food intake and possibly marginal intake of health-enhancing substances not found in supplements. However, this fear has not been supported by the research, which shows that most people tend to eat better, not worse, when they take a supplement. In all cases, consult your physician before taking any pill, including a supplement, during pregnancy.

## Pregnancy Complications Related to Diet

Most pregnancies come with a few bumps along the way, from morning sickness and heartburn to water retention and insomnia. In a few cases, more serious health problems develop, such as preeclampsia and pregnancy-induced diabetes. While I can't promise eating well will sidestep all these problems every time, in all cases it will help.

*Morning Sickness:* Morning sickness or nausea is common in the first trimester. Avoiding food limits your intake of critical nutrients, while excessive vomiting might result in vitamin and mineral deficiencies. The traditional approach to morning sickness includes eating frequent small meals and munching on Saltine crackers prior to rising in the morning. Vitamin B$_6$ supplements are successful in some cases. Drink fluids between meals, rather than with them. However, learning to recognize what foods trigger nausea (and avoiding them) and what foods sound, and smell, palatable (and eating those) is more important than any hard rules about what to eat during nausea. If sucking on a lemon soothes the stomach or carrots dipped in vinegar go down without coming back up, then do it!

*Heartburn:* Heartburn is common during the latter months of pregnancy and is caused by the pressure of the baby and the enlarged uterus on the stomach. The symptoms of heartburn are reduced if frequent, small, low-fat meals are consumed, rather than large meals. Also, eat slowly, wear loose-fitting clothes, remain in a sitting position after eating, consume small meals in the evening, and consult a physician about the use of antacids.

---

**TABLE 10.4     A Sample Prenatal Supplement**

Three to four tablets daily will provide the following nutrients.

| NUTRIENT | OPTIMAL AMOUNTS |
| --- | --- |
| Vitamin A | 800 RE*/4,000 IU |
| Beta Carotene | 10 mg |
| Vitamin D | 5–10 mcg |
| Vitamin E | 60 mg |
| Vitamin $B_1$ | 2.0 mg |
| Vitamin $B_2$ | 2.0 mg |
| Niacin | 20 mg |
| Vitamin $B_6$ | 2.0 mg |
| Folic Acid | 400–800 mcg |
| Vitamin $B_{12}$ | 2.2 mcg |
| Vitamin C | 100 mg |
| Calcium | 1,000 mg |
| Chromium | 100 mcg |
| Copper | 1.5 mg |
| Fluoride | 2.0 mg[†] |
| Iodine | 75 mcg |
| Iron | 30–60 mg[‡] |
| Magnesium | 320 mg |
| Manganese | 3.0 mg |
| Molybdenum | 100 mcg |
| Selenium | 65 mcg |
| Zinc | 15 mg |

*RE: Retinol Equivalents. 1 RE = 1 mcg of retinol or 6 mcg of beta carotene.

[†]No need for fluoride if your water is fluoridated.

[‡]Iron, in amounts greater than 18 mg, should be approved by a physician. The amount of supplemental iron often is high because this form of iron is poorly absorbed.

*Constipation:* To alleviate constipation during pregnancy, drink at least two to three quarts of water every day; eat plenty of fresh fruits and vegetables, legumes, and whole grains; and stay active every day. Avoid laxatives unless recommended by a physician.

*Eclampsia:* Once called toxemia, preeclampsia or pregnancy-induced hypertension (PIH) are general terms for a serious condition that develops in middle to late pregnancy and is characterized by edema, protein in the urine, and high blood pressure. The condition can occur anytime after the twentieth to twenty-fourth week of pregnancy, but is most common in the later months, has an unpredictable onset, and develops in stages. The causes of preeclampsia, PIH, or the more serious eclampsia are unknown; however, the syndrome is associated with poor diet and inadequate vitamin and mineral intake. For example,

- Calcium supplementation shows promise in preventing preeclampsia or reducing the severity of this disorder when it occurs.
- Magnesium supplementation has been used to prevent both hypertension and the seizures associated with preeclampsia.
- Preliminary evidence suggests that evening primrose oil, fish oils, or linoleic acid (a fatty acid in safflower oil) might help prevent preeclampsia or edema associated with preeclampsia. In contrast, trans fatty acids in processed fats might increase risk.
- Vitamins E and C also show promise in lowering risk. In a study of 283 women at high risk for preeclampsia, those who took these two vitamins between the sixteenth and twenty-second weeks of their pregnancies had a 76 percent lower risk of preeclampsia than those who took placebos. Researchers suspect that free radicals damage cells in the placenta, thus contributing to the initiation and progression of preeclampsia. If this proves true, antioxidant nutrients would help offset that effect.

Women with preeclampsia who do not respond to nutrient-dense, moderate-salt diets plus bed rest might need to be hospitalized or their physicians might recommend antihypertensive medications, such as diuretics, as a last resort. At this time no proven preventions for preeclampsia exist. But with careful monitoring by a physician, the condition can be successfully treated.

*Diabetes:* Diabetes during pregnancy, called gestational diabetes, is a high-risk situation. Diabetic women who are closely monitored by their physicians and who take extra care and stay committed during their pregnancy have a good chance of having a successful pregnancy and a healthy baby. Ideally, a woman with diabetes who wants to have a baby should first achieve the best possible blood sugar control before conception. The diet of a pregnant woman with diabetes is similar to the Healthy Woman's Diet and is high in whole-grain breads and pasta, legumes, and vegetables; moderate in protein (20 percent of total calorie intake); and low in fat (25 to 30 percent of total calories with fewer than 10 percent coming from saturated fat). Snacks and spacing meals are important, as are daily exercise and plenty of rest. Take advantage of sugar substitutes in moderation, since sugary foods should be limited.

*Insomnia:* As your pregnancy proceeds you might experience sleep problems caused by the need to urinate or the discomfort of a bulging tummy. However, there are a few dietary tricks to getting a good night's sleep, including:

- Keep the evening meal light and low-fat.
- Cut out spicy foods or gas-causing foods.
- Have a small all-carbohydrate snack an hour before bed such as half a toasted English muffin topped with honey or jam (this boosts a nerve chemical called serotonin that helps you sleep).
- Exercise. Physical activity helps a woman cope with daily stress and tires the body so it is ready to sleep at night.
- Try a warm bath before bedtime and when sleeping, try lying on your side with a pillow supporting your abdomen and another supporting your legs.

## Breast-Feeding: Staying Nourished

If you choose to breast-feed, your food and calorie intake will be at an all-time high. As during pregnancy, you remain the sole source of nutrition for your baby and your diet influences the nutritional quality of your breast milk. Skipping even one meal can reduce milk production! You'll need more of some nutrients, such as vitamins A and D, the B vitamins, calcium, and magnesium. Iron is still important, since you are restocking from blood loss during delivery and the depletion of body stores during pregnancy. Continued supplementation for two to three months, often up to one year, after the baby is born may be advisable if your iron is low (the blood tests called serum ferritin and total iron binding capacity or TIBC are the more sensitive blood tests for iron status).

## What Should You Eat while Breast-Feeding?

After nine months of eating well, you should have no trouble continuing the healthy diet while breast-feeding! Here are the basics:

- Your calorie intake should average approximately 2,200 to 2,700 calories a day (more if you exercise).
- Include three to four servings of calcium-rich low- or nonfat milk products or fortified soy milk.
- Continue to eat eight to ten fruits and vegetables every day, preferably the colorful ones, such as dark green leafies, carrots and sweet potatoes, strawberries, blueberries, prunes, and broccoli.
- Add a few extra servings of whole grains, for a total of at least eight per day.
- Protein-rich servings of extra-lean meat, chicken breast, fish, and legumes should average three servings daily.
- Drink lots of water to replenish fluids lost in breast milk.

Steer clear of fad diets. You can lose weight very gradually (i.e., one pound a week or less) to slowly return to prepregnancy weight, but don't crash diet. Severe or restrictive weight loss diets will jeopardize your health and the quality of your breast milk.

Watch what you eat. Many compounds, from nicotine in tobacco and caffeine in coffee and colas to aspirin, marijuana, morphine, oral contraceptives, alcohol, and hormones, are excreted from the body through breast milk. Avoid these substances and all medications unless prescribed by a physician.

Don't despair if you retain a little extra weight. This weight will drop off quickly when your baby switches from breast milk to solid foods. In fact, studies show that increased fat stores are used up by the end of the nursing period, while women who do not breast-feed retain the extra body fat and are likely to gain increasingly more body fat with the next pregnancy. In short, women who do not breast-feed remain heavier for a longer period of time than do women who nurse.

## *The Postpregnancy Diet*

For many women, the main agenda after pregnancy and breast-feeding is to slip back into that little black dress or those sexy jeans worn before pregnancy. When the weight doesn't come off as easily as they expect, they are discouraged. However, the best and most successful way to lose pregnancy weight is to do it slowly—no more than one pound a week while breast-feeding and no more than two pounds a week after that. Slow weight loss ensures you're losing the right kind of weight— fat weight. It also encourages you to select an eating style you can stick with for life. Remember, it took nine or more months to gain the weight and it is likely to take at least that long to lose it. You want to lose the weight for good and you want to renew and nourish your body after the nine-month ordeal of pregnancy.

---

**TABLE 10.5     The Vegetarian Mom's Weight-Loss Plan**

Planning a successful weight-loss diet remains the same for the vegetarian as it does for the meat eater, with the exception that the two to three daily servings from the protein-rich meat group must come from cooked dried beans and peas, nuts and seeds, and/or eggs. Base the diet on whole grains, fruits, legumes, and vegetables, with three to four servings of low-fat milk products or fortified soy milk and limited intake of sugars, oils, and alcohol. As with any diet, avoid or limit fried foods; instead, bake, broil, and steam foods. To boost the nutritional value of your vegetarian diet:

- Add tofu and beans for protein, iron, and zinc.
- Drink soy milk fortified with calcium, vitamin D, and vitamins $B_2$ and $B_{12}$.
- Include at least one whole grain and two fruits and/or vegetables at every meal and snack.
- Replace iceberg lettuce with leaf lettuce or spinach in salads and add toppings such as nuts, low-fat cheese, kidney beans, and winter pears.
- Avoid drinking tea or coffee with meals, since compounds called tannins in these beverages inhibit iron absorption by up to 75 percent.
- Take a daily moderate-dose multiple supplement that supplies 100 percent of the Daily Value for a broad range of vitamins and minerals.

---

Expect to lose between ten and thirty pounds within the first two weeks following delivery. (The higher weight loss reflects greater water retention during pregnancy.) To lose the remaining extra pounds, a non-breast-feeding woman should follow the Healthy Woman's Diet, combined with daily exercise (structured exercise of at least thirty minutes or more, not just chasing the kids around the house!). Include several glasses of water daily and avoid alcohol, low-nutrient junk foods high in sugar or fat. Now that you're not breast-feeding, what you eat doesn't directly affect your baby. Moderate amounts of coffee, tea, or diet colas can be included in the diet.

What you eat indirectly affects your growing child, since the example you set is a strong influence on the eating patterns your child will develop. Healthful eating habits are much easier to establish when a child is young, than they are later in life when unhealthful, but firmly entrenched, habits must first be recognized, stopped, and then replaced with healthful ones. Let your baby see you eating a whole-grain cereal with fruit at breakfast, lean turkey sandwiches and salads at lunch, fresh vegetables every night at the dinner table, and snacking on yogurt and nuts, not chips and soda pop. Also set an example by taking your baby with you when you exercise every day. Once your baby can walk, encourage her to move, rather than sit idly in a stroller.

## *Eating for the Next Baby*

It is never too early to start nourishing the next baby. Since one in every two babies is planned and the other half are surprises, maintaining optimal nutritional status during the childbearing years is an essential part of being a mother. The Healthy Woman's Diet provides an opportunity to build nutritional reserves, to alleviate nutritional deficiencies before a baby places additional demands on them, and to adapt dietary habits while there is time and less pressure to change. The best time to make dietary changes that will benefit both you and your future new baby is prior to morning sickness, heartburn, and other pregnancy-related problems!

If you're planning another baby, to resume an exercise program, or even to survive the additional stress of juggling family, work, and home, then the eating habits you establish during pregnancy are guidelines for a lifetime.

# CHAPTER 11

# *The Mature Woman*

Turning fifty, sixty, seventy, or more is not what it used to be. Women in their second fifty years are taking up mountain climbing, biking across the country, returning to college to finish a degree, traveling the world, starting their own business, and much more. We've come a long way from the days when women didn't outlive their ovaries, let alone consider living as many years after, as they had lived before, menopause.

While our grandmothers might have weathered age-related changes in silence, today women are vocally taking charge of their health. Take, for example, menopause, a major milestone in a woman's life that in recent years has been yanked out of the closet and into boardrooms and offices, into magazines and onto book covers, and made the topic of nationwide television talk shows. Not only is the topic of menopause no longer taboo, but many of the symptoms that women once suffered in silence are now preventable, or at least can be lessened, by a few simple changes in diet and activity.

## *What Is Menopause?*

The term menopause means the cessation of menstruation. You must be menstruation free for twelve months to qualify as being menopausal, so by the time you are officially diagnosed, the experience is over. Of course, a woman knows long before this that something is amiss. This premenopause stage is called perimenopause and the stage after menopause is called postmenopause.

The classic symptom of perimenopause is the hot flash (also called the hot flush) during the day. Night sweats are a hot flash in the evening. Both are a sudden rise in body temperature accompanied by sometimes intense perspiration, a flushing of the skin, waves of heat that can range from mild to tormenting. You also might experience a variety of other symptoms, including changes in:

| | | |
|---|---|---|
| skin | energy level | memory |
| mood | appetite | sleep habits |
| sexual drive | headaches | vaginal lubrication |
| weight | urination | |

Of course, the symptoms are as varied as the women who experience them. Eight out of every 100 women pass the menopause milestone before age forty, while some women are pregnant at age fifty-seven. The average woman is postmenopausal by age fifty-two. Some women say they were in a constant hot flash during perimenopause, while others slide through without breaking a sweat.

---

**TABLE 11.1     Solutions to Menopause Problems**

**MOOD: FROM ANXIETY TO DEPRESSION**

*Diet:* Divide your food intake into minimeals and snacks. Include some complex carbohydrates at each meal/snack. Avoid sugar, alcohol, and caffeine.

*Supplements:* Consider a multiple vitamin and mineral. Also, take a magnesium supplement if daily intake of dark green leafy vegetables, whole grains, legumes, wheat germ, and other magnesium-rich foods is low.

*Exercise:* Include regular aerobic exercise, such as walking, jogging, aerobic dance, or bicycling.

*Habits:* Reserve at least twenty minutes a day for relaxing, i.e., a hot bath, meditation, or deep-breathing exercises. Avoid tobacco. Replace negative thoughts with more nurturing ones. Avoid taking on too many tasks and responsibilities.

**LOW ENERGY**

*Diet:* Eat breakfast and divide daily food intake into evenly spaced five to six small meals and snacks. Avoid caffeine, sugar, and alcohol.

*Supplements:* A moderate-dose multiple vitamin and mineral. If a blood test identifies you as iron deficient, your physician might prescribe iron supplements.

*Exercise:* Daily exercise that includes either aerobic and anaerobic exercise, such as weight lifting, can help boost energy levels.

*Habits:* Get at least seven to eight hours of sleep nightly. Take afternoon naps if possible. Prioritize your life and avoid wasting emotional or physical energy on needless activities.

## INSOMNIA

*Diet:* Avoid caffeine, alcohol, and sugar, especially after noon. Eat a light, all-carbohydrate snack before bedtime. Avoid large evening meals, spicy or gassy foods at dinner.

*Exercise:* Exercise daily, including some aerobic and some anaerobic activity. Exercise in the morning or early afternoon, but not late at night.

*Habits:* Avoid tobacco. Take time to relax before bedtime. Develop a routine before bed that conditions the body for sleep.

*Other:* Herbs, such as catnip, chamomile, and valerian, might help to improve sleep.

## MEMORY AND CONCENTRATION

*Diet:* Consume a low-fat, high-fiber diet that is rich in fruits, vegetables, whole grains, and nonfat dairy foods. Include fish in the weekly menu. Drink caffeinated beverages in moderation and only in the morning. Avoid sugar and alcohol.

*Supplements:* Take a moderate-dose multiple vitamin and mineral that includes 5 mcg vitamin $B_{12}$, 400 mcg folic acid, and 5 mg vitamin $B_6$.

*Exercise:* Exercise should include some form of aerobic activity for at least thirty minutes daily.

*Habits:* Avoid tobacco. Sleep seven to eight hours nightly. Organize and use lists. Relax.

---

# Diet and Menopause

Most of the symptoms can be traced to the ebb and flow of hormones, which resemble Mr. Toad's Wild Ride during perimenopause. Your ovaries are the manufacturing hub for the female hormone estrogen. As the ovaries shut down, estrogen levels surge, fluctuate, and eventually decline. Here is where diet can help.

Anything that levels the surges in estrogen will help curb the symptoms of the menopause. While hormone replacement therapy (HRT) is by far the most effective at balancing estrogen swells, diet and exercise also can play important roles.

If you begin to question your sanity, feel out of touch with your body, or suspect you might have entered perimenopause, you can verify suspicions by a test that measures hormone levels, especially the female hormone called FSH (follicle stimulating hormone), which rises as estrogen levels fall.

## Soy to the Rescue

Estrogen-like compounds, called phytoestrogens (meaning plant estrogens), found in soybeans can help offset the drop in estrogen that accompanies menopause. While not exactly like estrogen, phytoestrogens act much like the female hormone, binding to the body's estrogen receptors and supplementing the effects of estrogen when levels are low.

This link between food and flush was first suspected when researchers noted the dramatic difference in the incidence of hot flashes across cultures. As few as 14 percent of women living in Asia experience hot flashes, while eight in every ten perimenopausal women in the United States and Europe suffer from night sweats and/or hot flashes. The only dietary difference the researchers have found to explain these dramatic differences is that women living in Japan and China include soy in their diets daily and excrete up to a thousand times more phytoestrogens in their urine. Add soy to American women's diet and some experience up to a 40 percent reduction in hot flashes. An extra health bonus is that soy also reduces your risk for heart disease, osteoporosis, and possibly breast cancer.

How much soy do you need to curb menopausal symptoms? No one is quite sure, but preliminary evidence suggests that as little as two glasses of soy milk or two to four ounces of tofu daily might be all you need. Don't take concentrated pills or powders; stick to real soy foods, since excessive intake (more than 50 mg of phytoestrogens) might increase, rather than decrease cancer risk.

Except for soy, few other alternative treatments have proven worthwhile, according to researchers at Toronto Hospital in Canada who investigated the effectiveness of these alternative therapies got mixed results. More than 200 studies were reviewed, covering topics such as nutritional supplements, herbal remedies, homeopathic remedies, and physical approaches. They found no supportive evidence for any of these treatments.

## What You Eat Affects How You Think and Feel

You might notice a change in your mood as you approach menopause. As estrogen fluctuates, so does brain chemistry, including a nerve chemical called serotonin. Peri- and postmenopausal women who struggle with mild depression might have lower serotonin levels than do other women. When serotonin levels are low, a woman is more likely to crave sweets and feel grumpy, while a rise in serotonin curbs the cravings and restores a more agreeable mood.

If serotonin is at the root of the mood swings, then including a carbohydrate-rich snack, such as a toasted English muffin with honey or a small bowl of peach sorbet with a vanilla wafer, could be all it takes to boost serotonin levels and mood. Make sure your diet is loaded with antioxidant-rich fruits and vegetables to stem the memory loss that sometimes accompanies menopause. Gingko biloba and phosphatidylserine (PS) are two supplements that show promise in boosting mental function.

---

**BOX 11.1    Mood-Boosting Snacks and Meals**

To raise serotonin levels, you need an all-carbohydrate snack. To prevent blood sugar swells caused by sugar, you need a quality, whole-grain carbohydrate that supplies a steady, slow release of sugar into the bloodstream. Here are a few of the best snacks to boost mood and energy.

- A bowl of air-popped popcorn
- Half a whole-wheat cinnamon bagel topped with all-fruit jam and/or fat-free cream cheese
- Fat-free, whole-wheat crackers and fruit
- A bowl of oatmeal topped with brown sugar
- Pretzels and orange juice
- Fresh fruit salad topped with candied ginger and served with a slice of cinnamon toast
- A low-fat carrot muffin topped with apple butter
- A whole-wheat toaster waffle topped with apricot syrup

## *Osteoporosis: Boning Up on Calcium*

Once you hit the second fifty years, osteoporosis becomes a daily topic of conversation. If you enter perimenopause having consumed daily the calcium-equivalent of three glasses of milk and exercised vigorously for years, then you probably have strong bones and a low risk of developing osteoporosis. If you are like most women, however, you should take stock of your lifestyle and make up for lost time and lost bone. One out of every two postmenopausal women consumes less than half the recommended calcium and very few women exercise enough, thus seriously escalating risk for bone loss and osteoporosis.

Your calcium intake is important for more than just your bones. The North American Menopause Society reports that while calcium's main function is to maintain optimal bone density, this mineral also might lower your risk for hypertension, colorectal cancer, obesity, and kidney stones. Optimal intakes are at least 1,200 mg, but no more than 2,500 mg. To ensure optimal calcium absorption, the committee recommends women also get 400 to 600 IU of vitamin D, either through sun exposure or through diet and/or supplements.

Since no good test is available to monitor calcium status, women must focus on prevention by consuming enough calcium throughout life to meet these recommended levels. You need at least three glasses of milk or fortified soy milk to meet your quota for calcium and vitamin D. If you can't meet this goal, take a supplement that contains at least 600 mg of calcium, 400 IU of vitamin D, and 240 mg of magnesium.

Calcium also is important in protecting your nervous system. A study from the University of North Carolina at Chapel Hill found that lead, which accumulates gradually in the bones throughout life, is released as minerals dissolve out of the bones after menopause. This places a woman at increased risk for high blood lead levels, a condition associated with nerve damage, anemia, muscle wastage, and mental impairment. Consuming ample amounts of calcium during the early years inhibits lead absorption, so less of this harmful metal is deposited into the bones. During and after menopause, optimal calcium and magnesium intake can slow or stop the loss of calcium from the bones, which may help curb the release of lead from these tissues.

## *Heart Disease: Women's Number One Health Threat*

One in every two women will die from heart disease. Your heart-disease risk escalates quickly as estrogen levels drop during and after menopause. A recent Gallup survey sponsored by 8th Continent Soymilk found that most women are seriously misinformed about heart disease. They think they know the symptoms of heart disease, when in fact women's symptoms, if any, can be very different from men's symptoms. You might have the traditional pains down the left arm and chest. Or you might have some abdominal discomfort or lower back pain and not realize this also could be a symptom of advanced heart disease. In many cases, you'll have no symptoms at all until your first heart attack. Many of those are fatal.

According to a study conducted at Harvard Medical School in Boston on 84,129 women, there is much you can do to lower, if not entirely eliminate, your risk. While very few women in the study took care of themselves (only 3 percent of the population), when they did, they almost eliminated the threat of heart disease. Women could lower their disease risk by 83 percent if they did not smoke, maintained a desirable body weight, consumed at least one-half serving of an alcoholic beverage daily, engaged in moderate to vigorous physical activity for at least half an hour every day, and consumed diets rich in fiber, omega-3 fatty acids, and folic acid, while low in saturated fats and trans fatty acids.

The sooner you adopt the Healthy Woman's Diet the greater the benefits to your heart. Cutting total dietary fat and sugar also will help maintain your figure, which is important for the prevention of heart disease.

## *Breast Cancer after Menopause*

Breast cancer is top on women's health-concerns list. One in eight women will battle breast cancer in her lifetime. While this number pales compared to one in every two women dying from heart disease, breast cancer is still a real and serious threat.

Most cases of breast cancer occur in women who are fifty years or older and the risk factors for this disease include a high intake of fat, especially saturated fat, low intake of fruits and vegetables, excess body weight, and alcohol consumption. Switching to the low-fat, nutrient-dense Healthy Woman's Diet with less than 25 percent fat calories and more than 55 percent of calories coming from high-quality, fiber-rich carbohydrates will help lower breast cancer risk. Fiber helps curb estrogen, which often is the trigger for breast cancer. Soy products also might lower breast cancer risk. (See pages 256 to 262 for more on breast cancer.)

## Is Weight Gain Inevitable?

Women typically gain weight after menopause and tend to deposit more fat in the tummy and hips. This body reshaping from a pear shape to more of an apple shape increases a woman's risk for diabetes, heart disease, cancer, and hypertension.

Women after menopause typically have 20 percent more body fat than premenopausal women; they also have more above-the-waist fat. Abdominal fat is divided into two compartments: subcutaneous fat just under the skin (the fat that makes up love handles) and visceral fat that is deeper, firmer, and closer to internal organs. It is this visceral fat that results in a "metabolic syndrome," which raises blood levels of glucose, triglycerides and cholesterol, and certain hormones that increase your risk for disease.

Yet weight gain, often called middle-age spread, is not inevitable. Women who engage in vigorous activity throughout life maintain their muscle mass. Since muscle is metabolically active tissue that burns calories even at rest, these women don't experience the metabolic slowdown that sedentary women do. Consequently, they don't gain weight as they age, nor do they become increasingly more feeble and frail with age. They maintain their balance, their health, their mental stamina, and a lively energy level. They look younger and eat more without worrying about gaining weight. In addition, women who are on hormone replacement therapy (HRT) also appear to gain less weight after menopause compared to women who avoid HRT, say researchers at the University of Pisa in Italy.

The Women's Healthy Lifestyle Project conducted at the University of Pittsburgh set out to see if reducing saturated fat and cholesterol, curbing calories and fat intake, and boosting exercise could lower disease risk and weight gain in women from perimenopause to postmenopause. After fifty-four months, LDL-cholesterol levels in the control group had risen almost three times as much as the LDL levels in the treatment group. Weight decreased by 0.2 pounds in the treatment group compared with a 5.2 pound increase in the controls. The researchers proved that eating well and exercising keeps you young and fit.

The bottom line is that it might take more effort to maintain your girlish figure in the second fifty years, but weight gain is inevitable only if you put down the bar bells and jump rope in favor of the couch.

## *Supplements in the Second Fifty Years*

Should you consider a supplement at this stage in your life? Yes. Approximately one in every two middle-aged women does not consume even two-thirds of the recommended amounts for many vitamins, including the B vitamins, vitamins C and D, and many minerals. Poor intake of these nutrients is linked to many mental, emotional, and physical problems associated with menopause, including memory loss, mood swings, depression, irritability, osteoporosis, and more.

The guidelines are simple.

1. Take a moderate-dose, broad-range multiple vitamin and mineral. You probably won't need iron once you've stopped menstruating, but make sure the multiple contains:

   - 400 IU to 600 IU of vitamin D (your requirement for this vitamin increases as you get older),
   - 400 mcg of folic acid (to protect against heart disease, cancer risk, and memory loss),
   - 5 mcg of vitamin $B_{12}$ (to protect against heart disease and memory loss, and because you don't absorb this vitamin as well as you used to),
   - 5 mg of vitamin $B_6$ (to aid in mood regulation and reduce heart-disease risk),
   - 200 mcg of chromium, preferably chromium picolinate or nicotinate or chromium-rich yeast (to help prevent diabetes and heart disease), and
   - 70 mcg of selenium, an important antioxidant that slows premature aging.

2. Take a calcium-magnesium supplement if you do not consume the calcium equivalent of three glasses of nonfat milk or fortified soy milk

every day and several servings daily of magnesium-rich whole grains, dark green leafy vegetables, and soybeans. Look for a product that supplies about 500 mg to 600 mg of calcium and 250 mg to 300 mg of magnesium.

3. Consider taking extra antioxidants. Numerous studies show that antioxidants, such as vitamins E and C, lower heart disease and cancer risk, improve memory, and prolong the healthy middle years. (See chapter 14 for more on antioxidants.) Along with eight to ten servings daily of antioxidant-rich fruits and vegetables, consider taking a natural vitamin E supplement that contains 100 IU to 400 IU of vitamin E and/or a vitamin C supplement of 250 mg.

## Fine-Tune the Healthy Woman's Diet

Menopause is a new beginning, not the end of an era. If you eat well and exercise regularly, it is very likely you'll be fifty years old at menopause with another seventy years of healthful living yet to go! The Healthy Woman's Diet is the foundation for looking and feeling your best. It is low in fat, saturated fat, salt, and sugar, and high in fiber, phytochemicals, and the nutrients that protect against mood swings and age-related disease. The only adjustment is to add one to two servings of soy to the diet daily. You also might consider increasing your intake of flaxseed, which modulates estrogen metabolism and might have a cancer-preventing effect in postmenopausal women, according to researchers at the University of Minnesota. To further tame the menopausal hot flash:

- Avoid coffee, chocolate, alcohol, and spicy foods, all of which alter blood flow and can increase the symptoms of hot flashes.
- Eat small meals and snacks regularly throughout the day. Large meals increase body temperature and might aggravate a hot flash.
- Place a glass of ice water by the bed at night to drink at the first sign of an approaching night sweat. Also try opening the bedroom window to keep the cool air flowing, use 100 percent cotton sheets, and try using a small fan by the bed.
- Be careful of what herb teas you drink. Some herbs, such as black cohosh or dong quai, cause blood vessel dilation and could aggravate a hot flash.

- Try vitamins E and C. Some women report these vitamins helped improve symptoms of hot flashes; however, this evidence is sketchy at best.
- Dress in layers, so you can add or subtract clothes as your body's temperature fluctuates.

## Get Serious about Exercise

Women who exercise in their second fifty years not only slow the aging process, they even reverse it. Never has regular exercise been so important! You need to combine a weight-bearing endurance activity, such as walking or jogging, with strength training, such as lifting weights. This combined approach to exercise improves cardiovascular health, strengthens bones to prevent osteoporosis, maintains muscle mass to prevent weight gain and progressive frailty, and lowers breast and colon cancer risk. In fact, an unfit woman at any age can reduce her risk of dying prematurely by up to 50 percent by becoming fit, and, health wise, active women are two decades younger than couch potatoes.

## The Best Years of Your Life

Life begins at fifty! This is the time when many women report feeling more self-confident and at peace with themselves. Many women after menopause are more emotionally stable than women in their twenties and thirties. They are more sure of themselves and happier with their lives than their younger counterparts, especially if they have taken care of and nurtured their physical and emotional health. Now, that's something to look forward to!

# CHAPTER 12

# Nutrition after Sixty-Five: The Antiaging Lifestyle

Take a minute and visualize what old age looks like to you. Close your eyes and picture what an old person looks like. What does old age feel like? How does that person act? Think? Move? What can't that person do now that she used to love doing?

If you are like most people, you probably conjured up the stooped, gray-haired, forgetful old lady. Your image might be wrinkled, weak, fragile, or mentally not so sharp. You also might assume disease escalates as we age; old women are likely to have heart disease, cancer, diabetes, hypertension, cataracts, loss of mental function. Old age often equates with being debilitated, dependent on others, confused, withered, over the hill, senile.

Well, forget all of that. The belief that aging is inevitable is a myth. A wealth of research is showing us that it's not age, but years of abuse and neglect that wear down our bodies. Most aspects of aging can be slowed or completely avoided—from sun spots and wrinkles to age-related diseases such as heart disease, diabetes, hypertension, and osteoporosis to memory loss and the frailty, feebleness, and loss of independence that so many of us fear—by making a few simple changes in what we eat, when we move, and how we think. There is every reason to expect we can live robustly, passionately, vitally into our nineties, and beyond one hundred! In fact, by following the advice in this chapter, you can expect to look, act, and feel at least twenty years younger. Not bad for a start!

According to the latest statistics, only 15 to 20 percent of aging is genetically predetermined. The rest—that's right, between 80 and 85 percent—is within our control. For example,

- 70 percent of cancers are diet and lifestyle related.
- 50 percent of heart disease is diet related.
- 80 percent of sun spots and wrinkling is caused by sun exposure.
- Middle-age spread is activity related, not age related.
- Frailty, feebleness, and disability are entirely preventable with exercise.
- Only 10 percent of seniors develop dementia, and new research shows that even many of these cases can be prevented, or at least slowed, with diet, exercise, and supplements.

We expect people over the age of eighty-five to be the most debilitated, but people who take care of themselves and have followed healthy eating and exercise habits live into their nineties and beyond, are mentally sharp, healthier, and more agile than younger folks. And it doesn't take major changes in how you eat or resorting to weird eating habits. In some cases, all it takes is eating a little more of what you're already eating. For example, researchers from the University of Naples in Italy studied people between the ages of seventy and one hundred plus years and found that those living the longest also were living the healthiest. Their secret? They ate lots more fruits and vegetables than their younger, less healthy friends.

## When Does Aging Start?

Aging doesn't happen overnight. It begins much earlier than you think, as early as your late teens. It's just that the accumulation of damage doesn't begin to show outwardly until you hit your thirties or forties. The sooner you jump on the anti-aging bandwagon and start supplying your body with all the nutrients it needs to stay young, the more likely you will hold on to that youthful health, sidestep the slow demise of aging, enjoy life to its fullest, and dramatically reduce medical costs later in life.

### Antiaging in a Nutshell

The three antiaging areas are:

- *Diet:* The antiaging diet is one filled with fresh fruits and vegetables, whole grains, legumes, and low-fat milk. You also will need to supplement this healthy diet with the right dose of the right nutrients.

- *Exercise:* You need to move a lot more, but it will be worth it! Your exercise plan must include some form of aerobic workout, like walking, bicycling, or using the StairMaster at the gym, combined with strength training. But, don't worry, whatever I ask you to do is no more than any healthy ninety-seven-year-old can do!!
- *Attitude:* Even if you could make it to 120 years old on diet and exercise alone it wouldn't be worth it unless you were enjoying the extra years, living them passionately and vitally. That's why attitude is essential to nurturing vitality. Talk to people over the age of ninety and you'll find they have robust, passionate attitudes toward life. They advise you to live in the present, think positive, be good to people, don't take yourself too seriously, never retire, learn something new every day, spend your time with happy people, don't blame others, take risks, and never give up!

The sooner you start to antiage your body the better, but it's never too late to reap the rewards. As Lily Tomlin once said, "I always wanted to be somebody, but I should have been more specific." Here are the guidelines you need to follow to be more specific about how well, and even if, you age.

---

### TABLE 12.1    The Antiaging Diet

| WHAT | WHY |
|---|---|
| Eight to ten fruits and vegetables daily | Supply antioxidants, fiber, vitamins, minerals, and phytochemicals. Help maintain a desirable weight. |
| a. Two dark green leafy vegetables daily | Supply folic acid to prevent memory loss, heart disease, and cancer. |
| b. One citrus fruit daily | Supplies vitamin C to protect against cataracts, heart disease, and cancer. |

| | |
|---|---|
| Six or more servings whole grains daily | Supply fiber, phytochemicals, vitamins, and trace minerals. Help lower risks for colon cancer, stroke, heart disease, diabetes, and obesity. |
| Three plus servings nonfat milk or fortified soy milk | Supply calcium and vitamin D for strong bones, reduce risk for hypertension and colon cancer. |
| Two servings legumes or fish daily | Legumes supply B vitamins, fiber, trace minerals. Fish supplies omega-3 fatty acids to lower risk for memory loss, heart disease, cancer, and possibly arthritis. |
| Garlic, one to three cloves daily | Supplies sulfur-containing phytochemicals that lower risk for cancer, heart disease, infection, and disease. |
| Eight or more glasses of water daily | Prevent fatigue, maintain normal body functions. |
| Eliminate unnecessary calories | Reduced calories increase life span. |

Supplement responsibly with:
    A moderate-dose multiple vitamin/mineral
    A calcium-magnesium supplement
    Extra antioxidants

## Why Do We Age?

Reduced to the simplest explanation, aging is the result of accumulating loss of functioning cells. Dwindling numbers of functional cells result in loss of tissue and organ function. These effects are most noticeable in muscle and nerve cells since they are limited in their capacities to regenerate.

Numerous theories try to explain this gradual decline in cell function. One of the most promising theories on aging is the antioxidant, or free radical, theory. Tiny oxygen fragments called free radicals, found in air pollution, cigarette smoke, fried foods, and pesticides, attack and damage cells, their genetic code, and their protective coatings called a membrane. Free radicals also impair energy production by damaging the cells' powerhouse centers (called the mitochondria). (See chapter 14 for more on free radicals and disease.)

With thousands of free radical attacks on each cell every day, over the course of decades the process results in fewer functioning cells and more damaged or abnormal cells. Because free radicals also attack the immune system, the body gradually loses its resistance to colds, infections, and disease. Eventually the cell dies, leaving an accumulating buildup of cellular debris that further escalates the aging process. The body is exposed to free radicals throughout life, but the damage seems to escalate as we age.

## *Antioxidants and Aging*

Luckily the body has an antioxidant system, comprised of vitamins, minerals, enzymes, phytochemicals, and other compounds that sweep up and deactivate free radicals. Stockpiling a strong antioxidant defense and minimizing anything that generates free radicals help slow or even halt free radical damage to the tissues, thus helping prevent premature aging and age-related diseases, such as heart disease, cancer, arthritis, skin wrinkling, cancer, and cataracts.

A wealth of evidence shows that the antioxidant nutrients, including vitamins C and E, the carotenoids, selenium, and the thousands of phytochemicals,

- Help prevent age-related diseases.
- Stimulate the immune system, thus protecting the body from disease and infection.
- Protect the nervous system and brain from free radical damage associated with age-related memory loss and loss of mental function.
- Work at the basis of the body's biological clock, preventing or at least slowing the aging process.

Since the 1970s, thousands of studies have shown that the consumption of diets rich in antioxidants prevents disease and possibly premature aging. Many of those studies show a protective effect from antioxidants in fruits, vegetables, and their antioxidants in preventing numerous types of cancers, including cancers of the bladder, breast, pancreas, esophagus, lungs, larynx, oral cavity, cervix, stomach, ovary, endometrium, colon, and rectum.

Your antioxidant defenses must keep pace with your free radical levels to prevent aging and disease. Research supports this link and shows that people who maintain the highest blood levels of antioxidant nutrients are also the ones most likely to live long and healthy.

## Eat Your Vegetables

Think back over what you ate today. If you are like most people you could double, even triple, your current intake of fruits and vegetables and still barely meet the amount needed to slow the aging process. Americans typically consume far too few fruits and vegetables, thus escalating their aging and diseases processes.

- The U.S. Department of Agriculture (U.S.D.A.), author of the Food Guide Pyramid, released an index called the Healthy Eating Index, which graded diet quality from 1 to 100, with 100 equaling an "A." Most people score in the "barely passing" range with a "D" average of 63.9. The average score for fruits was "F" at 40 percent. Vegetables barely made a score of "D," 60 percent.
- A dietary intake survey of almost 3,000 adults conducted by researchers at the University of Michigan found that the average intake of fruits and vegetables is only three and a half servings daily, which is a far cry from the eight to ten recommended in the Healthy Woman's Diet.

Fruits and vegetables are the most antioxidant-rich foods in your diet. They supply all of the vitamin C and beta carotene you need and are rich in thousands of phytochemicals that are as potent, and in some cases more potent, than antioxidant vitamins like vitamin E in protecting against age-related disease. If you did nothing else except double your current intake of fruits and vegetables, you will be well on your way to living longer and healthier.

How do you boost fruit and vegetable intake?

- Consume two fruits and/or vegetables at every meal and snack.
- Snack on precut vegetables and baby carrots or frozen berries.

- Add corn or green chilies to corn bread and muffin batters, and grated carrots or zucchini to spaghetti sauce and chili.
- Drink your vegetables: Juice carrots, apple, spinach, and a slice of fresh ginger. No juicer? Then blend canned plum tomatoes, cooked carrots, peeled cucumber slices, roasted red pepper, orange juice, and a dash of tabasco.
- Add minced garlic and fresh herbs to dips, stews, sauces, sautéed vegetables, wraps, casseroles, and marinades.
- Eat more meal salads. Top a big bowl of baby spinach with grilled chicken or Cajun salmon.
- Mix fruit with vegetables. Add winter pears, raspberries, sliced peaches, or orange sections to tossed salads.
- Try one new fruit or vegetable every week.

### Take an Antioxidant Supplement

To adequately protect tissues from free radical damage, consume an antioxidant-rich diet loaded with fruits, vegetables, whole grains, legumes, nuts, and other real foods. Then consider taking extra vitamin E and possibly vitamin C. A conservative recommended dose for vitamin E is 100 IU to 400 IU daily, preferably as natural d-alpha tocopherol. A daily dose of 250 mg, but no more than 1,000 mg, of vitamin C also is important. Combined with dietary intake, this should be ample to defend the body against aging.

## *Cut Calories and Live Longer*

There's a possible dietary trick to help you live healthy past 120 years! If the abundance of research on animals showing that cutting calories increases life span can be applied to people, then reducing your food intake by a third for the rest of your life is all it would take to make you the healthiest centenarian in your family.

Calorie restriction is the only diet trick known to improve both life expectancy and life span. Every mouse, rat, and monkey that researchers have studied increased their life span from 50 percent to fourfold when calorie intake was cut by 30 percent of what the animals usually ate to feel satisfied and full. If the fat was cut at the same time, the animals lived even longer.

The benefits of cutting calories far exceed just living longer. Animals fed low-calorie diets also are disease free. Every age-related disease, from heart disease, diabetes, and cancer to memory loss and dwindling immunity, seems to vanish. Blood levels of the stress hormones and disease-causing free radicals also drop when calories are curtailed.

The secret is undernutrition, not malnutrition, which means reducing calories, while still providing all the vitamins and minerals in optimal amounts for health. Every mouthful must be nutrient-packed, while every mouthful in excess of basic calorie needs increases the risk for disease and aging. The good news is that it's never too late to cut back, since even older animals placed on calorie-restrictive diets live longer and age more slowly than their full-fed friends. Granted, people aren't rats or monkeys. But a wealth of indirect evidence shows that humans are similar to other mammals and could successfully trade a lot less food for a little more high-quality life.

## Cut Back without Feeling Deprived

You are not likely to jump at the chance to eat like a starved monkey, but even a modest reduction in calories—say cutting calories from 2,500 down to 2,000 daily—could significantly boost the chances (depending of course on your genes) of your making it to age ninety or more in great health.

To maximize the benefits of calorie restriction, while minimizing the deprivation and possible harm, your best bet is to achieve a lean and fit weight in the early years and then maintain that weight throughout life, i.e., strive for a healthy weight and avoid drastic changes in weight. Both being too skinny or too fat increases the risk of dying early.

Cut back on useless calories, such as fatty processed, convenience, and fast foods. Limit your intake of processed sugary foods. Americans are currently eating 20 percent of their calories as sugar, or up to forty teaspoons of sugar daily. Even if sugar isn't directly linked to heart disease or obesity, every time you reach for something processed or sweet you're not reaching for vegetables, fruits, whole grains, and other antiaging foods. To cut sugar:

- Avoid sticky, sweet foods, such as processed fruit bars, candy, and caramel, since they are the worst offenders of tooth decay.
- Limit soft drinks to three cans a week, or cut them out altogether.
- Cut back on sweets, such as doughnuts, pies, cakes, cookies, and ice

cream, since these foods are doubly harmful because of their high sugar and high fat content.

- Read labels. A teaspoon of sugar is equivalent to 4 grams of sugar. However, if the grams or percentage of sugar calories are not listed, you can get an idea of the sugar content by reading the ingredients list. A food is too sweet if sugar is one of the first three ingredients or if the list includes several sources of sugar. Keep in mind that sugar comes in a variety of names from glucose, brown sugar, and high-fructose corn syrup to corn syrup, dextrose, and fructose. Also, watch out for honey; it has little nutritional value other than calories. (It would take 1,200 tablespoons of honey for a total of 76,800 calories to supply a day's requirement for calcium or 100 tablespoons and 6,400 calories to supply enough iron.)
- Use more spices. Cinnamon, vanilla, spearmint, and anise provide a sweet taste to foods without adding sugar or calories.

Another way to maximize your nutrients for the least amount of calories is to focus on whole grains. Many women overeat refined grains, which contributes to weight problems. In contrast, whole grains fill you up before they fill you out, so you eat fewer calories yet feel satisfied.

Switching from meat to cooked dried beans and peas several times a week is another way to cut calories, while maximizing nutrients. Phytosterols in beans slow the progression or even prevent colon cancer. Phytoestrogens, such as daidzein and genistein, in soy products alter estrogen production, which might reduce the risk for developing breast cancer and lessen the symptoms of menopause. Saponins, another group of phytochemicals in beans, interfere with the process by which DNA reproduces, which might prevent cancer cells from multiplying. Saponins also might lower blood cholesterol, thus lowering heart-disease risk. Easy ways to increase your intake of beans are to

- Add beans to canned soups, stews, and salads.
- Snack on roasted soy nuts, replace peanut butter with soy nut butter, use whipped silken tofu as a replacement for milk when making pumpkin pie or creamed soups, experiment with different soy cheeses, and crumble firm tofu into your favorite wrap or burrito.
- Make it a goal to replace meat with beans at least five times a week in lunches or dinners.

## *Protect Your Memory*

Your diet has a profound effect on how clearly you think and concentrate, on your intelligence level, and even on how well you remember today and in the future. Every nerve cell, the chemicals (called neurotransmitters) that relay information from one nerve to the next, and the circulatory system that carries oxygen to the brain depend on a constant supply of nutrients to function properly throughout your entire life.

But don't take feeling fine as a sign of thinking good. In most cases, your mental function is affected long before you notice physical problems. Consequently, vague yet profound changes, such as cloudy thinking, mental fatigue, or reduced memory, can progress undetected because you otherwise feel OK.

### B Vitamins and Your Mind

B vitamins speed nerve transmission by maintaining the insulating sheath around nerve cells; they convert energy to a useable form for the brain; and they regulate the neurotransmitters that allow brain cells to communicate. Poor dietary intake of any B vitamin literally starves the brain for energy and leads to abnormal brain waves, confusion, irritability, and impaired thinking, concentration, memory, reaction time, and mental clarity.

For example, in a study from the University of Swansea in Wales, 120 women daily took either a placebo or vitamin $B_1$ supplements. After two months, the supplementers reported they were more clearheaded, composed, and energetic. Reaction times also improved after supplementation. Other studies, such as a study from the University of New Mexico School of Medicine in Albuquerque, also report that people who consume a diet rich in B vitamins score higher on tests measuring memory than do people who eat poorly.

You don't need to gulp brewer's yeast smoothies or swallow handfuls of vitamin pills to nourish your brain. Just include several servings daily of B-vitamin-rich foods, including nonfat milk and yogurt, fortified soy milk, wheat germ, bananas, seafood, whole grains, and green peas.

### Antioxidants and Brain Power

The brain consumes more oxygen than any other body tissue, which exposes it to a huge daily dose of oxygen fragments called free radicals. Free radicals are trouble-makers, attacking, damaging, and destroying every brain cell in sight. The wear and tear after decades of free radical attacks is thought to contribute to the gradual loss of memory and thinking associated with aging, even Alzheimer's disease.

That's where the antioxidants come in. The research on antioxidants and mental function is preliminary; however, the results of several studies look promising. For example, a study from Erasmus University Medical School in the Netherlands found that thinking ability remained high throughout life when people consumed the most antioxidant-rich foods. To keep your antioxidant defenses strong, consume daily at least eight to ten servings of orange juice, strawberries, carrots, spinach, cantaloupe, and other fresh fruits and vegetables.

### Other Memory-Boosting Diet Tips

Why put up with "getting by" when you can think and remember at your best with just a few simple dietary guidelines!?

1. Take time to eat breakfast. This meal needn't be big or complicated, but it should be nutritious. Make sure to include at least one fruit, one grain, and a protein-rich source such as nonfat milk or egg beaters. For example, a whole-wheat English muffin with peanut butter, an orange, and a glass of nonfat milk. Breakfast is essential for restocking drained glucose stores, the brain's main fuel.
2. Eat every three to four hours and always include complex carbohydrates like whole grains, starchy vegetables, or legumes for brain fuel with a little protein to sustain energy and alertness.
3. Keep all meals light. Avoid high-fat or heavy meals that contain more than 1,000 calories, which divert the blood supply to the digestive tract and away from the brain, leaving you feeling sluggish and sleepy.
4. Make sure you consume daily at least six servings of whole-grain breads or cereals, eight to ten servings of fruits and vegetables (with at least two dark green leafy vegetables and one citrus fruit), three servings of calcium-rich foods such as nonfat milk or fortified soy milk, two servings of

legumes or fish, and one to two servings of choline-rich foods such as wheat germ, brewer's yeast, or soybeans. These foods supply the B vitamins, antioxidants such as beta carotene and vitamin C, minerals such as magnesium and calcium, and trace minerals such as iron and zinc that help maintain a healthy nervous and circulatory system.

5. Take a moderate-dose multiple vitamin and mineral with extra antioxidants such as vitamins C and E.

6. Avoid or limit intake of alcohol and nicotine, which are either toxic to the brain or constrict blood vessels and interfere with circulation (and oxygen flow) to the brain. A cup of coffee might kick start the day and even temporarily improve memory, but more than three cups during the day can interfere with mental processes and give you the coffee jitters.

7. Avoid exposure to mercury, lead, and other toxic metals that damage brain and nervous tissue and are associated with subtle neurological and psychological disorders, including learning disabilities, reduced attention span, poor reasoning and concentration skills, and reduced IQ. (See pages 347 to 353 for more on diet and memory.)

## Beyond Diet: You Must Exercise to Stay Young

Are you out of breath after sprinting across the street to make a light? Do you grunt when getting up from a low chair? Has your back ever gone out when all you did was bend over? Do you take the escalator, rather than the stairs? Do you use your body weight to help open heavy doors? Have you gained some weight around the middle? If so, you've started to age. Not because you have to, but because you're not keeping your muscles and joints young by exercising them every day.

### What Happens If You Don't Exercise

Being a couch potato won't do you in when you're a teenager or young adult. But your muscles will take a nosedive in your thirties. Women lose approximately 1 to 2 percent of muscle mass every year after this point, which equates to a five to ten pound loss of muscle every decade. You probably won't notice the loss until your fifties, when you find that standing up after sitting cross-legged on the floor requires a grunt and maybe some help or you drive one block rather than walk from store to store. But that's just the beginning.

Your body loses muscle and accumulates fat as it ages. Fat tissue is relatively inactive, so you need fewer calories to maintain your body weight. In comparison, muscle is metabolically active tissue that burns calories even when you're resting. Consequently, as you trade muscle for fat, your metabolism slows. Now it takes fewer calories to keep you going, so you'll gain weight if you eat like a thirty-year-old. The gradual fitness meltdown also contributes to bone loss and osteoporosis, elevated blood cholesterol and glucose, elevated blood pressure, and increased insulin resistance, which increases your risk for most age-related degenerative diseases, from heart disease and diabetes to hypertension and cancer.

Over decades your body becomes less fit. It takes more effort to accomplish even simple daily tasks; so you do less and less. If you live long enough, you reach a point where you can't get up out of a chair without help or even pick up the groceries, let alone your grandchild. The changes are so gradual that most people blame aging as the cause, rather than putting the blame squarely where it belongs—years of inactivity. It's not a pretty picture and it doesn't have to happen!

## What Happens If You Do Exercise

Hundreds of studies spanning decades of research consistently show that people who continue to exercise throughout life remain strong, flexible, independent, and less prone to disease.

Compared to inactive older women, seniors who regularly exercise

- Have lower blood pressure, lower blood cholesterol, higher HDL cholesterol (the good cholesterol), and as much as a 40 percent lower risk of developing, and an even lower risk of dying from, heart disease.
- Have lower body weight and body fat and improved insulin sensitivity, thus lowering their risk of high blood pressure and diabetes.
- Are less likely to experience colon cancer, stroke, or even back injuries.
- Have stronger bones and are at lower risk of developing osteoporosis.
- Are less likely to injure themselves or even fall compared to unfit older people.

- Are happier, more satisfied with their lives, and less prone to depression, anxiety, and stress.
- Live longer.

---

**TABLE 12.2    The Exercise Guidelines to Stay Young**

Move every day for at least 45 minutes:

1. Engage in some form of aerobic activity, such as walking, swimming, or jogging, at least four hours a week.
2. Do some form of strength training, such as lifting weights or calisthenics like sit-ups, at least twice a week.
3. Warm up and cool down before and after each exercise session.

---

The sooner you take charge of the aging process the better, although it's never too late to reap the rewards. Aging is a continuum not a sudden event. You don't wake up one morning to discover you're old. The same nutrition issues related to seniors—from heart disease to osteoporosis—have their beginnings in the early to middle adult years. It's just that the stakes get higher as we age. If you take charge of your health today, pay attention to the quality of the food that fuels your body, and start moving daily as your body was made to move, you'll be stacking the deck in favor of enjoying your grandchildren and great-grandchildren and of living long, healthy, and vitally well past one hundred years young.

# CHAPTER 13

# *Women, Nutrition, and Medications*

Would you caution a friend against taking tetracycline with a glass of milk? Do you wonder if taking two aspirins every day will affect your red blood cells? Do you worry that your neighbor who takes birth control pills might not be eating enough dark green leafy vegetables? Are you concerned that the diuretics your boss takes for hypertension could possibly cause a magnesium deficiency? These concerns might seem strange, but the effect that foods and drugs have on one another can influence whether the body receives the nutrients it needs and whether a medication is effective, or even toxic.

## *Medication Use and Nutritional Status*

The widespread use of prescription and over-the-counter (OTC) medications has resulted in a growing interest in how medications affect a woman's health and nutritional status. Long-term use of many common medications, such as birth control pills, aspirin, cholesterol-lowering medications, or hormone replacement therapy (HRT), might pose serious concerns for a woman's nutritional status. Even short-term use of some medications can have a temporary influence on how the body handles certain nutrients.

A woman's nutritional status also can affect the desired outcome of medication therapy. Prescription and OTC medications can affect a woman's nutritional status by increasing or decreasing appetite, altering the absorption of nutrients in the intestines, affecting how the body uses nutrients, and increasing the excretion of certain vitamins or minerals. For example, drinking grapefruit juice while tak-

---

**TABLE 13.1    Eating When You're Not Hungry**

Some medications cause a temporary loss of appetite and could result in poor nutrient intake. The following suggestions help counteract drug-induced appetite changes.

- Eat when hungry, regardless of the time.
- Schedule small nutritious snacks throughout the day.
- Have nutritious snacks available, such as fresh fruit, crisp vegetables, dried fruits, cottage cheese, or sliced meat.
- Sip on nutritious beverages, such as milk shakes, juices, or milk.
- Make food appetizing. Vary the color, shape, and texture of foods.
- Eat with friends and family.
- Have nutritious snacks by the bed, such as nuts and dried fruit.
- Try new recipes.
- Exercise before eating.
- Catch up on food intake on days when eating is enjoyable.
- Take a moderate-dose multiple vitamin/mineral supplement with consent of your physician.
- Talk to your physician if poor appetite persists.

---

ing certain medications, such as calcium-channel blockers, antihistamines, sleeping pills, cyclosporine, allergy medications, or even some hormones, can increase absorption of the medication up to threefold, resulting in potential toxicities. High-protein diets, on the other hand, help eliminate certain drugs like phenazone and theophylline from the body.

## Take a Pill, Eat More or Less

Some medications increase appetite and food intake and even increase food cravings, especially for sweets. Long-term use of medications, such as some antidepressants, could increase the risk for weight problems and degenerative diseases related to obesity, such as cardiovascular disease, cancer, diabetes mellitus, and high blood pressure.

Other medications reduce appetite and result in weight loss. This might sound attractive if you are trying to lose weight, but loss of appetite (anorexia) means reduced food and nutrient intake and the potential for nutrient deficiencies, malnutrition, and loss of lean body mass. Many drugs alter taste, which reduces your interest in eating. Other medications alter mood, which reduces the desire to eat. Often weight loss occurs in women who already are underweight, thus compounding borderline malnutrition. Poor nutrition also suppresses the immune system, which interferes with the body's ability to defend itself against disease.

## Pills That Increase Nutrient Losses

Medications can interfere with nutrient absorption in numerous ways. For example, they can

- Bind to a nutrient in the intestinal tract and limit its absorption. Mineral oil binds to the fat-soluble vitamins, such as vitamins A, D, E, and K, and limits absorption. Secondary deficiencies of these vitamins are a side effect of long-term mineral oil use.
- Increase urinary loss of nutrients, such as potassium, with use of some high blood pressure medications.
- Speed movement of food through the intestines, thus limiting the absorption time of nutrients. For example, drugs that increase intestinal movement, such as laxatives, might decrease the absorption of vitamins $B_2$ and $B_{12}$.
- Change the structure or function of a nutrient so it is not absorbed in the intestines. Drugs, such as OTC antacids or some medications for gastroesophageal reflux disorder (GERD), change the acidity of the intestinal tract and might interfere with the absorption of nutrients, such as iron and vitamin $B_{12}$, that depend on a specific acidity for absorption.
- Physically or chemically block absorption sites in the digestive tract or reduce the absorption capabilities of the intestinal lining. For example, neomycin alters the intestinal lining and blocks the absorption of vitamins A and $B_{12}$.
- Interfere with the digestive juices, such as bile salts, so that dietary fat and the fat-soluble vitamins, which require these emulsifiers for absorption, are poorly absorbed.
- Interfere with the functioning of the pancreas and its digestive enzymes that are required for the absorption of other nutrients, such as protein and carbohydrate.

- Increase the urinary excretion of nutrients, especially minerals. Since minerals coexist in a delicate balance with one another, loss of one mineral could result in secondary deficiencies of other minerals.

## Pills Change How the Body Uses Nutrients

How medications affect nutrients within the body is complicated and poorly understood. Some drugs mimic the shape of a vitamin. In the body, these drugs are mistaken for the vitamin, bind to enzymes or enter into metabolic reactions, and block the real vitamin from doing its job. The drug, however, has no nutritional activity and, thus, halts or hinders metabolic processes. In other cases, receptor sites on cells might not recognize a nutrient when the inside body is bathed in a medication.

---

**TABLE 13.2     Who Is at Risk for Drug-Induced Nutrient Deficiencies?**

Although every woman should be aware of how medications affect her nutritional status, there are some women who are at greater risk for drug-induced deficiencies. These include:

- *Seniors:* They use the most medications and often are taking medications long-term. Seniors also are most prone to poor diets and reduced nutrient absorption, so the combination of medication use and poor nutritional status can result in malnutrition.
- *Women who frequently drink alcohol:* Alcohol reduces nutrient absorption, increases nutrient needs, reduces appetite and food intake, and often is accompanied by a poor diet.
- *Women with long-term health problems:* Diseases, such as cancer, diabetes, epilepsy, disorders of the digestive tract, emotional disorders, or heart disease, require long-term use or multiple use of medications. High-dose therapies also affect nutritional status more than low-dose therapies.
- *Women who frequently diet:* Anyone on restricted diets, from strict vegetarians and women who eat sporadically to pregnant or breast-feeding women with high nutritional needs who also must take medication, should be extra careful to ensure optimal nutrient intake.

---

In short, a woman's nutritional status is affected by long-term or multiple use of medications. The consequences will vary depending on many factors: a woman's nutrient stores; her age, size, and medical condition; the nutritional adequacy of her diet; and how much or how many medications she is taking and for how long.

It is always best to take medications for the prescribed amount of time and no longer. In addition, optimal nutrition prior to, during, and following long-term use of medications minimizes the potential drug-induced effects on a woman's nutritional status. In contrast, a woman who is marginally nourished prior to taking a medication, continues to consume a nutrient-poor diet while on the medication, and who takes several medications or takes one medication for long periods of time is placing herself at risk for developing medication-induced malnutrition.

## *Alcohol*

Malnutrition is a common result of alcohol abuse. Alcohol either replaces other nutritious foods and limits nutrient intake or is consumed along with a normal diet, adding extra calories and increasing your chances of weight gain. Alcohol also increases a woman's requirements for several nutrients, including the B vitamins, that aid in detoxification in the liver. Alcohol is suspected to increase free radical damage to tissues, which increases the body's need for the antioxidant nutrients to repair and rebuild damaged tissues. (See chapter 14 for information on free radicals and antioxidants.)

Alcohol irritates and damages the digestive tract and inhibits the absorption of several nutrients, including vitamins C, $B_1$, $B_{12}$, folic acid, the fat-soluble vitamins, protein, calcium, and other nutrients. Deficiencies of these nutrients affect the absorptive capability of the digestive tract and can contribute to malnutrition.

Alcohol interferes with the body's use of many nutrients, so even if the diet is adequate, the nutrients are unavailable for normal metabolic processes. Consequently, symptoms of malnutrition develop. For example, excessive alcohol intake interferes with the conversion of vitamins D, $B_1$, and $B_6$, and folic acid to their biologically active forms, so malnutrition develops even when dietary intake of these nutrients is adequate.

Excessive alcohol intake also depletes the body's tissue stores of several nutrients, including vitamin A, selenium, and vitamin E. Many of these nutrients function as antioxidants and alcohol-induced depletion of these nutrients can leave the body defenseless against disease and infection.

Women might suffer the effects of alcohol more than men. Compared to men, women maintain higher blood levels of alcohol after drinking the same amount of alcohol. The lining of a man's stomach has higher concentrations of enzymes to inactivate alcohol, while more alcohol remains intact in a woman's stomach and enters the bloodstream. These higher blood levels of alcohol in women over time could place women at higher risk for liver disease, pancreas problems, nerve damage, and nutritional deficiencies.

The best thing a woman can do for her health is to drink alcohol in moderation or not at all, as well as follow the guidelines of the Healthy Woman's Diet. Moderation is defined as one drink or less a day. One drink is a 6-ounce glass of wine, a 12-ounce glass of beer, or 1 ounce of liquor.

Even the best diet combined with vitamin-mineral supplements cannot protect the body's organs from the damage caused by alcohol abuse. However, diet and supplementation might help replenish lost nutrients and, thus, slow the progression of some nutritional problems related to alcoholism. Also, do not combine alcohol with certain herbs, such as valerian and kava, since these herbs add to the drowsy effects of alcohol and cause oversedation.

## *Antacids*

Antacids might provide quick relief for stomach discomfort and an easy source of calcium. They also could contribute to nutrient deficiencies if consumed in excess.

Antacids that contain magnesium or aluminum hydroxides inhibit calcium absorption and increase the risk of developing bone disorders and osteoporosis. Aluminum is toxic to the nerves and bones and absorption of this metal from antacids could pose a problem if they are consumed with citrus fruits or juices, such as grapefruit or orange juice. Sodium bicarbonate (baking soda) used as a stomach settler also interferes with calcium absorption; however, a woman is only at risk if she drinks a sodium bicarbonate mixture daily while also eating a low-calcium diet. Consuming calcium-rich milk products within two hours before or one hour after taking this antacid might cause kidney damage over long-term use.

Antacids reduce stomach acidity, which is useful to someone with excessive stomach acid or a nervous stomach, but could result in anemia or nutrient deficiencies if they are consumed frequently and for long periods of time. Neutralizing stomach acid reduces the absorption of the vitamins and minerals, such as iron, calcium, folic acid, vitamin A, and vitamin $B_{12}$, that require an acid digestive system for maximum absorption. This effect can be minimized if the antacid is taken on an empty stomach, rather than with meals or with vitamin/mineral supplements where it can interact with dietary nutrients.

## Antibiotics

Antibiotics indiscriminately destroy both harmful and beneficial bacteria that help maintain health. Several nutrients are manufactured by bacteria in the large intestine, including biotin, vitamin K, and other vitamins. Antibiotics upset the delicate balance in the digestive tract and reduce or halt the manufacture of these nutrients.

Long-term use of antibiotics can produce a vitamin K deficiency and might deplete the small amount of vitamin C stored in the body. In addition, consuming some antibiotics, such as tetracycline, with a meal or with milk reduces the absorption of both the medication and several minerals, including calcium, iron, and magnesium. Reduced absorption of vitamin $B_{12}$ and potassium also have been reported with long-term antibiotic use. These deficiencies are prevented when the guidelines for the Healthy Woman's Diet are followed and if antibiotic therapy is temporary. A side effect of tetracycline is an increased sensitivity to the sun. This effect is worsened by also taking the herb Saint-John's-wort.

In contrast, vitamin C might reduce bacterial resistance to antibiotic therapy and improve recovery from infection, according to researchers at Harvard School of Public Health in Boston. In this study, the combined effect of vitamin C and antibiotics was more effective in destroying bacteria than medication alone. In fact, the effective antibiotic dose could be reduced when vitamin C intake was increased.

## Antidepressants

Some women on long-term antidepressant medications lose their desire to eat, stop eating or eat sporadically, choose nutrient-poor foods, and experience reduced absorption or increased urinary excretion of several nutrients, including calcium, magnesium, the B vitamins, and vitamin C. Some antidepressant medications produce nausea, dry mouth, diarrhea, reduced salivation, or stomach upsets that also interfere with optimal nutrition. In fact, some patients on long-term antidepressant medication therapy show low blood levels of B vitamins and respond favorably with improvements in mood and anxiety levels when vitamin supplements are added to the diet.

The monoamine oxidase inhibitors (MAOI) used in the treatment of depression can cause several unpleasant and potentially harmful effects, including hypertension, when consumed with foods that contain a substance called tyramine. Aged and fermented cheeses, sour cream, fermented sausages, beer, red wine, and soy sauce are a few examples of tyramine-containing foods. These foods should be limited or avoided when taking MAOI medications. The effectiveness of the antidepressant doxepin is reduced when it is mixed with carbonated beverages or grape juice.

## TABLE 13.3    Selected Drug-Nutrient Interactions

| DRUG | POTENTIAL NUTRIENT DEFICIENCY |
| --- | --- |
| Colchicine | Vitamin $B_{12}$ |
| Proton pump inhibitors, i.e., Prilosec, Nexium, Aciphex | Vitamins A and $B_{12}$, iron, calcium, and folic acid |
| Oral contraceptives | Vitamin $B_6$ |
| Hydralazine | Vitamin $B_6$ |
| Isoniazid | Vitamin $B_6$ |
| Penicillamine | Vitamin $B_6$ |
| Salicylates | Vitamin C |
| Alcohol | Vitamin C |
| Cathartics | Vitamin D |
| Glutethimide | Vitamin D |
| Digoxin | Vitamin D |
| Anticonvulsants | Vitamin K |
| Dicumarol, warfarinVitamin K | Vitamin K |
| Cholestyramine | Vitamins A, D, E, K, and $B_{12}$ |
| Clofibrate | Vitamin $B_{12}$, iron, beta carotene |
| Tetracycline | Calcium, magnesium, zinc, vitamins $B_6$ and $B_{12}$ |
| Neomycin | Calcium, magnesium, iron, potassium, vitamins A, $B_{12}$, and K |

Several herbs alter the effectiveness of antidepressants. Ginseng and psyllium block the activity of amitriptyline HCL, chlordiazepoxide (Librium), and lithium carbonate. Some herbs, such as kava, ma huang, yohimbe, and Saint-John's-wort, enhance activity of these medications, and should not be taken at the same time.

Nutrient deficiencies are rare, even when therapy continues for some time, as long as a woman consumes the Healthy Woman's Diet and takes a moderate-dose vitamin-mineral supplement when dietary intake is poor.

## *Arthritis Medications*

A common medication used in the treatment of rheumatoid arthritis is d-penicillamine, or Cuprimine. This medication sometimes reduces food intake by producing nausea, mouth sores, stomach pain, and tongue inflammation and also reduces the absorption of several nutrients, including zinc, iron, and other minerals. The drug-nutrient interactions are minimized if this medication is taken on an empty stomach one to two hours following a meal. Vitamin $B_6$ requirements also might increase when taking this medication. Any vitamin or mineral supplement should be taken at least two or more hours before or after the medication and always should be monitored by a physician.

Corticosteroids are powerful drugs that help reduce the pain and inflammation associated with rheumatoid arthritis. They also cause bone loss, leading to osteoporosis. Long-term users of these medications should discuss with their physicians the need to take 1,500 mg of calcium and 800 IU of vitamin D daily.

## *Aspirin and Anticoagulants*

Aspirin is used for everything from headaches and athletic injuries to the treatment of heart disease. However, this panacea-like over-the-counter medication also can increase a woman's risk for developing nutrient deficiencies if taken repetitively and for long periods of time.

Since aspirin can cause bleeding in the digestive tract, long-term use could result in iron deficiency, reduced formation of red blood cells, and anemia, especially in women with preexisting stomach problems. Long-term use of aspirin also might cause deficiencies of folic acid, vitamin $B_{12}$, and vitamin C, which can be prevented by consuming more foods rich in these nutrients or by taking a moderate-dose multiple vitamin and mineral supplement at opposite times of the day from aspirin intake.

Another pain killer called acetaminophen can cause liver damage if taken in large amounts over long periods of time. Discuss with your physician the possibility of increasing your intake of orange and dark green vegetables, since carotenes in these foods show promise in protecting the liver from damage.

Prescription anticoagulants, such as warfarin, interact with several herbs and taking both at the same time could produce harmful effects, possibly triggering bleeding or a stroke in susceptible people. These herbs include chamomile, bromelain, feverfew, ginseng, ginger, ginkgo, and seaweed. Garlic also is a blood thinner. Although some physicians recommend avoiding all vitamin K–rich foods when taking warfarin, many people can continue to eat their regular diets as long as vitamin K intake remains reasonably constant over time. Vitamin K aids in blood clotting and warfarin (also called Coumadin) works by opposing this action. Discuss medication dosages with your physician if you increase your typical intake of vitamin K–rich greens.

## *Birth Control Pills*

Long-term use of birth control pills can affect the absorption and use of several nutrients. Birth control pills are associated with weight gain, increased appetite, reduced absorption of folic acid and other vitamins, and altered distribution of several nutrients within the body's tissues.

High blood levels of some nutrients, such as vitamin A, copper, and iron, are noted in some women, while low blood levels of vitamins E, C, $B_1$, $B_2$, and $B_6$, folic acid, iron, and zinc, are noted in other women on birth control pills. Although increased dietary intake of foods rich in these nutrients and taking a moderate-dose vitamin and mineral supplement are practical approaches to the prevention of drug-induced deficiencies, there is no evidence that large supplemental doses of these nutrients improve nutritional status in women taking birth control pills.

Birth control pills lower blood and tissue levels and increase the dietary requirements for vitamin $B_6$. This nutrient is particularly interesting, since even moderate deficiencies of vitamin $B_6$ produce many of the mood disorders associated with the use of birth control pills, such as depression, irritability, and insomnia. Vitamin $B_6$ is an essential component in the production of the brain chemical serotonin that regulates pain, mood, some eating behaviors, and sleep. Low vitamin $B_6$ levels reduce serotonin levels, which could produce mild depression and the other symptoms mentioned above. Birth control pills only affect vitamin $B_6$ status in women who are already consuming a marginal amount of this vitamin in their diets. In these women, improvements in mood and sleep are reported when vitamin $B_6$ intake is increased. Often all that is needed to ensure optimal nutrient intake and reduced mood or sleep problems are improved dietary habits and increased dietary intake of vitamin $B_6$–rich foods, such as chicken breast, fish, bananas, whole grains, nuts, and legumes.

## Cigarettes and Tobacco

Tobacco smoke is harmful to both the smoker and the people forced to inhale other people's smoke (passive smokers). Tobacco smoke

- Depletes the tissues and blood of vitamin C, increasing the daily requirement from 60 mg to as much as 200 mg per day.
- Increases daily requirements for vitamin A and beta carotene.
- Alters vitamin $B_6$ metabolism, and the residual effects might last as long as two years after cessation of smoking. One study found that blood levels of vitamin $B_6$ and its active enzyme form in the body were significantly lower in smokers than in nonsmokers.
- Increases the daily need for folic acid and vitamin $B_{12}$.

The best advice is to stop smoking and avoid all forms of tobacco smoke, including cigarette, pipe, chewing tobacco, and cigars. Since women who smoke during pregnancy have low blood zinc levels and are more likely than nonsmokers to give birth to zinc-deficient babies who are at high risk for birth defects and disease, it is even more important that any woman who is considering pregnancy should avoid cigarette smoke from all sources.

## *Heart Disease Medications*

Most medications that lower your risk for heart disease aim at lowering blood cholesterol levels. Some of these medications, such as cholestyramine, block cholesterol absorption in the digestive tract. They also block other fat-soluble substances, including vitamins A, D, E, and K. Make sure you eat additional servings of foods rich in these nutrients and take a moderate-dose supplement to counter the drug's effects. Drugs that regulate the heartbeat, such as digitoxin and digoxin, should not be taken with herbs that enhance the drug's effectiveness, including senna, Siberian ginseng, dandelion, hydrangea, Saint-John's-wort, uva ursa or bearberry, and rauwolfia.

## *High Blood Pressure Medications and Diuretics*

Diuretic medications used in the treatment of high blood pressure increase urinary loss of several minerals, including potassium and magnesium, which might increase a woman's resistance to medication therapy and the risk for heart disease. One in every two people treated with the blood pressure–lowering medications, such as thiazides and furosemide, have low blood levels of potassium and magnesium and require higher doses of medication to keep their condition under control. In one study, supplementing the diets of these patients with magnesium lowered blood pressure and allowed the patients to take lower medication dosages. Do not take natural laxatives, such as aloe, dandelion, senna, or cascara sagrada, when taking diuretic medications, since severe loss of potassium can cause confusion, weakness, irregular heartbeat, and even death.

Other links of diuretics, blood pressure medications, and nutrition include:

- Two hypertensive medications called captopril and enalapril might reduce zinc levels. One study reported that these medications, especially captopril, increased urinary loss of zinc and reduced zinc levels in red blood cells. Depletion of zinc from the tissue could compromise immune function, reduce a woman's resistance to colds and infection, and delay wound healing.
- Diuretic medications, such as clopamide, used in the treatment of hypertension alter tissue levels of copper and zinc. On the other

hand, taking potassium supplements with these blood pressure medications, which are called potassium-sparing medications, might increase the risk of heart problems caused by excessive blood potassium levels.

- Licorice in its natural form and yohimbe raise blood pressure, which would counteract the effectiveness of drugs used to treat hypertension.
- Vitamin $B_1$ supplements should be considered for patients taking the diuretic furosemide, according to a study from Tel Aviv University.

## Hormone Replacement Therapy (HRT)

HRT might affect nutritional status. Some women taking HRT retain salt and water and complain of weight gain. HRT also can affect dietary intake if a woman experiences abdominal cramping, loss of appetite, diarrhea, or nausea. These side effects can reduce food and nutrient intake. HRT might also increase a woman's risk for several nutrient deficiencies, including folic acid and vitamins $B_6$ and $B_{12}$. Other estrogen-containing drugs, such as birth control pills, lower blood levels of B vitamins and raise blood levels of vitamin A, iron, and other minerals. However, it is poorly understood whether HRT also affects these nutrients.

## Stimulants and Diet Pills

Phenylpropanolamine (PPA) is an over-the-counter appetite suppressant with inconsistent effects on weight loss. Many studies report this drug produces minimal weight loss, while the side effects, such as hypertension, can be serious. One study reported a slight improvement in weight loss when people combined PPA with a low-calorie diet; however, the drug did not reduce appetite, so it is unclear what effect it had on weight loss.

Stimulants can cause problems when taken in combination. For example, some over-the-counter drugs, such as Excedrin and the decongestant pseudoephedrine contain caffeine, and should not be taken with herbs that have a stimulant effect, such as yohimbe, guarana, yerba mate, and Asian ginseng. The combined effects of the drug ephedrine (found in the herb ma huang) and caffeine might help weight-loss efforts, according to a study conducted at Harvard Medical School in Boston. However, ephedrine causes heart and blood pressure abnormalities that could be fatal. The possible, but minimal, effects on weight loss obviously are not worth the risk! Taking a double dose of stimulants can aggravate anxiety, insomnia, high blood pressure, and rapid heartbeat. Herbal stimulants also interfere with medications that lower blood pressure or help regulate heartbeat.

## A Final Word

Throughout this chapter I've recommended that you discuss nutrition with your physician when medications are prescribed. Keep in mind, however, that most physicians haven't a clue when it comes to drug-diet interactions; even fewer discuss these issues with their patients. According to a study conducted at Cornell University, most doctors report they have little or no formal training in drug-nutrient interactions in medical school or residency, even though up to 89 percent of doctors believe it is their responsibility to inform patients about potential adverse interactions.

That means it's up to you to stay informed. In short, you can't take any medication, even something as simple as aspirin, without realizing it is affecting your overall nutritional status. Be your own health advocate; investigate how a pill will affect your health before you put it in your mouth by asking questions of your physician and pharmacist.

· PART III ·

# *Health Issues*

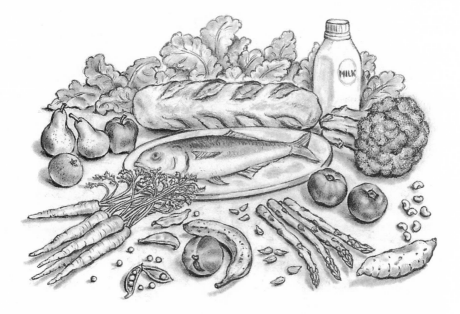

# CHAPTER 14

# What Causes Disease?

Why do we get sick? How can a body so brilliantly made that it can grow from a tiny cell into a multiorgan, thinking, feeling, and imagining miracle of life, succumb to disease caused by something as tiny as a virus? Why do some people battle one cold or one illness after another, while others seem to glide through life untouched by disease?

Perhaps the key word here is "disease," or dis-ease. Your body has an amazing ability to handle daily onslaughts of bacteria, viruses, environmental chemicals, and more. A symphony of systems rallies to defend tissues against damage, infection, and abnormal cell growth. These systems only work at their best when supplied with the necessary building blocks, many of which are nutrients and substances obtained from the diet. When your body is not supplied with these necessary substances, it is unable to work at its peak. Put another way, the body is in dis-ease much like a multigeared engine supplied with inadequate or dirty fuel. The key to health is to supply the body with a constant source of all the building blocks it needs to do its job of keeping you healthy, youthful, and vital.

## Free Radicals, Antioxidants, and Other Liberators

Free radicals. These cellular "rebels" wage war on health and could be the fundamental cause of numerous diseases from cancer to heart disease, reduced resistance to colds and infection, and compromised athletic ability.

### What Are Free Radicals?

Free radicals are highly reactive oxygen fragments. They are found in air pollution, cigarette smoke, fried foods, and are generated by radiation and chemicals, such as pesticides. Even if you lived in a pristine world, your body would make free radicals (also called oxidants) during normal metabolic processes. To stabilize themselves, free radicals seek out and grab on to fats, proteins, and the genetic material in your body's cells. Unfortunately, this initial attack, while stabilizing the first free radical, damages the cell and generates a new free radical—producing a destructive chain reaction.

The fatty membranes that surround every cell in your body are the prime targets for free radical attack. The shape and function of the polyunsaturated fats in membranes are changed by a free radical attack. The damaged membrane is unable to transport nutrients, oxygen, and water into the cell or regulate the removal of waste products out of the cell. Extensive free radical damage causes the membrane to rupture and release cellular components into surrounding tissues, which further damages tissues and generates additional free radicals. In effect, free radical attacks on cell membranes result in damage to the cell, destroy important cell enzymes, and often cause cell mutation and death.

Free radicals also attack the fats floating in the blood. For example, free radicals react with low-density lipoproteins (LDL), the carriers of blood cholesterol associated with an increased risk for atherosclerosis and heart disease. Free radical–damaged LDLs linger longer in the blood and raise LDL levels. In addition, "oxidized" LDLs are more damaging than normal LDLs, which further increase the risk for developing atherosclerosis and heart disease.

The powerhouses of the cell are surrounded by a cell membrane comprised of polyunsaturated fats that are vulnerable to free radical attack. These powerhouses, called mitochondria, are the site of the cell's energy production. Free radical damage to these centers shuts down energy production and protein synthesis. The cell dies and only a cell remnant, or clinker, remains in the body. The age of tissues is determined by the number of clinkers present, thus linking free radical damage to premature aging.

Free radicals attack and alter cellular enzymes, the catalysts that speed all metabolic processes. The damaged enzyme is inactivated, which slows or halts all processes dependent on that enzyme. Other protein compounds in the body, in addition to enzymes, also are altered by free radical attack. In addition, free radicals activate dormant enzymes that, in turn, cause tissue damage and disease, such

---

**TABLE 14.1    Free Radicals and Disease**

Free radical damage to the body is implicated in the initiation and progression of numerous diseases, including:

- Destruction of the cells that line the blood vessels, which increases the risk for developing atherosclerosis, hypertension, and cardiovascular disease.
- Suppressed immune function, increasing a person's risk for colds, infections, and disease.
- The inflammatory response observed in rheumatoid arthritis.
- Lung injury, irreversible respiratory damage, and asthma.
- The initiation and progression of cancer.
- Eye damage, associated with cataracts and macular degeneration.
- Premature aging.
- Duodenal ulcers and other digestive tract disorders.
- Liver damage.
- Multiple sclerosis.

---

as emphysema. Free radicals also release neurotoxins that affect nerve and brain function.

The cell's genetic code or DNA is susceptible to free radical damage, causing "breaks" or "tears" in the DNA. DNA regulates cell reproduction and the growth and repair of all body processes. These breaks have important implications in the development of disease because they must be repaired or the cell cannot function properly. At best, the cell dies when the genetic code is so altered that its messages can no longer be read by the cell. Excessive cell death is associated with premature aging. At worst, the cell mutates and begins a line of renegade cells that could be cancerous or at least disease-promoting. The enzymes that repair damaged DNA are not accurate and there is a high probability that the wrong DNA unit will be incorporated into the repaired DNA strand. This alters the cell's blueprint and increases the risk for abnormal cell growth and cancer.

## The Antioxidants: Armed Forces against Free Radicals

Fortunately, the body has a complex defense system against free radicals. If it were not for this system, the chain reactions generated from free radical attacks might quickly cripple and destroy the body. This defense system is called the body's antioxidant system and includes enzymes, such as superoxide dismutase (SOD) and xanthine oxidase; scavengers; vitamins, such as beta carotene, vitamin C, and vitamin E; and minerals, such as selenium, manganese, and zinc. In addition, thousands of phytochemicals in fruits, vegetables, whole grains, green tea, and legumes have antioxidant capabilities.

Vitamin E is the first line of defense, destroying free radicals when they first attack cell membranes. Optimal vitamin E intake protects against ozone-generated free radicals in smog and protects the fatty portions of all tissues from most forms of free radical damage. Inadequate vitamin E intake increases the risk for disease because it leaves cells vulnerable to unchecked free radical damage.

Vitamin C is the primary antioxidant in the body's watery compartments. Vitamin C reduces the risk of developing numerous free radical–associated diseases from cataracts to cancer. The carotenoids, including beta carotene, also are potent antioxidants. The carotenoids are especially effective in preventing free radicals from forming and strengthen the immune system, which might explain the effectiveness of these nutrients in helping prevent cancer.

The antioxidants function as teams to deactivate free radicals. Vitamin E and the enzyme superoxide dismutase intercede at the first stage when free radicals attack polyunsaturated fats and convert them to more free radicals. Any free radicals that escape this attack are recognized by the combined efforts of selenium and the enzyme glutathione peroxidase and are converted back into polyunsaturated fats before they can attack other fat molecules. Some antioxidants, such as vitamin C or glutathione, protect other antioxidants, such as vitamin E, from premature destruction and, therefore, strengthen and self-preserve the antioxidant system.

Thousands of studies show that elevated intakes or blood levels of antioxidants reduce the risk of free radical damage to tissues and lower a person's risk for numerous diseases. For example, optimal dietary intake or supplementation with selenium, vitamin C, and vitamin E improves the antioxidant capabilities of patients with multiple sclerosis. People who consume diets filled with antioxidant-rich fruits and vegetables are at lowest risk for all age-related diseases and live long, healthy lives. In contrast, low levels of antioxidants are found in diseased organs and tissues and increase a person's risk for developing disease, including cancer, cardiovascular disease, duodenal ulcer, lung disease, and hyperthyroidism. The role of antioxidants in the prevention and treatment of specific diseases will be discussed in detail in the chapters that follow.

# *Your Immune System*

If you seldom get a cold, have never had a serious illness, and bounce back quickly even when you are sick, chances are your body has built up a strong defense system against invading bacteria, viruses, and other hostile microorganisms. You also probably eat a healthy diet. In contrast, marginal nutrient deficiencies compromise the body's fundamental ability to defend itself against infection and disease, which has profound and far-reaching effects on health and the quality of life.

The body is under constant attack. Air, water, food, other people, and any aspect of the environment expose a person to bacteria, viruses, and other microorganisms that either aid in the maintenance of health or are potentially harmful. However, the body is not as much a victim as an accomplice to disease and infection.

The immune system, a complex system that includes numerous specialized chemicals, cells, tissues, and organs, is the body's fundamental defense against both invasion by foreign substances that cause infection and internal generation of abnormal cell growth, such as cancer. A well-functioning immune system successfully combats the repeated onslaught of disease-causing microorganisms; a poorly functioning immune system cannot fight off infection and can unleash a variety of diseases from allergies and arthritis to cancer and the common cold.

## The Immune System: A Brief Overview

The immune system is composed of millions of cells that pass information back and forth. This complex defense system provides constant feedback on the "state of the union." The result is a sensitive and intricate system of checks and balances that, in the presence of optimal nutrient intake and moderate to low stress, guarantees an immune response that is efficient, quick, and specific.

Your skin and the mucous linings in the nose and lungs are the body's first lines of defense against routine invasions from bacteria, viruses, and other microorganisms. Within the body, the immune system includes several specific organs strategically located throughout the body and generally referred to as "lymphoid organs." Lymphoid organs include the bone marrow, the thymus, the lymph nodes, the spleen, the tonsils, the appendix, and clusters of lymphoid tissue in the small intestine called Peyer's patches.

The immune system stockpiles an enormous arsenal of weapons and signals for fighting foreign invasion by bacteria, viruses, and more. Specialized white blood cells, called B-cells, are the hub of the immune system outside the body's cells. They circulate in the blood and other body fluids where they neutralize the toxins produced by bacteria. B-cells secrete chemicals called antibodies. In contrast, T-cells are the hub of immune function within the cells. Among other things, T-cells produce chemicals called lymphokines, such as interferon (a protein that defends cells from viruses). Other specialized cells in the immune system include natural killer cells, macrophages, monocytes, and other white blood cells.

## Nutrition and Immunity

Your diet is the single most important determinant of immune function. Nutrition affects almost every aspect of the body's resistance to disease. Even mild deficiencies of zinc, selenium, iron, copper, vitamin A, vitamin C, vitamin E, vitamin $B_6$, or folic acid can have important consequences on your body's ability to defend itself against disease. Deficiencies of these nutrients are found in a large segment of the population, including at least one-third of seniors. Immunological status is one of the most sensitive markers of nutritional adequacy; consequently, certain immune indices should be used to monitor nutritional status, according to Dr. Ranjit Kumar Chandra, a well-known authority on nutritional immunology at Memorial University of Newfoundland and the World Health Organization Centre for Nutritional Immunology in Canada.

Even marginal deficiencies of a vitamin or mineral can affect your body's ability to defend itself against disease. For example, a person's resistance to disease declines with age. At the same time, nutrient deficiencies often develop that coincide with depressed immune function. When seniors eat better, their immune systems often are restored. Marginal nutrient deficiencies can depress immune function long before clinical signs of deficiency have developed.

*The Antioxidants:* Almost every vitamin and mineral plays a role in the immune system. However, some nutrients appear to have a more important role than others. The antioxidant nutrients, such as vitamin E, vitamin C, and the carotenoids, are especially important in maintaining optimal immune function. For example, the initiation of the immune response probably occurs at the cell membrane. Vitamin E, the primary fat-soluble antioxidant, is an essential component of all membranes found in cells including the outer cell membrane and the membranes that surround the cell's nucleus (which houses the genetic material) and the cell's powerhouse centers called mitochondria. Vitamin E and other antioxidants prevent free radical damage to, and help maintain, the normal structure and function of immune cells and tissues.

Beta carotene in carrots and other dark green or orange produce is a powerful immune-enhancing nutrient that affects both the activity of immune cells and acts directly on abnormal cell growth (tumors) to inhibit their growth. Optimal intake of beta carotene increases the production and activity of both B- and T-cells, macrophages, and natural killer cells, and slows or halts the growth of tumors.

Even a marginal intake of vitamin C can have far-reaching effects on your resistance to infection and disease. Vitamin C strengthens the immune system by increasing the production and activity of lymphocytes and other white blood cells. This antioxidant vitamin also

- increases the ability of white blood cells to destroy disease-causing microorganisms,
- stimulates the speed and aggressiveness of white blood cells,
- deactivates harmful substances produced when immune cells attack bacteria, and
- increases the production of interferon.

In contrast, white blood cell formation and wound healing are suppressed when vitamin C intake is poor.

Selenium is another antioxidant that strengthens the immune system. Optimal selenium intake increases antibody production, accelerates the production and effectiveness of white blood cells to attack and destroy harmful microorganisms, and strengthens the body's surveillance against abnormal cell growth and cancer.

*Other Vitamins and Minerals:* Other vitamins and minerals, in addition to the antioxidants, also strengthen the body's resistance to infection and disease. These nutrients include the B vitamins, vitamins $B_1$, $B_2$, $B_6$, $B_{12}$, niacin, folic acid, biotin, pantothenic acid; vitamin D; and the minerals copper, iron, magnesium, and zinc.

For example, marginal dietary intake of vitamin $B_6$ reduces resistance to infection and disease, while increasing vitamin $B_6$ intake strengthens the immune response. People diagnosed with impaired immunity have low blood levels of zinc. When these people increase zinc intake, their immune response improves.

*Other Dietary Factors:* An increasingly large number of dietary factors, other than vitamins, minerals, and protein, alter immunity. For example, garlic contains compounds, including allicin, the substance responsible for garlic's smell, that kill or inhibit the growth of bacteria, fungi, and yeast. Garlic extracts also enhance immune function and strengthen the body's defense against cancer. Citrus fruits contain flavonoids, yogurt contains *Lacto-bacillus acidophilus,* and the herb echinacea contains compounds that also boost immunity.

A low-fat diet stimulates the immune system, while high-fat diets increase a person's susceptibility to infection and disease. The type of fat also influences immune function. For example, the polyunsaturated fats in vegetable oils (linoleic acid) might suppress immunity when consumed in large amounts. Other aspects of a healthful lifestyle, such as maintaining desirable weight, moderate exercise, and effective stress management, also improve your resistance to infection and disease.

*More Is Not Better:* While moderate doses of most nutrients stimulate the body's defense system, larger doses might impair the immune response. For example, two grams of vitamin C taken daily impaired the immune system's ability to kill bacteria in one study. Immune function returned to normal within four weeks of discontinuing the megadose therapy. Zinc, in doses greater than 50 mg, also might interfere with immune function.

Mineral interactions enhance or suppress immune function, depending on how much of what is supplied. Magnesium functions in the development, distribution, and function of immune cells. Because it is involved in more than 300 enzymatic reactions, magnesium influences the metabolism and activity of other minerals, especially calcium, potassium, sodium, and phosphorus. For example, normal functioning of leukocytes in the immune system requires a balanced supply of magnesium, calcium, and manganese. High intakes of any one of these minerals in the absence of the other two could result in secondary deficiencies that would suppress a critical step in the immune process.

*How Much Is Enough?* The optimal range of nutrient intakes to maximize the body's defense system is unknown. In most cases, consuming recommended levels of a nutrient is sufficient to strengthen immunity. However, in some cases, as with vitamin E, immune function progressively improves with increasing amounts of a nutrient, even to amounts far in excess of recommended levels. Until more is known about vitamin and mineral tolerances and the effects of these nutrients on immunity, it is best to stay within the safe zone and limit dietary intake of most nutrients to within 300 percent of the Daily Values as listed on supplement labels.

At this time, there are no inexpensive, accurate, or accessible tests that determine a person's unique nutritional status. Hair analysis is just one of several tests touted as a way to assess your nutritional status. None of these have proven accurate. Traditionally, poor nutrition was assessed by overt clinical symptoms, such as a low value on a hematocrit test (indicator of advanced iron deficiency). These measures are crude and incomplete. More importantly, immunity can be strikingly affected by even marginal nutrient status long before clinical deficiency symptoms are detected. Since even marginal nutrient deficiencies uniformly depress specific aspects of the immune system, it is likely that immune function tests some day will serve as indicators of nutritional status and disease susceptibility.

## *Eat Your Medicine*

The antioxidant and immune systems are just two of several systems that, if maintained, protect your body against disease and even aging. Other systems include the cell communication system that allows cells to recognize abnormal cell growth, and the cell suicide system that encourages destruction of abnormal cell growth.

More is unknown than is known about how food affects your risk for disease. However, the good news is that research repeatedly and consistently shows that what you eat has a strong and far-reaching effect on your health today and your risks for disease and premature aging in the future. Eat in tune with your body's rhythm and needs and it runs in balance and harmony. Fuel your day on highly processed junk food and you will pay the price at some point in reduced health and premature aging.

An optimal diet such as the Healthy Woman's Diet, not just an adequate one, provides all the building blocks your body needs to stay healthy and counteracts many of the processes once thought to be the inevitable consequence of disease and aging. Even a minor nuisance, such as the common cold or flu, might be prevented or at least the severity reduced with proper diet. Nutrition has grown far beyond the balanced diet. Eating really well and supplementing responsibly can maximize your body's health potential.

# CHAPTER 15

# *Women's Main Health Concerns*

A ny health issue that you personally face is the most important condition for you, whether it is a serious life-threatening problem such as heart disease or an aggravating, but painful, wart. However, the following four conditions are most women's greatest health threats: anemia, cancer, heart disease, and osteoporosis.

## *Anemia*

At least one in every ten women is at risk for anemia, while some reports place the numbers closer to eight in every ten premenopausal women. More than one in every five women are anemic after pregnancy, according to a study from the University of North Carolina School of Public Health.

Most people think of iron-poor blood when you mention anemia. Iron is a major player in this condition, especially for women, but it doesn't work alone. Other nutrients, such as folic acid, copper, zinc, and vitamins C, $B_{12}$, and E, also contribute to healthy circulation.

### What Is Anemia?

Anemia occurs when there is something wrong with your red blood cells, and they don't carry adequate oxygen to the tissues. The blood cells might be too small, too few, or contain too little hemoglobin, oxygen-carrying proteins within each red blood cell. Without a hefty supply of oxygen, every cell, tissue, and organ in your body essentially suffocates.

All symptoms of anemia are related to the reduced oxygen-carrying capacity of the blood. You might feel tired, have trouble concentrating, be forgetful and more susceptible to colds and infections. Your work performance is compromised or you are out of breath after walking up a flight of stairs. Athletes battling anemia can't improve in their exercise performance. Many of these symptoms are subtle, but become more pronounced during times of stress, such as when you take an airplane trip, become pregnant, vacation at high altitudes, or compete in a 10K race. Only then do you experience unusual shortness of breath, weakness, or other symptoms of anemia.

## Your Diet and Anemia

Anemia can result from numerous conditions, including blood loss, infection and inflammation, and kidney disease. By far the most common causes are nutritional, and include low intake or absorption of iron, protein, B vitamins (i.e., vitamin $B_{12}$, folic acid, vitamin $B_6$), vitamin C, vitamin E, copper, and/or zinc.

*Iron:* Iron deficiency is the most common cause of anemia. In fact, iron-deficiency anemia is the number one deficiency in women. Women who eat low-calorie or fad diets, who exercise, have had a baby in the past two years, who drink coffee or tea, or who are vegetarian are at highest risk, but everyone who menstruates and many women past menopause are at risk.

Within each red blood cell are protein molecules called hemoglobin. Embedded in each hemoglobin are four iron particles. This iron binds to oxygen in the lungs, carrying it in the blood, and releasing it to the tissues. Iron also is the active component of a hemoglobin-like molecule within the muscle cells called myoglobin. Here iron is responsible for storing and transporting oxygen within the cells of the heart and working muscles. Low iron levels reduce production of red blood cells and myoglobin. Red blood cells that do form are small with less hemoglobin and a limited ability to carry oxygen.

*The Best Tests for Iron:* Anemia is the final stage of iron deficiency. For weeks, months, years, even decades, a woman can be low in iron without being anemic. The symptoms of low iron and anemia are the same but proceed unnoticed in the preanemic stage, since iron deficiency doesn't show up on routine blood tests, such as the hemoglobin and hematocrit tests. These tests check only for anemia. Up to

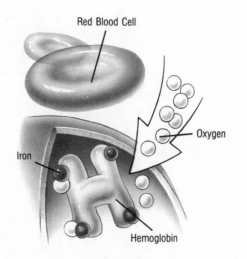

**FIGURE 15.1  The Red Blood Cell**

80 percent of women put up with feeling "under the weather" or "not up to par." They are told their tiredness is "all in their heads" or that they are "doing too much." They grab a cup of coffee to stay awake, when they should be eating more iron-rich foods.

The serum ferritin and total iron binding capacity (TIBC) tests are the best and most sensitive tests, detecting iron deficiency before it progresses to anemia. For example, a value less than 20 mcg/L on a serum ferritin test or a TIBC above 360 mcg/dl are red flags you are iron deficient. Also ask your physician about a new test called the serum transferrin receptor (sTfR) concentration. Tested in a group of marginally iron-deficient women at Cornell University, this test quickly reflected changes in iron status. Iron levels vary from day to day, so the average values from multiple tests provide the most reliable information on iron status. (See chapter 16 for more information on marginal iron deficiency and the common cold, emotions and moods, fatigue, headaches, skin, and stress.)

*Why Women?* Women are more susceptible than men to iron deficiency because we menstruate. Every month we lose blood, which means we lose iron. Unless we replenish that loss, deficiency is inevitable. Women also eat less food than men. The average diet supplies about 6 mg of iron for every 1,000 calories. A menstruating woman must consume at least 2,500 to 3,000 calories a day to meet her iron needs of 15 mg to 18 mg. Most women don't eat anywhere near this

---

**BOX 15.1    Iron Might Be All You Need to Feel Good Again**

---

Many women during their childbearing years unnecessarily put up with feeling under the weather. According to a study from the University of Newcastle in New South Wales, Australia, increased intake of iron might be all these women need to feel good again. Women diagnosed with iron deficiency and women with adequate iron status were compared for mental health, fatigue, and vitality. The iron-deficient women scored significantly lower on mental health and vitality and much higher on fatigue compared to optimally nourished women. After twelve weeks on either iron supplements or iron-rich diets, these women showed marked improvement in iron status (as measured by serum ferritin levels), mental health, vitality, and energy levels.

---

much. If you menstruate heavily or use the IUD as a birth control device, your daily iron needs could be two to four times higher than the regular recommendation. In contrast, women on the birth control pill need closer to 15 mg, since this form of birth control often reduces menstrual flow.

*Iron Is Poorly Absorbed:* The iron in meats (called "heme" iron) is best absorbed; about 20 to 34 percent actually enters the bloodstream. Iron in plants, such as grains, vegetables, and cooked dried beans and peas, is called nonheme or inorganic iron. Only 2 to 5 percent of this type of iron is absorbed. The average iron absorption from a mixed diet containing heme and nonheme iron is estimated at only 10 percent of total intake. You can boost iron absorption from plant sources if you:

- Combine a vitamin C–rich food such as orange juice with an iron-rich food like legumes or whole grains.
- Mix a small amount of heme iron (lean red meat) with a large amount of nonheme iron (cooked dried beans and peas), such as chili with meat and beans.
- Don't drink milk with your iron-rich meals, since calcium reduces iron absorption.
- Limit coffee, tea (black, decaffeinated, and green), and cocoa to between meals, since compounds called tannins in these beverages, as well as in some herbs such as peppermint and chamomile, reduce iron absorption by as much as 75 percent.

*Vitamin B$_{12}$:* Insufficient intake or poor absorption of vitamin B$_{12}$ results in a form of anemia called macrocytic (large cell) or megaloblastic anemia. As compared to the small, pale red blood cells in iron-deficiency anemia, the cells in this form of anemia are large, fragile, misshaped, and few in number. The symptoms are the same and include lethargy, weakness, and poor concentration. A high intake of folic acid masks vitamin B$_{12}$ anemia. However, this problem is avoided if women take supplements that contain both folic acid and vitamin B$_{12}$.

Vitamin B$_{12}$ is found only in meats, milk products, and fermented foods such as miso. The amount required to maintain health is very small, only 2 mcg to 5 mcg a day, so even small amounts of lean meat or fish (i.e., 3 ounces of tuna or 2 cups of milk/yogurt) usually meet a woman's daily need. Strict vegetarians who avoid all animal products could develop a vitamin B$_{12}$ deficiency unless fortified soy milk, fortified ready-to-eat cereals, and fermented soy foods are included in the daily diet, or a supplement that contains vitamin B$_{12}$ is taken daily. Low blood levels of vitamin B$_{12}$, however, also are found in nonvegetarians and older women.

As a woman ages, poor absorption, not dietary intake, often causes B$_{12}$ deficiencies. In this case, the condition is called pernicious anemia. Vitamin B$_{12}$ requires a substance in digestive juices called intrinsic factor as well as adequate stomach acid for absorption. People produce less of these necessary digestive aids as they age and so become at increasingly higher risk for deficiency. Overt vitamin B$_{12}$ deficiency affects 10 to 15 percent of seniors. Many of these people show no classic symptoms of B$_{12}$ deficiency, such as anemia, so the deficiency progresses undetected, according to researchers at U.S.D.A. Human Nutrition Research Center on Aging at Tufts University. The vitamin is better absorbed from supplements than from food, so women after menopause should consider taking a daily supplement that contains 5 mcg or more of vitamin B$_{12}$. Nasal spray administration of vitamin B$_{12}$ is a quick, effective way to maximize absorption and might be a convenient alternative to monthly injections or large supplemental doses for seniors.

*Folic Acid:* Folic acid is essential for the normal development and maintenance of red blood cells, so a deficiency produces macrocytic anemia similar to that noted in vitamin B$_{12}$ deficiency. The most common causes of folic acid–induced anemia are poor dietary habits; reduced absorption; prolonged use of folic acid–competing medications such as anticonvulsants, aspirin, and birth control pills; and/or increased requirements during growth periods such as pregnancy. (See chapter 13 for more information on how medications affect folic acid status and chapter 10 for information on folic acid and pregnancy.)

Women typically don't consume enough folic acid–rich foods. Since the

1970s, national surveys repeatedly report that most women are more likely to snack on chips than green leafy vegetables, legumes, and other folic acid–rich foods, consuming only half the recommended daily amounts for this B vitamin. Poor handling or overcooking of foods further reduces the amount of folic acid in the diet. Processing removes as much as 68 percent of the folic acid in foods. Refined grains, such as white bread, are now fortified with this B vitamin, which helps, but is not a replacement for including at least two folic acid–rich greens in the daily diet. Folic acid also is better absorbed from supplements than from food, so all women should consider taking daily a multiple that contains 400 mcg of folic acid.

*Vitamin E:* Several hereditary diseases, including sickle cell anemia, are characterized by destruction of red blood cells, a condition called hemolytic anemia. Vitamin E protects cell membranes from destructive oxygen fragments, called free radicals, that contribute to this form of anemia. Vitamin E supplements often effectively treat hemolytic anemia.

Interestingly, high iron intake for the treatment of iron-deficiency anemia and/or substituting vegetable oils for saturated fats increases free radical damage and creates increased demands for vitamin E. Both iron and vegetable oils in large quantities generate free radicals; therefore, a diet or supplemental program that is high in either vegetable oils and fried foods or iron increases the daily requirement for vitamin E.

*Vitamin B$_6$:* Iron levels in the blood are normal, but hemoglobin and red blood cells are not formed properly in the absence of optimal vitamin B$_6$ intake. The anemia that develops resembles iron-deficiency anemia. Treatment requires a physician's supervision and usually includes therapeutic doses of 50 mg to 200 mg of vitamin B$_6$ daily, with symptoms subsiding within a few weeks.

*Vitamin C:* This vitamin is necessary for proper absorption and function of iron. One of the symptoms of vitamin C deficiency is anemia related to the vitamin's role in iron metabolism.

*Copper:* Anemia was the first identified symptom of copper deficiency. Copper stimulates hemoglobin synthesis, while poor copper intake results in impaired red blood cell formation even in the presence of adequate iron intake. Copper also releases iron from storage and increases intestinal absorption of iron when the two minerals are consumed in moderate amounts.

*Protein:* Protein is essential for the normal formation of hemoglobin and red blood cells. Protein deficiency is rare in the United States; in fact, people are much more likely to consume too much protein. A deficiency does occur in elderly women who do not eat properly (i.e., the "tea-and-toast" syndrome) or who suffer from long-standing illnesses that interfere with optimal dietary intake.

### Anemia: Diet Advice

During the childbearing years, a woman who battles fatigue or any symptom of iron deficiency should request a serum ferritin test from her physician. Ask for the value, since less than 20 mcg/L is a sign of deficiency; often women are told, "you're fine," when their values are lower than this. If the test confirms that you are deficient, your physician will prescribe iron supplements.

*The Best Iron Supplements:* The best absorbed forms of iron supplements are ferrous succinate and ferrous sulfate. Other iron compounds that are absorbed well include ferrous lactate, fumarate, glycine sulfate, glutamate, and gluconate. Iron is best absorbed on an empty stomach; however, large supplemental doses of iron can cause digestive tract upset, diarrhea, or constipation in some women. These symptoms might subside by starting with a small dose and increasing the dose over several days or weeks, or by taking the supplement in divided doses throughout the day.

Although time-release supplements reduce stomach upset, they might not be absorbed as well as traditional forms of iron. The optimal dose will depend on the severity of the anemia and other compounding factors, and always should be determined after proper diagnostic tests and consultation with a physician. Iron supplementation usually produces improvements within one to three weeks, but should be continued for six to twelve months to ensure that tissue iron levels are restored. A study from the University of California, Berkeley, confirmed that women do best taking moderate-dose iron supplements long-term to correct iron deficiency.

*Iron-Rich Foods:* In addition to iron supplements, the nutrient content of the diet should be carefully reviewed. Several servings daily of iron-rich foods should be included in the Healthy Woman's Diet, preferably combining extra-lean meats and vitamin C–rich foods with iron-rich plants. Women consuming less than 2,500 calories daily, especially women using the IUD or who menstruate heavily, are likely candidates for iron depletion and deficiency and should be particularly aggressive in their iron intakes.

One of the best sources of dietary iron is to cook in cast-iron skillets. Replacing coated or glass cookware with cast iron increases the iron content of a meal by

**TABLE 15.1    Iron-Rich Foods**

| FOOD | AMOUNT | TOTAL IRON (MG) | HEME IRON (MG) | NONHEME IRON (MG) |
|------|--------|------------------|----------------|-------------------|
| Meatless spaghetti sauce (cooked in cast-iron skillet) | 6 ounces | 11.5 | - | 11.5 |
| Applesauce (homemade in cast-iron skillet) | ½ cup | 9.8 | - | 9.8 |
| Beef, lean | 3 ounces | 2.7 | 1.1 | 1.6 |
| Apricots, dried | ½ cup | 3.6 | - | 3.6 |
| Molasses, blackstrap | 1 tbsp. | 3.2 | - | 3.2 |
| Beans, cooked | ½ cup | 2.6 | - | 2.6 |
| Raisins | ½ cup | 2.6 | - | 2.6 |
| Prune juice | ¼ cup | 2.6 | - | 2.6 |
| Chicken, meat only | 3.5 ounces | 1.5 | 0.8 | 0.7 |
| Meatless spaghetti sauce (cooked in non-iron skillet) | 6 ounces | 1.4 | - | 1.4 |
| Greens, mustard | ½ cup | 1.3 | - | 1.3 |
| Strawberries | ¾ cup | 1.1 | - | 1.1 |
| Bread, whole wheat | 1 slice | 0.8 | - | 0.8 |
| Broccoli | ⅔ cup | 0.9 | - | 0.9 |
| Peanut butter | 2 tbsp. | 0.6 | - | 0.6 |
| Applesauce | ½ cup | 0.4 | - | 0.4 |

as much as twenty-six-fold. Acidic foods, such as spaghetti sauce, chili with meat and beans, and beef-vegetable stew, are especially good at leaching the iron out of the pot into the food. In addition, the longer the food simmers, the higher its iron content. In contrast, the iron in fortified foods, such as ready-to-eat cereals and enriched bread, is poorly absorbed, but is better than no iron at all.

*Boost Vitamin B$_{12}$ and Folic Acid:* Pernicious anemia is treated by vitamin B$_{12}$ injections, which bypass the intestinal failure to absorb it. Macrocytic or megaloblastic anemia associated with poor dietary intake of either vitamin B$_{12}$ or folic acid is treated with improved diet and oral supplements. Symptoms may improve, such as increased alertness and improved appetite, before changes are noted in the blood.

Several servings of vitamin B$_{12}$ and folic acid–rich foods should be included daily in the Healthy Woman's Diet. Two to three servings daily of protein-rich foods from animal sources will supply ample amounts of vitamin B$_{12}$. Folic acid is found primarily in dark green leafy vegetables (foliage), orange juice, and wheat germ. This B vitamin is destroyed by heat, prolonged storage, and reheating of leftovers. For example, spinach stored in the refrigerator for three or four days, overcooked or reheated, or allowed to sit on a serving table for long periods of time (i.e., cafeteria style) contains little or no folic acid by the time it is eaten.

Fruits and vegetables should be chosen fresh or frozen, stored for limited amounts of time, eaten raw when possible or only slightly cooked, and prepared in a minimum amount of water. Finally, select minimally processed foods to ensure optimal dietary intake of vitamin E, trace minerals such as copper, and vitamin B$_{6}$.

*Precautions:* Concerns about iron overload (also called "hemochromatosis") in women appear to be unfounded. This condition is most likely to occur in men after age fifty. Researchers at Memorial Sloan Kettering Cancer Center in New York investigated the effects of meat consumption and supplement use on serum ferritin levels in middle-aged women and found no risk for iron overload in women. Iron supplements do not cause other health concerns, such as heart disease, especially when they supplement an excellent diet rich in antioxidants, such as vitamins E and C.

Large supplemental doses of iron for prolonged periods of time could result in secondary deficiencies of other trace minerals, such as zinc or copper. To help avoid this potential interaction, iron supplements should be taken alone and/or zinc and copper intake should be increased slightly, either by increased consumption of foods high in these nutrients or by low- to moderate-dose supplementation taken at opposite times from the iron supplement.

Anemia can result from more serious problems than just a nutrient deficiency. Ulcers, colon polyps, or anything that causes internal bleeding will result in a shortage of red blood cells. Always seek medical advice if you feel unusually tired.

# Cancer

Cancer is an umbrella term for a variety of diseases all characterized by the uncontrolled growth and spread of abnormal cells. Women fear cancer more than any other disease, yet some news about these dreaded diseases is good. For example,

- While one in every eight women will develop breast cancer in her life, up to 85 percent of those women will survive the cancer for at least five years.
- According to the American Cancer Society, only 5 to 10 percent of breast cancer cases are attributable to inherited factors, which means up to 95 percent of breast cancer might be prevented with changes in lifestyle.
- Many women's cancers can be cured if detected and treated promptly.

**GRAPH 15.1     Women's Cancer Rates in Perspective**

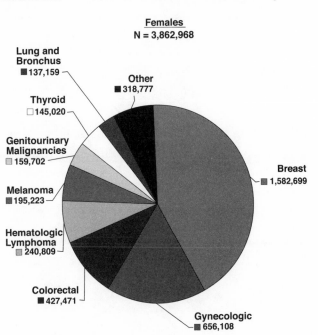

Estimated number of women in the United States diagnosed with cancer in the past twenty years, by site.

Source: National Cancer Institute.

## What Causes Cancer?

The causes of cancer are only partially understood. Both environmental factors (i.e., chemicals, radiation, and viruses) and internal factors (i.e., hormones, immune conditions, and inherited mutations) are suspected to contribute to cancer risk. After exposure to these factors, either acting alone or working together, it may take ten or more years before clinical signs of cancer develop.

Under normal conditions, cell growth is monitored so that cell death balances cell growth. The random cell that mutates is identified and destroyed by the immune and antioxidant systems or by signals from adjacent cells. Cancer cells ignore all these systems, setting up their own rules, growing and spreading uncontrollably.

The cancer process consists of two stages: the initiation stage and the promotion stage. Initially, a normal cell is exposed to a cancer-promoting substance called a mutagen or a carcinogen that converts it into an abnormal cell. During the promotion stage, the abnormal cell is encouraged to multiply and spread into surrounding tissues. Both stages must be present for a normal cell to develop into cancer. Other processes also are necessary for cancer development, such as a compromised immune system, since many normal cells convert to abnormal cells but are recognized and removed before they can cause harm.

## Breast Cancer

Breast cancer is the leading type of cancer and the second leading cause of cancer deaths in women (second to lung cancer). Despite those dismal statistics, up to 85 percent of women survive their disease.

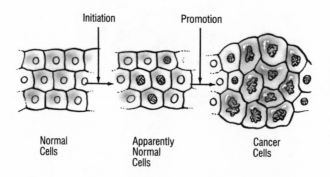

Normal Cells — Apparently Normal Cells — Cancer Cells

**FIGURE 15.2  The Two Stages of Cancer Growth Are Initiation and Promotion**

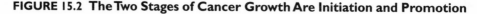

Many factors beyond a woman's control contribute to risk, including having a mother or sister with breast cancer, having a first child after age thirty, beginning menstruation at an early age, or having a special type of fibrocystic breast disease (FBD) called atypical hyperplasia. (See pages 322 to 325 for more information on FBD.) Early detection and prompt treatment have greatly reduced mortality rates for breast cancer in this country.

*Body Fat:* No one really knows what percentage of breast cancer cases are caused from diet, but most experts agree that excess calories lead to excess body fat and this contributes to breast cancer risk. Body fat generates its own estrogen, increasing levels of the hormone in the blood. An elevated blood estrogen level is a marker for breast cancer risk. Staying lean by exercising and eating a low-fat diet helps blunt this rise in estrogen. Gaining weight early in life, especially before and during puberty, is particularly harmful. So keep your daughters lean, but not too thin, by encouraging exercise and healthy eating habits.

Excess body fat increases both a woman's risk for developing breast cancer and for cancer to progress to more serious stages. It is where the fat is deposited that has the greatest impact on health. A woman who carries most of her extra fat above the waist in her abdomen and chest (an apple-shaped body) has up to a 34 percent greater risk for breast cancer than does a woman with hefty thighs and hips (a pear-shaped body). Losing weight lowers what is called the "waist-to-hip ratio" (WHR), that is the proportion of fat above the waist compared to the fat at hip and thigh level (an apple has a high WHR, while a pear has a low WHR). When it comes to health, the good news is "apples" derive the greatest benefits from weight loss, because they lose more weight from the upper body; even a 10 percent reduction in weight significantly decreases the "apple's" risk for developing breast cancer. According to the American Health Foundation, women's risk for breast cancer decreases considerably when they keep their weight below a BMI of 27.

*Dietary Fat:* High-fat diets favor fat accumulation in breast tissue and increase estrogen, which explains why they promote cancer formation. Fat also might suppress the body's immune system so the body fails to reject abnormal cells. Another set of hormonelike compounds, called prostaglandins, might stimulate the growth of cancer and are regulated by dietary fat intake.

The more fat and animal protein a woman consumes, the greater is her risk for breast cancer. Both total dietary fat (that includes fat from meats and most vegetable oils) and saturated fat from meats and dairy products increase breast cancer risk. For example, women living in Japan consume only 11 to 15 percent of calories from fat and have one-tenth the breast cancer risk of American women. When Japanese women migrate to the United States and adopt typical American diets containing 40 percent fat calories, their children's breast cancer death rates skyrocket, eventually equaling that of other Americans. In the United States, young women who consume low-fat, meatless diets have hormone levels associated with low risks for later breast cancer. Risk appears to increase as women age, with postmenopausal women who consume high-fat diets more likely than younger women to develop breast cancer. This correlates with breast cancer rates, since more than two-thirds of all cancers occur in women past age fifty.

The link between breast cancer and dietary fat is not clearly defined. But the weight of the evidence does suggest that:

- Saturated fat in red meat and fatty dairy products and polyunsaturated fats in vegetable oils such as safflower and corn oils, increase cancer risk, especially when fiber intake is low.
- Monounsaturated fats in olive oil and nuts and the omega-3 fats in fish protect against cancer.

Restricting total dietary fat to less than 25 percent of calories also lowers blood estrogen levels by about 13 percent. Currently, most American women consume more than 34 percent of calories from fat. Since the Healthy Woman's Diet is low-fat, helps you maintain a desirable weight, and lowers heart-disease risk, it is a safe habit to adopt and might lower breast cancer risk, too.

*Soy:* The humble soybean might lower a woman's risk for cancer. However, the link is not clear-cut and some researchers caution that soy is a double-edged sword.

Estrogen is the link between soy and cancer. Both epidemiological and clinical data show that exposure to estrogen increases breast cancer risk by encouraging the growth of malignant breast cells. Asian women living in Asia have a 40 percent lower blood estrogen level compared to Caucasian women living in the United States, and they consume more phytoestrogens in soy products. Some studies show that adding soy to the diet reduces blood estrogen levels in premenopausal women. Compounds in soy inhibit blood supply to cancer cells and curb the spread of breast cancer. Phytoestrogens also have a structure similar to estrogen, but their binding affinity is severalfold weaker than that of a woman's normal estrogen, so they should curb estrogen's effects on initiating cancer.

The confusion arises from the limited evidence that soy also might increase breast cancer risk because it adds more estrogen to a body already sensitive to the effects of this hormone. Whether soy increases or decreases breast cancer risk might be dose, tissue, and time dependent. Estrogen production varies dramatically throughout a woman's life span. It is possible that the phytoestrogens have varying effects on the breast in the presence of high estrogen (during pregnancy), moderate estrogen levels (during premenopause), and low estrogen (during childhood and postmenopause). One reason why women living in Asia have low breast cancer risk is that lifetime exposure to soy provides the protective effect. It is also possible that soy contains other factors other than the phytoestrogens that oppose the estrogenic effects of phytoestrogens and thereby reduce breast cancer risk. Or perhaps other environmental factors might be related more to low cancer rates in Asian women than increased soy consumption.

The bottom line? Moderate intake of minimally processed soy products, such as tofu and soy milk, are safe and possibly beneficial in the prevention of numerous diseases, including breast cancer. Until more is known, excessive intake of highly processed soy constituents, such as soy powders or phytoestrogen pills, especially in women with a family or personal history of breast cancer, should be viewed with a cautionary eye.

*Fiber and Vegetables:* Fiber is another natural way to lower estrogen levels and help prevent breast cancer. Within two months of consuming a high-fiber diet, blood estrogen levels fall. The combined effect of raising fiber and lowering fat intake is most effective in reducing breast cancer risk.

---

**TABLE 15.2    Where's the Soy?**

*Dry Soybeans:* Use as any dried bean in soups, chili, casseroles, salads, and stews. Isoflavones make up 0.1–0.3 grams/100 grams of soybeans.

*Soy Milk:* Pour on cereal, stir into hot drinks, drink cold, or use in any recipe that calls for milk. Comes in plain, vanilla, chocolate, and other flavors.

*Tofu or Bean Curd:* Silken tofu is best for blending into dips and milk shakes. Soft tofu is best in Oriental soups or in combination with light mayonnaise. Firm tofu is best for stir-frys.

*Tempeh:* A cultured soy cake made from whole, cooked soybeans. It can be used in soups, casseroles, and salads.

Other soy products include miso, soy flour, edamame (green soybeans), and soy grits.

---

Women who consume several servings daily of fresh fruits and vegetables have up to a tenfold lower risk for breast cancer compared to women who eat too few of these foods. One study found that the more vegetables, fruit, fiber, vitamins C and E, lycopene (a carotenoid found in tomatoes), folic acid, and phytosterols (typically consumed in legumes) women eat, the lower is their risk for developing breast cancer. It is unclear why fruits and vegetables are protective; however, the high fiber and vitamin content, as well as the phytochemicals such as lycopene, definitely contribute to reduced risk.

*Antioxidants:* As vitamin C intake increases, breast cancer risk decreases. In fact, some researchers speculate that as many as 25 percent of breast cancer cases are preventable by eating more fiber- and vitamin C–rich fruits and vegetables.

Both vitamin A and beta carotene (the building block for vitamin A found in fruits and vegetables) help protect against breast cancer; however, the two nutrients provide different means of protection and both should be consumed in the diet. Beta carotene also stimulates the immune system and might have a secondary effect in cancer prevention. Daily intake of beta carotene–rich foods is necessary since blood levels of beta carotene drop quickly when dietary intake is inadequate.

A deficiency of vitamin E increases the incidence of mammary (breast) tumors in animals. Tumor formation, tumor growth, and the number of tumors decrease when animals are given supplements of this fat-soluble vitamin. They also live longer. In studies on humans, women with low blood levels of vitamin E have a fivefold increase in risk for breast cancer compared to women with normal or high blood levels of the vitamin, while women with breast cancer show improvements when diets are supplemented with vitamin E.

Women with low blood selenium levels have two times the cancer risk of women with high selenium levels. The link between selenium intake and breast cancer is not conclusive and more research is needed. It could be that selenium works in conjunction with vitamin E and vitamin C for maximum effectiveness. Selenium is potentially toxic and total intake from diet and supplements should not exceed 200 mcg per day.

*Calcium and Vitamin D:* According to a review from Rockefeller University, poor intake of vitamin D and calcium, in the presence of a high-fat diet, might increase breast cancer risk. In contrast, increased intake of these two nutrients might inhibit the development of breast cancer, as will increased exposure to sunlight, which helps the body manufacture vitamin D. The researchers state that this fat-soluble vitamin helps protect breast cancer cells from turning cancerous,

---

### BOX 15.2    And Your Credentials Are?

---

If you're looking for sound health information, the local health-food store might not be your best bet. Researchers from the Cancer Research Center at the University of Hawaii posed as daughters of breast cancer patients and asked local health-food store personnel to recommend products for cancer care. The number one suggestion was for shark cartilage, with the cost for recommended dosages varying multifold from one store and brand to another.

Shark cartilage, made from ground-up shark skeletons, has been touted as an anticancer treatment. However, studies on this supplement found that it does not effectively treat cancer, and, in fact, in one study on patients with advanced cancers, more patients in the group supplementing with shark cartilage died and many had to stop taking the supplements because of nausea and vomiting. Shark cartilage had no effect on quality of life, weakness, fatigue, or other symptoms of cancer.

---

which might explain why women with tumors that responded to vitamin D have longer disease-free survival time than other breast cancer patients.

*Alcohol:* Women who consume more than one alcoholic beverage a day have an increased risk for cancer. "Alcohol may raise estrogen levels, which would help explain its underlying connection to breast cancer," says Walter Willett, M.D., Dr.P.H., professor at Harvard School of Public Health. Alcohol alters both hormone balance and the menstrual cycle similar to patterns characteristic of aggressive cancer progression.

Alcohol might be related to folic acid when it comes to breast cancer. In a study of more than 3,000 women with breast cancer, the risk from alcohol was strongest in women who consumed less than 300 mcg of folic acid a day. Those taking at least 460 mcg a day from supplements had the lowest risk. Alcohol also has been linked to an increased risk for esophageal and bladder cancers. However, moderate intake of red wine lowers heart-disease risk, so each woman must weigh the evidence and decide which risk is more important to her.

*Pesticides:* The evidence is not conclusive, but does suggest that pesticides might contribute to breast cancer risk. For example, human breast tissue is directly exposed to environmental chemicals that are known to cause mammary cancer in female rats, warn researchers at the University of Guelph in Ontario. It is probably wise to reduce your intake of these chemicals by washing and peeling produce or purchasing organic varieties when possible.

*Flax:* You might consider adding a little flax to your diet. Premenopausal women who supplement their diets with flaxseed improve their estrogen ratio in favor of a lower risk for developing breast cancer, according to researchers at the University of Minnesota.

## Colorectal Cancer

Although not exclusively a disease of women, colorectal cancer is the third most common form of cancer in women, after breast and lung cancers. This form of cancer is responsible for more than 11 percent of all deaths from cancer in women. A family history of colorectal cancer is a risk factor. However, diet plays a big role in the development and progression of this disease.

*Body Fat:* According to an accumulating body of evidence, people who consume too many calories and gain excess body fat develop insulin resistance with increased circulating levels of insulin and blood fats. These circulating levels trigger cell growth in the colon and expose these cells to free radicals, which in the long run cause cancer. These processes are inhibited by a variety of compounds, including antioxidants.

*Meat and Dietary Fat:* Your risk for developing colon or rectal cancer is directly proportional to how much fat you consume. Dietary fat enhances cholesterol and bile acid production by the liver and results in greater amounts of these substances in the colon. Bacteria in the colon convert these fatty substances into cancer-causing compounds. Bile acids and other fats in the intestine also damage the lining of the colon and increase abnormal cell growth. The following fatty foods also escalate colon cancer risk:

- Processed fats, called trans fatty acids (TFAs), in hydrogenated vegetable oils found in margarine, shortening, and snack foods.
- Charred meat cooked on a barbecue or broiler.
- The combination of a high-fat diet with low fiber and/or little exercise. According to the National Cancer Institute, couch potatoes who eat meat more than twice a day have the highest risk for developing colon cancer. In fact, a high-fat diet combined with a seden-

tary lifestyle might be responsible for as much as 40 percent of the colorectal cancer rate in women.

Researchers at the American Health Foundation in New York report that the dietary recommendations to lower cancer risk are similar to those for most chronic diseases and include lowering fat to no more than 25 percent of calories, increasing intake of monounsaturated fats in olive oil and omega-3 fats in fish, 20 to 30 grams of fiber daily, and up to ten servings daily of fruits and vegetables.

*Fiber:* A fiber-rich diet, comprised primarily of whole-grain breads and cereals, fresh fruits and vegetables, legumes, and other fiber foods, reduces a woman's risk for developing precancerous polyps and colorectal cancer. A high-fiber diet speeds the removal of cancer-causing substances, such as bile acid and cholesterol by-products, and reduces the risk for developing colorectal cancer.

*Whole Grains:* Whole grains exert their health-protecting effects in a variety of ways. They contain compounds, such as fiber and oligosaccharides, that alter the gut environment in favor of health. They are also rich in antioxidants, such as trace minerals and phenolic compounds, and hormone-modulating phytoestrogens. Whole grains bind cancer-causing substances in the gut. The less processed the whole grain, the greater its health benefits. Aim for at least 25 to 35 grams of fiber from a variety of sources every day.

*Fruits and Vegetables:* You've probably heard enough about how important it is to eat your fruits and vegetables! Just in case you're still not convinced, researchers at Harvard Medical School report that people who don't take that message seriously and eat too few servings of produce are at the highest risk for developing colorectal cancer.

*Calcium:* Drinking milk or taking a supplement that contains calcium and vitamin D reduces a woman's risk for developing colon cancer. Tumor incidence is 50 to 75 percent lower in women who consume high-calcium diets, possibly because calcium binds to cancer-causing fats in the colon and converts them into harmless substances that the body excretes. Vitamin D might aid in destroying cancer cells. In addition,

- Compounds in milk called sphingolipids might lower cholesterol and help prevent colon cancer.
- Yogurt contains healthful bacteria called probiotics that lower cancer-causing substances in the colon, further reducing the risk for colon

cancer. Probiotics crowd out or kill off disease-causing bacteria, produce natural antibiotics, and possibly switch off an enzyme that triggers colon cancer.

The optimal calcium intake is unknown; however, researchers at Rutgers University College of Pharmacy recommend intakes of 1,500 mg to 1,800 mg per day for maximum benefit. Vitamin D can be toxic, so limit daily intake to no more than 800 IU from all sources.

*Meat and Beans:* Dietary protein from animal sources increases colorectal cancer risk. In one study, protein increased risk two- to threefold. The risk is highest in women who eat approximately 5 ounces or more of red meat daily, while women who limit red meat to no more than 2 ounces per day have a much lower risk. The less the better. Women who eat red meat infrequently, such as once a week, still have a 40 percent higher risk of colon cancer than do women who eat meat less than once a month.

While meat increases, beans lower colon cancer risk. Phytosterols are compounds in legumes that resemble cholesterol, but have a protective, rather than a harmful, effect on the digestive tract. They possibly increase the excretion of cholesterol, inhibit the conversion of cholesterol to cancer-causing substances, and reduce cancer initiation and growth in the colon. Nondigestible oligosaccharides, carbohydrate-like compounds found in soybeans, are prebiotics that influence bacteria levels in the colon and might help lower colon cancer risk.

*Calories and Sugar:* People with colorectal cancer consume more calories and more sugar than do healthy people. A high-sugar diet alone doubles a person's risk for colon cancer. Highly refined carbohydrates might be fermented by bacteria in the colon and these by-products might contribute to the development or progression of cancer. In addition, women tend to eat too much when they eat refined grains and the excessive calories cause weight gain. As body fat increases above desirable levels, colorectal cancer risk also increases.

*Antioxidants:* The antioxidants protect against colon cancer. Whether it is antioxidant vitamins such as vitamins C and E or phytochemicals such as beta carotene, lycopene from tomatoes, and lutein from spinach, women who eat antioxidant-rich diets and supplement their diets with extra antioxidants show fewer precancerous conditions in the colon. The antioxidant vitamins are most effective when consumed with a low-fat, high-fiber diet. Green tea also contains antioxidants that lower colon cancer risk.

*Garlic:* Including garlic in your daily diet also might lower colon cancer risk. Sulfur-containing compounds in garlic block tumor growth, including colon cancer. Garlic fights cancer at both the initiation and promotion phases of cancer development, as well as in altering DNA repair and enhancing immune response, thus boosting the body's own defense systems against abnormal cell growth.

*Alcohol and Folic Acid:* Women are at lower risk for developing colon cancer when they include lots of folic acid–rich foods in their diets. In a study from New York University School of Medicine, colon cancer risk in people with high folic acid levels was half that of people with the lowest levels. Colon cancer risk also was twice as high in people with above average alcohol intakes and with folic acid levels below average. Other studies show the risk for developing colorectal neoplasia decreases up to 40 percent when women consume diets high in folic acid. However, blood levels of the vitamin are not indicative of cancer risk, since even a mild folic acid deficiency, with blood levels within the lower end of normal, can increase cancer risk.

## Cervical and Endometrial Cancers

*Cervical Cancer:* Cervical cancer rates are on the decline as a result of improved early diagnostic and treatment techniques, yet this cancer still is worrisome. In the United States, the American Cancer Society estimated that 13,000 new cases of invasive cervical cancer would be diagnosed and 4,100 women would die of this cancer in 2002. Invasive cervical cancer develops from early lesions of the cervix called cervical intraepithelial neoplasia (CIN). While millions of women are diagnosed with low-grade cervical abnormalities every year, cervical cancer is one of the most successfully treatable cancers with a five-year survival rate of 92 percent when the condition is caught in its early stages. Left undetected, the condition progresses to invasive cervical cancer by increasing grades of cervical dysplasia.

The most significant risk factor for CIN is infection with the sexually acquired virus called human papillomavirus (HPV). DNA from this virus is found in 90 percent of cervical tumors. However, HPV infection is not the sole cause of CIN or its progression to cervical dysplasia and cancer. In fact, only 28 percent of women infected with HPV develop CIN. Other modifying factors must contribute to the progression of lesions to cancer.

*Endometrial Cancer:* Endometrial cancer is cancer in the lining (endometrium) of the uterus. It is the fourth leading cancer in women, yet 83 percent of women survive the disease for at least five years. Endometrial cancer risk increases if a woman has a history of infertility, fails to ovulate, is obese, or has been on prolonged estrogen therapy. Accumulation of excess body fat in the upper body (giving the woman an apple-shaped figure) significantly increases a woman's risk for endometrial cancer.

*Fruits, Vegetables, and Milk:* Blood levels of the antioxidant nutrients, including beta carotene and vitamins C and E, are inversely related to cervical cancer risk. Women with cervical cancer have low levels of these nutrients in blood and cervical tissue compared to healthy women. Women with HVP and low vitamin A levels are at especially high risk. Women who smoke cigarettes (a risk factor for cervical cancer) also have lower blood levels of vitamin C and beta carotene, thus further increasing their risk for developing cervical cancer. The low blood levels reflect poor dietary intake, since women at risk for cervical cancer also typically consume fewer fruits and vegetables, such as carrots, spinach, broccoli, cantaloupe, and leaf lettuce, that are high in these nutrients. According to researchers at the University of Pennsylvania School of Medicine, women with high intakes of lycopene-rich foods have one-fourth the risk of developing cervical dysplasia compared to women with low lycopene intakes. Calcium intake is low in women with endometrial cancer, while frequent consumption of yogurt is associated with a reduced risk.

Low intake of several B vitamins, including vitamins $B_{12}$ and $B_6$ and folic acid, raises blood levels of a compound called homocysteine. While most attention has been paid to this compound's effect on increasing heart-disease risk, researchers at the University of Alabama report homocysteine also increases a woman's risk for developing cervical dysplasia, a precancerous condition. Homocysteine levels are significantly higher in women with dysplasia and appear to increase the risk for other factors associated with cervical dysplasia, such as increasing the risk for HPV and escalating the harmfulness of cigarette smoking.

Numerous studies have investigated the link between folic acid intake, cervical tissue levels of folic acid, and CIN. Folic acid is essential for the synthesis and replication of cellular DNA, while low tissue levels of this B vitamin result in fragile sites along the DNA, increased carcinogenic damage to DNA, and reduced DNA repair. Abnormal cervical tissue often is low in folic acid; however, folic acid supplementation does not always prevent CIN or cause it to regress. Folic acid deficiency probably is a cocarcinogen during the initiation of cervical cancer (combined with HPV, a folic acid deficiency increases CIN risk sevenfold), but supplements are less likely to alter the course of preexisting disease.

*Body Fat and Calories:* Body weight is associated with postmenopausal endometrial cancer and also might be associated with cancer in younger women. Women with high body fat percentages have increased levels of a type of estrogen that is very "biologically active" and is associated with elevated cancer risk. Women who gain weight later in life are at highest risk for developing endometrial cancer after age sixty, while cutting back on unnecessary calories reduces the risk for breast and uterine cancers.

## Ovarian Cancer

Ovarian cancer accounts for only 4 percent of all cancers among women, yet ranks second in gynecologic cancer, following cancer of the uterus (endometrial cancer). Its rates are decreasing each year. Risk increases with age, in women who

- have never had children.
- experience an early age of first pregnancy or menopause.
- have a family history of ovarian cancer or colon cancer.
- live in industrialized countries, other than Japan.
- are obese.
- have had breast cancer.

Pregnancy and the use of birth control pills lower ovarian cancer risk. Unfortunately, the disease typically remains silent until advanced stages, making treatment difficult and prognosis poor. When ovarian cancer is diagnosed and treated early, 95 percent of women live five years or longer; however, only about one-quarter of all cases are detected early.

*Dietary Fat:* Diet is loosely linked to ovarian cancer risk. Women who eat high-fat, high-meat, high-whole-milk diets have a slightly higher risk for the disease than do women who eat low-fat, fiber- and vegetable-rich diets. A high intake of eggs and fried foods also might increase risk.

*Fruits and Vegetables:* In nearly 90 percent of cases, cancer originates in the lining or epithelial tissue of the ovaries. Vitamin A helps maintain these tissues, including the lining of the ovaries. This might explain why women who eat lots of vitamin A–rich fruits and vegetables and maintain the highest blood levels of vitamin A and beta carotene are at lowest risk for developing ovarian cancer.

*Coffee and Caffeine:* Coffee and caffeine might increase ovarian cancer risk in some women. Granted the link is not confirmed, but a study from the Harvard

School of Public Health did find that women who consumed caffeine from coffee or other sources were at higher risk than women who did not consume caffeinated beverages.

## Cancer: Diet Advice

The most important dietary changes you can make to protect against cancer are:

- Maintain a desirable weight.
- Include eight to ten fruits and vegetables in your daily diet. Make sure two to three vegetables are orange or green to ensure optimal phytochemical and vitamin A intake and consume two or more vitamin C–rich foods, such as citrus fruits, to guarantee at least 200 mg of this vitamin daily.
- The cruciferous vegetables, including brussels sprouts, broccoli, cabbage, asparagus, and kohlrabi, contain additional anticancer substances, called indoles. Include three or more servings of these vegetables in the weekly menu.
- Cut back on fat to 25 percent or less of total calories, and saturated fat to less than 8 percent of calories. Less is better. Limit red meat to once a month (or avoid altogether) and replace with more servings of fish and legumes.
- Include more whole grains than refined grains in your daily diet. Ideally, eliminate refined grains from the menu.
- Cut back on coffee and caffeine if you drink too much.
- Limit exposure to pesticides.
- Add a few servings of soy to your weekly diet, such as fortified soy milk or tofu.
- Take a moderate-dose multiple vitamin and mineral with extra antioxidants.

Beyond diet, other lifestyle factors help reduce cancer risk. Relaxation and stress management, monthly breast self-exams, daily vigorous exercise, avoidance of tobacco smoke, moderate alcohol intake, and routine screening, such as a mammography and Pap smear, are essential in the prevention of cancer.

# *Heart Disease*

While most women fear cancer, it is heart disease that is the biggest health risk. One in two women will eventually die of heart disease or stroke, compared with one in twenty-seven who will eventually die of breast cancer. Yet, the news is good when it comes to heart disease. You have a lot to say about whether or not you battle heart disease or stroke. Eat well, exercise daily, and make a few simple changes in your lifestyle and there is every reason to believe your heart will stay strong and healthy throughout life.

## A Perception Problem

Why are women so misinformed about this number one health threat?

- Many women hold to a common misconception that heart disease is a man's problem. Yet more women than men die from heart disease.
- Women often think of heart disease as something that happens later in life. But heart disease is a "now" problem (the underlying cause of heart disease is atherosclerosis and it begins in adolescence). Later might be too late.
- A national Gallup survey funded by 8th Continent Soymilk found that fewer than half of all women surveyed reported that their health-care provider had ever talked with them about heart disease and its prevention.

Even more frightening is that most women report they are confident they would recognize the symptoms of heart disease, even though few have been told what to look for and many think symptoms are the same as for men, such as chest pain and shooting pains down the left arm. In fact, women's symptoms can be very different from men's. Sudden fatigue, dizziness, indigestion, abdominal pain, and rapid heartbeat are incorrectly thought to be flu, so women don't seek immediate treatment and are more likely to die from a heart attack as a result.

The symptoms of heart disease don't usually surface until a woman is past menopause. That is when cholesterol levels begin to rise and HDL cholesterol (the good cholesterol) plummets. The lower risk prior to menopause suggests that the female hormone estrogen provides protection against heart disease. Younger women with risk factors such as smoking, diabetes, hypertension, high cholesterol, or a family history of heart disease also are targets for premature heart disease.

You don't suddenly develop heart disease. The arteries begin to accumulate fatty plaque in your teens if you've been following a typical American diet. It's only when the disease advances to later stages that symptoms develop, if you're lucky. Sometimes the first symptom is a fatal heart attack.

## What Causes Heart Disease?

Heart disease begins in early childhood and progresses at varying rates throughout a woman's life. Clogged arteries, called atherosclerosis, are the underlying cause and blood cholesterol and triglyceride levels are the primary indicators of

**FIGURE 15.3  A Possible Theory for the Beginning of Atherosclerosis**

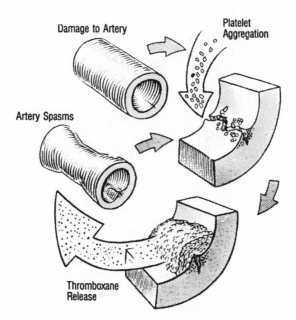

The damaged artery attracts blood cell fragments called platelets. These platelets release a substance called thromboxane that causes the artery to spasm, which causes more damage to the artery. A cycle develops that causes more and more damage to the artery, the accumulation of cholesterol, and the development of atherosclerosis.

risk. Elevated levels of a compound called homocysteine also signal heart disease, even if cholesterol is low.

In the blood, cholesterol is packaged in water-soluble "bubbles" called lipoproteins. The more total cholesterol packaged in low-density lipoproteins (LDL cholesterol or LDLs), the greater a woman's risk for developing atherosclerosis, heart disease, and stroke. The more total cholesterol packaged in high-density lipoproteins (HDL cholesterol or HDLs), the lower the risk.

---

**TABLE 15.3    What to Look for on the Lab Report**

Your risk for developing heart disease depends on your blood cholesterol levels, ratio of total cholesterol to HDL cholesterol, and age. The following blood cholesterol levels are guidelines for heart disease risk, based on data primarily gathered on men.

| AGE | MODERATE RISK | HIGH RISK |
|---|---|---|
| Less than 20 years | 170 mg/dl of blood | 185 mg/dl of blood |
| 20–39 | 200 | 220 |
| 30–39 | 220 | 240 |
| 40+ | 240 | 260 |

The amount of total cholesterol packaged in HDLs also is important in establishing risk. The information obtained from a blood cholesterol test can be used to determine the ratio of total cholesterol to HDL. A ratio of 3.5:1 reflects a very low risk for developing heart disease. A ratio of 4.5:1 to 6.5:1 is a moderate risk category, and a ratio greater than 6.6:1 reflects a high risk.

$$\frac{\text{TOTAL CHOLESTEROL (MG/DL)}}{\text{HDL CHOLESTEROL (MG/DL)}}$$

| | | |
|---|---|---|
| Example 1: | $\dfrac{260 \text{ mg/dl}}{40 \text{ mg/dl}}$ | = 6.5:1 or high risk |
| Example 2: | $\dfrac{180 \text{ mg/dl}}{55 \text{ mg/dl}}$ | = 3.3:1 or low risk |

---

If your cholesterol is above 200 mg/dl, doctors say you should worry about heart disease, unless you are a woman. The Lipid Research Clinics studied women between the ages of 50 and 69 and found that high HDLs were most protective against fatal heart attacks. Also, total cholesterol values didn't affect fatal heart disease. Women with HDL values less than 50 mg/dl were more than three times more likely to die from heart disease than those with higher HDL levels. In essence, a high HDL "wipes out" any increased risk from high total cholesterol or LDLs. However, women should watch all their blood cholesterol levels.

Women at low risk should repeat the blood test every five years, while women with high levels should be checked annually or even more frequently. HDL values are not routinely checked, so you should ask specifically for this test. More important, ask for a copy of the blood lipid panel sheet; do not settle for a vague answer, such as "Your cholesterol is normal." Remember, "normal" in the United States means you have a 50-50 chance of dying from heart disease!

## Diet and Your Heart

The most important piece in the diet-heart-disease puzzle is cholesterol. Any dietary habit that raises total cholesterol or LDLs and/or lowers HDLs increases your risk for developing heart disease.

*Saturated Fat:* Cutting back or cutting out saturated fat is the most important dietary habit you can adopt to lower your risk for heart disease. As saturated fat intake increases so does blood cholesterol, LDLs, and the risk for developing atherosclerosis and heart disease. As women reduce their saturated fat, their blood cholesterol levels and risk for heart disease drop.

*Fish Oils and Monounsaturated Fat:* Not all fat is bad. In fact, some fats, such as olive oil, canola oil, nuts, and fish oils, are even heart-healthy. These fats lower total blood cholesterol, do not lower HDLs, and slow the progression of atherosclerosis by generating a special kind of cholesterol that is resistant to free radical damage (see below). Fish oils also reduce platelet clumping, improve artery wall function, and decrease the production of a hormonelike compound called thromboxane that otherwise damages artery walls. Although not a panacea, fish combined with a low-fat, high-fiber diet is the most effective way to lower blood triglycerides and is very effective in reducing the risk of developing heart disease.

*Margarine and Shortening:* Hardened vegetable oils, such as margarine, shortening, and all processed foods made with these fats, contain altered fats called trans fatty acids (TFAs). TFAs act like saturated fats, increasing your risk for heart disease. These altered fats represent up to 15 percent of total fat intake and up to 50 percent of the fat in some individual foods, such as some margarines.

*Meat versus Soy:* Women, especially postmenopausal women, who love red meat are at higher risk for the disease than are vegetarians or women who eat meat only occasionally. Switching from meat to beans is your best bet, since legumes contain several compounds that lower cholesterol, and they are low-fat and high-fiber alternatives to meat. Legumes contain saponins that bind to cholesterol in the intestines and usher it out of the body. Soy products contain phytoestrogens that also are powerful heart-protecting compounds, lowering total cholesterol and improving the ratio of cholesterol to HDLs. Including a glass of soy milk or a serving of tofu in the daily diet is a wise choice for women at risk for this disease.

*Fiber and Whole Grains:* The insoluble fibers found in oat bran, psyllium, flaxseed, fruits, some vegetables, and cooked dried beans and peas lower blood cholesterol and LDL levels, thus reducing the risk of developing heart disease. Fiber is most effective when combined with other healthy diet habits, such as increased intake of antioxidants. The soluble fibers found in wheat bran have little effect on heart disease risk; however, switching from refined grains to whole grains lowers risk, so there must be more than fiber in whole grains that protects the heart.

*Body Weight:* Women who are overweight, especially if the excess fat accumulates in the chest and abdomen (called the apple-shaped body) are at high risk for developing heart disease. Being overweight is associated with 40 percent of all heart disease in women, and gaining an additional 20 pounds during adult life doubles the risk. Losing weight lowers blood cholesterol levels and reduces heart-disease risk.

*The Antioxidants:* Free radicals damage the cells that line artery walls, thus increasing the blood vessels' susceptibility to atherosclerosis. Maintaining an active antioxidant arsenal to protect arteries from free radical damage is essential to reducing the risk of developing atherosclerosis and heart disease. (See chapter 14 for a description of free radicals and the antioxidants.)

Women who supplement their diets with at least 100 IU of vitamin E lower their risk for heart disease by up to 39 percent, and lower their risk of dying from heart disease by almost 50 percent. A study from Cambridge University found that a woman could reduce her risk of dying from heart disease by half if she maintained high vitamin C levels. Another study found that women who increased their vitamin C intake by as little as 50 mg by eating more fruits and vegetables cut their risk of dying from heart disease by 20 percent. Other foods and nutrients that have antioxidant activity, such as green tea and coenzyme Q10, also might lower heart-disease risk.

---

**TABLE 15.4    A Fiber Quiz**

Test your fiber IQ by answering the following questions True or False.

_____  **1.** Only foods of plant origin, such as vegetables, grains, and nuts, have fiber.
_____  **2.** Fiber decreases the risk of heart disease by binding to blood cholesterol and removing it from the body.
_____  **3.** All of the fiber in a fruit is in the skin or the peel.
_____  **4.** Crunchiness is a good indicator of a food's fiber content.
_____  **5.** The terms "crude fiber," "dietary fiber," and "edible fiber" all refer to the total fiber content of the diet.
_____  **6.** Wheat bran is approximately 40 percent to 50 percent fiber and also contains protein and some starch, sugar, and fat.
_____  **7.** Vegetables and fruits should be eaten raw because cooking destroys fiber.
_____  **8.** Always check the label on commercial fiber foods since some products contain the equivalent of a pat of butter in highly saturated coconut oil per serving.
_____  **9.** When it comes to fiber, the old saying, "Just because something is good doesn't mean more is better," applies.

**Answers:**

  **1.** True.
  **2.** False. Fiber never enters the bloodstream, so it has no direct effect on blood cholesterol. Instead, fiber lowers blood cholesterol by binding to cholesterol-rich bile acids in the digestive tract, thus reducing their reabsorption and helping to drain cholesterol from the body.
  **3.** False. Although the skin and peel are rich sources of fiber, fiber is also in the rest of the fruit.
  **4.** False. Crunch does not always equate with fiber. The crunchy crust on French bread has no more fiber than plain white bread, while soft cooked carrots have the same fiber content as crunchy raw carrots.

**5.** False. Crude fiber is what remains after foods are chemically treated with strong acids or alkalis, but it is only a small portion of the fiber in foods. Dietary fiber includes all substances that are resistant to the body's digestive enzymes but does not include fiber compounds that are broken down by bacteria in the colon; it is therefore a low estimate of the total fiber intake. However, dietary fiber is a more precise measurement than crude fiber values and can be as much as three times higher. Edible fiber is difficult to measure but includes all fiber consumed in the diet.

**6.** True.

**7.** False. Cooking softens the cell walls of vegetables, but the fiber content remains the same.

**8.** True.

**9.** True. Excessive fiber intake (greater than 50 grams per day) is associated with diarrhea, bloating, and possibly a reduced absorption of minerals such as zinc, iron, and manganese.

---

Free radicals also play a role in cholesterol metabolism. Free radical–damaged LDLs, called oxidized LDLs or Ox-LDLs, in the blood are stickier and more likely to attach to blood vessels, causing atherosclerosis and heart disease than do normal LDLs. Ox-LDL also causes arteries to spasm and constrict, thus increasing artery damage and the risk for developing atherosclerosis. Vitamins C and E protect against the formation of Ox-LDL by preventing free radicals from damaging LDLs.

Free radicals also damage cholesterol in foods producing an altered type of dietary cholesterol called cholesterol oxides that are more likely to damage arteries and the heart. Cholesterol oxides are generated when fat, air, and heat come together in cooking, such as deep-fat-fried foods, scrambled eggs, and grilled hamburgers. In laboratory studies, cholesterol oxides injected into artery cells produced defects in the artery lining, platelet clumping, and cholesterol accumulation associated with the initiation of atherosclerosis. Avoiding exposure to these cholesterol oxides by sautéing in chicken broth instead of oil, baking not frying, and avoiding fatty foods combined with ample intake of antioxidant-rich foods, such as fruits and vegetables, is key in the prevention and treatment of heart disease.

*Fruits and Vegetables:* Fruits and vegetables lower heart-disease risk for more reasons than just their antioxidant vitamins. They also supply flavonoids that protect the heart and fiber that lowers cholesterol levels. The evidence is so strong that even the American Heart Association has added antioxidants to its list of heart-healthy dietary components, encouraging people to increase intakes of antioxidant-rich produce and vitamin E.

*Eggs:* For years, people were told not to eat eggs, which are the richest sources of cholesterol in the diet. But researchers at the Harvard School of Public Health say to go ahead and have an egg a day. In their study, eggs posed no cardiovascular problems except for diabetics. However, other studies show that as dietary cholesterol increases so does blood cholesterol, raising a person's risk for heart disease. Until the issue is settled, your best bet is to limit whole eggs, use egg whites and throw out the cholesterol-rich yolks, or use egg substitutes to your heart's content.

*Niacin:* As nicotinic acid, niacin lowers total cholesterol, raises HDL, thwarts the atherosclerotic process, and might aid in the regression of atherosclerosis. Niacin lowers blood fat levels, relaxes artery walls, reduces platelet clumping, and helps remove cholesterol from artery walls, thus aiding in the regression of atherosclerosis.

Therapeutic doses of niacin cause flushing, which is reduced if supplements are taken in divided doses throughout the day, one-half an aspirin is taken a half hour before the niacin, and the niacin dose begins small and is gradually increased during several weeks. Niacin in doses greater than 500 mg should be taken only with the supervision of a physician, since large doses can cause liver damage.

*Other B Vitamins:* Even if your blood cholesterol level is low, you could be at risk for heart disease if you have high circulating levels of a compound called homocysteine. Approximately one in every four women has elevated levels of this compound, but most respond favorably when they boost intakes of folic acid, vitamin $B_{12}$, and/or vitamin $B_6$, which lower homocysteine levels and heart-disease risk.

It might not be as accurate as a blood test, but researchers at the University of Bergen, Norway, report that there are a few indicators that can give you a rough estimate of your homocysteine levels. In their study, older people and people who smoke, consume little folate-rich foods, or drink coffee were the mostly likely candidates for elevated homocysteine levels.

*Chromium:* Chromium is an essential element in the regulation of fat metabolism and insufficient dietary chromium is linked to an increased risk of developing heart disease. Low chromium intake and blood chromium levels are associated with elevated blood cholesterol levels and increased risk for atherosclerosis. In contrast, increased intake of chromium lowers total cholesterol, LDLs, and plaque formation in the arteries, and increases HDLs.

Most women don't consume enough chromium. Researchers at U.S.D.A. Human Nutrition Research Center in Beltsville, Maryland, report that 90 percent of diets contain less than the recommended lower limit of 50 mcg (the upper limit is 200 mcg). Chromium intake averages 15 mcg per 1,000 calories, while dietary intakes average less than 1,600 calories for women. Consequently, most women are likely to be low in chromium, consuming less than 25 mcg each day unless they increase intakes of chromium-rich whole grains, vegetables, legumes, and extra-lean meats.

*Copper:* According to a review from U.S.D.A.'s Grand Forks Human Nutrition Research Center in North Dakota, low copper intakes increase a person's risk for abnormal fat metabolism, poor blood pressure control, abnormal electrocardiograms, and impaired glucose tolerance. Any or all of these problems contribute to an increased risk for developing heart disease and diabetes. The recommended daily intake of 3 mg of copper can be met by increasing intakes of whole grains, shellfish, nuts, cooked dried beans and peas, and dark green leafy vegetables and/or by making sure your multiple contains at least 2 mg of this essential trace mineral.

*Iron:* A few studies have reported that men with high blood iron levels are at increased risk for suffering a heart attack, so some researchers speculate that excessive iron generates free radicals that might predispose a person to increased risk for heart disease. If these findings are true, it is likely that the problem is not enough antioxidants rather than too much iron or it is the iron in meat not in plants and supplements that causes problems. Either way, the issue is specific only to men; there is no evidence that high iron levels in women increase the risk for heart disease.

*Magnesium:* A marginal magnesium deficiency might be a common contributor to heart disease. Magnesium deficiency is associated with irregular heartbeat, angina or chest pain associated with heart disease, heart muscle damage, coronary artery spasms, and increased risk for atherosclerosis and heart attack. Blood magnesium levels are low in patients suffering heart attacks and tissue levels of magnesium are suboptimal prior to, during, and following a heart attack. In contrast, increased magnesium intake normalizes the heartbeat, relaxes the coronary arteries, and reduces a person's likelihood of suffering a heart attack. Women who consume diets rich in magnesium and calcium have a 30 percent lower risk of dying from heart disease compared to women who don't consume enough of these minerals.

The ratio of calcium to magnesium is also important. Women who supplement with calcium, but fail to also increase magnesium intake, might increase their risk for heart damage. Consequently, if a woman chooses to supplement, the two minerals should be supplied together in a ratio of approximately two parts calcium to every one part magnesium (i.e., 1,000 mg of calcium and 500 mg magnesium).

*Zinc:* Poor intake of zinc is associated with elevated total blood cholesterol and LDL cholesterol and decreased HDL cholesterol, thus increasing a woman's heart-disease risk. In contrast, optimal zinc intake reduces total and LDL cholesterol and raises HDL cholesterol and is associated with a lowered heart-disease risk. Limited evidence also shows that zinc might strengthen the lining of the arteries so they are less susceptible to damage and atherosclerosis. As with copper, excessive zinc intake has the reverse effect of lowering HDLs and increasing the disease risk. Consequently, zinc intake should not exceed three times the recommended guidelines or between 15 mg and 45 mg per day.

*Garlic:* Garlic and garlic oil might protect the heart against disease. Garlic dissolves blood clots, inhibits clot formation, and lowers both total cholesterol and LDL levels. In rabbits, garlic even reverses atherosclerosis. A sulfur-containing compound in garlic called ajoene is at least partially responsible for garlic's ability to reduce platelet clumping and, thereby, reduce the risk for developing atherosclerosis and heart disease.

No one agrees on an optimal dose. LDLs were more resistant to free radical damage and thus less likely to contribute to atherosclerosis when people consumed 2.4 grams of aged garlic extract (AGE) in one study. Others think optimal dietary intake is as high as eight garlic cloves a day, while even modest daily consumption of two to three cloves or a high-quality garlic supplement is likely to produce beneficial effects.

*Coffee and Chocolate:* Some studies report coffee increases a woman's risk for developing heart disease, while other studies show no association. At Stanford University School of Medicine, researchers found that even decaffeinated coffee raised LDL levels, which suggests that another compound in coffee besides caffeine might affect heart disease risk. However, researchers at Harvard Medical School say the evidence on coffee just doesn't hold water. Using dietary intake data obtained from the Nurses' Health Study, which includes 85,747 women thirty-four to fifty-nine years old, the researchers investigated the ten-year incidence of heart disease and compared it to coffee consumption patterns. They found no evidence for any association between heart-disease risk and coffee consumption (up to six cups per day) or caffeine from all sources combined. The best advice at this point is to drink coffee in moderation.

Cocoa extract contains compounds called procyanidins that help relax artery walls, possibly reducing blood pressure or heart-disease risk, according to a study from the University of California, Davis. Procyanidins in chocolate also function as antioxidants to inhibit free radical damage of blood fats.

*A Glass of Wine:* An occasional glass of red wine lowers heart-disease risk, but women should limit intake to no more than one glass a day. You can get the same heart-healthy boost from alcohol-free red wine, which also increases the body's antioxidant defense systems.

*Yogurt:* Blood cholesterol levels dropped by up to 3.2 percent when yogurt fermented with *Lacto-bacillus acidophilus* was added to the diet in a study from the VA Medical Center in Lexington, Kentucky.

## Heart Disease: Diet Advice

Making a few changes in how you eat and live will have profound effects on whether or not you battle heart disease. In a study conducted on 84,129 women at the Harvard Medical School in Boston, only 3 percent of the women took good care of themselves. However, those few women almost eliminated the threat of heart disease. They lowered their disease risk by 83 percent by not smoking, maintaining lean figures, limiting alcohol to about one small serving daily, exercising vigorously for at least half an hour every day, and adopting diets rich in fiber, omega-3 fatty acids, and folic acid, but low in saturated fats and trans fatty acids.

The Healthy Woman's Diet, coupled with regular aerobic exercise, remains the primary defense. In addition to these low-fat, high-fiber guidelines,

- Use olive and canola oils, rather than other vegetable oils or processed oils, such as margarine or shortening.
- Cook with fresh garlic whenever possible.
- Limit eggs to five per week. Use egg whites and egg substitutes.
- Drink coffee and alcohol in moderation.
- Divide the day's food intake into four to six small meals and snacks throughout the day. Several minimeals as opposed to the three-square-meals-a-day food pattern lower blood cholesterol levels, help you maintain a desirable weight, and reduce the risk for developing heart disease.
- Take a broad-range, moderate-dose multiple vitamin and mineral supplement, plus extra antioxidants. Daily intakes of 500 to 1,000 mg of vitamin C might lower serum total cholesterol by approximately

10 percent in some people, while 100 IU to 400 IU of vitamin E also protect against heart disease and heart attacks.

Don't think you're off the hook by eating well. The best diet in the world won't make up for being sedentary. You must exercise to lower heart-disease risk, including some form of aerobic activity such walking, jogging, aerobic dance, or swimming. In addition, maintain a normal blood pressure, encourage loyal and lasting friendships and relationships with family, relax regularly, prevent or control hypertension and diabetes, and don't smoke. (Even living or working with a smoker can increase a nonsmoker's risk for heart disease!)

Your family history is an important factor. If you have an immediate family member who died from heart disease or is at high risk, you should pay close attention to the risk factors that are within your control. Keep in mind, you begin to lose your inborn protection against heart attacks after menopause, so risk increases in later years, making lifestyle choices even more important as you age.

## Osteoporosis

Osteoporosis is a condition, not a disease, where calcium gradually drains from the bones leaving them brittle, porous, and likely to fracture with even minimal trauma, such as a minor fall. In advanced osteoporosis, the bones of the spine collapse, giving a woman a stooped posture called dowager's hump. There are no symptoms of osteoporosis until a fracture occurs, indicating the condition is in the advanced stages with less likelihood of successful treatment. Only one in every three women who breaks a hip regains her independence. One in four dies within a year following the fracture. Almost half who survive cannot walk without help.

Most women are past sixty-five years when they suffer their first fracture, but the disease has been progressing undetected for decades. Preventing this disease also starts early—beginning in childhood.

### Why Are Women at Greatest Risk?

You have a one in six chance of fracturing a hip during your lifetime. Osteoporosis strikes women far more frequently than it does men because our bones are smaller than men's bones, so less calcium can be lost before obvious problems occur. We are more likely to follow low-calorie diets that supply inadequate amounts of dietary calcium and other nutrients essential for bone maintenance. Women also engage in fewer weight-bearing exercises, which place stress on the bones and help maintain their density.

## Diet and Your Bones

*Calcium:* Calcium is the foundation of any plan to prevent osteoporosis. Your need for this mineral begins at birth, since your greatest bone mass and density (called peak bone mass) are reached by your mid-thirties. Prior to this time, you are building bone density, which will serve as your bank account for calcium for the rest of your life. The more bone you build in your early years, the less likely you will battle osteoporosis later in life. Shortly after peak bone mass is reached, the bones begin to lose calcium at a rate of 1 percent a year until menopause. After menopause, the loss accelerates and in the spine it can reach 6 percent per year. High calcium intake (i.e., 1,500 mg/day), ample vitamin D, exercise, and hormone replacement therapy (HRT) help slow this bone loss.

**TABLE 15.5    Estimating Your Risk for Osteoporosis**

You are at greatest risk for osteoporosis if you:

- Have a mother, father, or sibling with a history of fractures, or you have fractured a bone in a fall after age fifty.
- Are Caucasian.
- Smoke cigarettes.
- Started menopause before age forty-five or are premenopausal but have not menstruated for more than one year.
- Weigh less than 127 pounds, especially if you are more than fifty years old.
- Consume few milk products.
- Exercise infrequently.
- Are more than sixty-five years old.
- Are frail or in poor health.

It is never too late to correct a calcium-poor diet, although the sooner you start, the better. Unfortunately, nothing can mend the damage caused when osteoporosis is allowed to progress unchecked to advanced stages. In short, calcium provides a protective effect in the development of bone loss and osteoporosis. Hip fracture risk is reduced by as much as 75 percent in persons who consume high-calcium diets, whereas people who consume low-calcium diets or don't supplement throughout life are at high risk for developing bone disorders.

*Salt:* A salty diet might interfere with calcium retention and increase the risk of developing osteoporosis. A high-salt diet increases calcium loss in the urine, which could reduce bone density if prolonged. In contrast, other dietary factors, such as lactose in milk, increase calcium absorption and help prevent osteoporosis.

*Vitamin D:* You can nibble and sip on calcium-rich foods your entire life, but if you're not also getting enough vitamin D, you are at risk for osteoporosis. This vitamin makes sure the calcium in your diet is absorbed and packed into bone tissue.

Sunlight on the skin and diet are the two sources of vitamin D. Our bodies gradually lose the ability to convert sunlight into vitamin D as we age, so dietary sources become increasingly more important during middle years and later years. Current recommendations are 200 IU of vitamin D for young women and 400 IU for women past fifty years old. But studies show that some older women show signs of deficiency even at intakes of 600 IU, suggesting that at least this amount, but no more than 1,000 IU of vitamin D, should be consumed in the senior years. It is difficult to reach this level unless you take a supplement.

*Supplements:* Calcium from nonfat milk products or fortified soy milk is the best absorbed source of calcium. Vegetables, such as the dark green leafy vegetables, are excellent sources of calcium, but the mineral is not as well absorbed as it is from milk. Calcium supplements also are best absorbed if taken with milk.

Several supplemental forms of calcium are well absorbed, including calcium carbonate, calcium citrate, and calcium citrate-malate. People with low stomach acid (a condition called achlorhydria) absorb calcium better from calcium citrate or calcium citrate/malate than from calcium carbonate.

Supplementing with calcium and vitamin D helps boost bone density and reduce bone turnover, but only if you continue to supplement. According to a study from U.S.D.A. Human Nutrition Research Center on Aging at Tufts University in Boston, seniors who discontinued their calcium and vitamin D supplements after three years of supplementing rapidly began to lose the bone they had accumulated. Within two years of not supplementing, their bones had returned to presupplement densities in the spine and femoral neck bones.

*Vitamin K:* For more than forty years, the only recognized role for vitamin K was in blood clotting. Vitamin K shed its outdated image when new research uncovered a diverse group of vitamin K–dependent proteins with no role in blood clotting, but essential in calcium metabolism, tissue mineralization, and bone maintenance. The two most prominent proteins are osteocalcin (OC) and matrix carboxyglutamic acid or Gla. Healthy bones require optimal vitamin K to ensure each osteocalcin molecule is filled to capacity with Gla groups. When vitamin K levels are low, the Gla groups can't attach to osteocalcin, resulting in a less active protein called undercarboxylated osteocalcin or ucOC. Bone mineralization slows as a result.

The link between vitamin K, osteocalcin, and hip fractures is strong. First, vitamin K intake decreases as people age, and older people with low vitamin K levels are most prone to broken bones. Second, blood levels of ucOC rise as bone density drops, thus a high ucOC is associated with weak bones and a high risk for hip fractures. Third, high blood levels of ucOC are found in people prone to vitamin K deficiency. The risk of future hip fractures is three to six times higher in people with an elevated ucOC level. The good news is that increasing dietary intake of vitamin K lowers ucOC levels, reduces calcium loss from the bones, improves bone mineralization, and possibly reduces the risk of later bone loss. The trick is knowing who might be deficient and how much vitamin K to recommend.

The current requirements for vitamin K were based solely on the now outdated belief that the vitamin's only role was in blood coagulation. Nailing down an optimal vitamin K intake to ensure healthy bones is difficult, partially because for years it was thought that the vitamin K manufactured by bacteria in the digestive tract made up for any dietary lack. However, the evidence supporting this assumption is sorely lacking. To further complicate the issue, researchers have yet to accurately identify the vitamin K content of foods, let alone how much vitamin K is absorbed. It appears that the vitamin is much better absorbed from supplements than from food.

So what is an optimal intake? No one really knows. Until more is known, include several servings daily of vitamin K–rich greens, such as spinach, kale, broccoli, collards, and mustard greens. On days when leafy vegetable intake falls short of optimal, consider taking a multiple vitamin and mineral supplement that contains 45 to 100 mcg of vitamin K.

*Magnesium:* Approximately 60 percent of the body's magnesium is in the bones. This mineral affects bone status from conception throughout life. Inadequate intake might contribute to the development of osteoporosis. People who eat magnesium-rich foods, such as nuts, whole grains, and dark green leafy vegetables, and people who supplement with this mineral show less bone loss and greater bone density compared to women whose intake is poor. In addition, magnesium and calcium absorption and metabolism are interrelated; increasing calcium intake without a concurrent increase in magnesium intake can reduce magnesium levels in bone and other tissues.

*Soy:* Optimal intake of phytoestrogens has a modest positive effect on improving bone mass. Soy might even be a viable alternative to hormone replacement therapy. Researchers at the University of Cincinnati College of Medicine found that phytoestrogens in soy reduce bone loss caused by estrogen deficiency. Whether these compounds are as good as estrogen or if the benefits of estrogen plus soy are even better than either one alone deserve further attention.

The tricky word here is "optimal." In Asian cultures where the women consume 40 mg of phytoestrogens daily (compared to Western intakes of 0 to 3 mg)

---

**TABLE 15.6     Beyond Calcium**

Calcium and magnesium work as a team with other nutrients in the maintenance of healthy bones.

- Poor intake of copper is associated with calcium loss from the bones, reduced bone formation, and bone deformities.
- Silicon improves bone mineral density, thus lowering a person's risk for osteoporosis, according to a study from Tufts University in Boston.
- Fluoride strengthens bones and teeth and women who live in areas where the water is fluoridated have a lower incidence of developing osteoporosis.
- Manganese also is important in bone growth and metabolism. A deficiency of this trace mineral increases calcium loss from the bone and the risk for fractures.
- Zinc intake is directly related to bone density; as zinc intake increases (up to recommended levels) bone loss decreases in women of all ages.
- Vitamin C is important in maintaining collagen, a key component of connective tissue in the bone matrix. Underdeveloped collagen results in weakened bone structure and increased susceptibility to fractures.

---

and excrete a thousand times the levels of phytoestrogens in their urine, bone fracture rates are a fraction of what they are in the United States and other Western
cultures.

*Fish Oils:* For hundreds of thousands of years our ancestors consumed diets
rich in both omega-3-rich plants and wild game, providing a ratio of plant oils
called omega-6 fatty acids (from seeds and nuts) to omega-3 fatty acids of somewhere between 4:1 and 1:1. Today, we include very little omega-3-rich fish and no
wild game in our daily diets, but lots of salad oils, fried or processed foods, and
margarine. Consequently, we consume eleven times more omega-6-rich oils than
we do omega-3 fats. Accumulating evidence shows that the high intake of omega-
6s with inadequate amounts of omega-3s, so common in industrialized countries,
contributes to the development of bone and joint disorders.

Fats play an important role in skeletal biology and bone health. They help
mineralize cartilage and support functions that build, tear down, and remodel
bone tissue. Frequent intake of the omega-3s helps maintain bone density in seniors and build bone density in children. Studies on animals also show that
increased intakes of omega-3s improve the rate of bone formation. It appears that
omega-3s transform the fatty acid composition of bone compartments, which
influence the local factors influencing bone formation. These fats also affect cartilage metabolism, which in turn influences bone modeling.

The best deterrent for osteoporosis is to build strong bones early in life and
maintain that bone density throughout life by exercising regularly and consuming diets rich in calcium, other factors, and omega-3 fats.

*Exercise:* A sedentary lifestyle results in substantial bone loss, while weight-
bearing and resistance or weight-training exercises increase bone mass and prevent osteoporosis. The combination of weight-bearing exercise, such as walking or
jogging, and calcium supplementation is more effective than calcium alone. In
one study, up to 64 percent of physically inactive women who consumed calcium-
poor diets had osteoporosis, while only 12 percent of women who consumed
ample calcium, exercized regularly, and maintained a low body weight had signs
of serious bone loss.

## Osteoporosis: Diet Advice

The Healthy Woman's Diet forms the foundation for the prevention and treatment
of osteoporosis. Consuming this low-fat, nutrient-packed diet with moderate

amounts of protein (high-protein diets increase calcium loss in the urine) will increase calcium absorption and reduce calcium loss, thus maximizing the amount of calcium available for bone growth and maintenance.

- Aim for at least 1,200 mg of calcium daily, 400 IU of vitamin D, 350 mg of magnesium, and 90 mcg of vitamin K. You'll need even more vitamin D if you are over sixty-five years old. While you can meet these needs by following the guidelines of the Healthy Woman's Diet, you'll probably need to supplement to reach this level of vitamin D, unless you consume four glasses daily of milk or fortified soy milk.
- Drink coffee in moderation. In the past, coffee was suspected to contribute to bone loss by increasing urinary loss of calcium; however, several recent studies found no effect from moderate coffee or caffeine intake. Adding a little milk to your coffee should more than offset any calcium lost.
- Avoid fad diets. Severely restricting calories in an effort to lose more than a pound or two a week can offset any of the gains you made from exercise in boosting bone density. Lose weight gradually so that you don't sacrifice your bones for your waistline. (See chapter 7 for tips on losing weight.)
- Skip the soft drinks. These beverages contain phosphates that increase calcium loss in the urine.

In addition to diet, avoid tobacco and increase weight-bearing exercise, such as walking, jogging, and jumping rope. Strength training also increases bone density and helps prevent osteoporosis. Since stress increases the loss of magnesium and other minerals in the urine, effective coping skills and relaxation also might be useful in preventing bone loss.

Hormone replacement therapy (HRT) and new antibone loss medications, such as biphosphonates (Fosamax and Actonel) and raloxifene (Evista), reduce fractures in both the spine and the femur (thighbone) and are likely to remain the therapy of choice for the treatment of osteoporosis, in combination with calcium supplementation and exercise.

**TABLE 15.7    Bone-Boosting Snacks**

- Spinach salad with blue cheese (vitamin K and calcium)
- Halibut ceviche with whole-wheat crackers (vitamin D and magnesium)
- Salmon patties made with canned salmon (calcium and vitamin D)
- Nonfat, plain yogurt with strawberries (calcium and vitamin C)
- A bowl of Total cereal topped with nuts and milk (vitamin D, magnesium, and calcium)
- Calcium-fortified orange juice with a small bowl of coleslaw (calcium and vitamin K)
- A glass of 8th Continent Chocolate Soymilk (calcium and vitamin D)
- Brown rice pudding made with nonfat milk or fortified vanilla soy milk (calcium and vitamin D)
- Whole-wheat tortilla filled with low-fat cheddar cheese, spinach, and salsa (magnesium, calcium, and vitamin K)

# CHAPTER 16

# *Other Health Conditions*

## *Arthritis*

The most common forms of arthritis are rheumatoid arthritis, osteoarthritis, and gout. Rheumatoid arthritis is the most serious because it is the most crippling of the three. Inflammation and thickening of the lining and tissues surrounding the joints damage the bones, causing deformity and disability. Although the cause is poorly understood, some scientists believe rheumatoid arthritis is linked to disruption of the body's immune system and/or free radical damage to the tissues surrounding joints. (See chapter 14 for more information on free radicals and antioxidants.)

Osteoarthritis is the "wear and tear" disease associated with degeneration of the cartilage that cushions the bones at the joints. Long-term irritation of the joints, caused from overweight, poor posture, injury, or strain, is the primary contributor to this form of arthritis. Women are more affected than are men, and older women are more prone to osteoarthritis than are younger women.

Gout is the easiest form of arthritis to diagnose and treat but is most common in men. In gout, uric acid accumulates and forms crystals that lodge in the joints.

### Diet and Arthritis

No diet or nutrient is known to prevent or cure rheumatoid arthritis. However, several dietary habits contribute to a person's optimal health and possibly reduce symptoms.

Women with rheumatoid arthritis often eat poor diets, have low blood levels of several vitamins and minerals, and are overweight. They often consume too few whole grains, vegetables, legumes, nonfat milk products, and other healthful foods. In turn, poor nutrition aggravates disease symptoms. For example, pain and stiffness increase when a woman is malnourished. Rheumatoid arthritis is an inflammatory disease that increases nutrient needs but, at the same time, alters the intestinal lining, which interferes with the absorption of nutrients. The disease and some medications used in its treatment also can cause peptic ulcers and gastritis, which further reduce digestion and a woman's desire to eat.

Deficiencies of folic acid, copper, iron, zinc, and vitamins D, $B_2$, and $B_6$ are frequently found in women with rheumatoid arthritis. Symptoms often improve when patients increase their intake of one or more of these nutrients. Some studies also show improvement when patients consume vitamin A, selenium-rich yeast, vitamin E, and calcium. Although altered levels of vitamins and minerals could be a result rather than a cause of the disease, maintaining optimal nutrition provides the immune system with tools to fend off infection and disease.

Nutrition also counteracts the adverse effects of medication. Steroids used in the treatment of rheumatoid arthritis can cause bone loss. Daily supplementation with calcium and vitamin D helps prevent this loss. Anti-inflammatory medications and aspirin increase vitamin C losses and can result in bruising, while adequate intake of this vitamin prevents these symptoms.

*The Antioxidants:* Several studies report that arthritis patients have much higher levels of free radicals in their blood and lower levels of antioxidant enzymes. This altered antioxidant status might affect the initiation and promotion of the disease. Since free radical damage to the immune system and joint tissues contributes to rheumatoid arthritis, optimal intake of the antioxidant nutrients might help counteract this tissue damage by deactivating free radicals, reducing inflammation, and strengthening the immune system. Numerous studies support this benefit:

- Both vitamin E and selenium supplements show promise in reducing pain and stiffness of arthritis.
- Vitamin C helps reduce the inflammation of rheumatoid arthritis, curbs cartilage loss, slows the progression of, and might lessen the pain associated with, osteoarthritis.
- Low dietary intake of vitamin C promotes the development of osteoarthritis in experimental animals and inhibits inflammation in

rheumatoid arthritis. Treatment of osteoarthritis with vitamin C might help slow the deterioration of cartilage, resulting in less pain and the unlikelihood of surgical intervention.

*Fat:* Two families of hormonelike substances called prostaglandins and leukotrienes regulate the inflammatory processes in rheumatoid arthritis. Dietary fats are building blocks for these compounds. While vegetable oils aggravate inflammation by encouraging the formation of harmful prostaglandins and leukotrienes, fish oils from either dietary sources or capsules curb the pain, stiffness, and swelling of rheumatoid arthritis by reducing levels of harmful prostaglandins, altering inflammatory processes, and strengthening the immune response. In addition, the dosage of anti-inflammatory medication is sometimes reduced when patients increase their consumption of fish oils. Fish oils are most effective when vegetable oil consumption is low. Olive oil, evening primrose oil, and borage oil also might help reduce arthritis symptoms.

*Vegetarian Diets:* Rheumatoid arthritis symptoms improve when people fast, which strongly suggests a diet-related component to the disease. In addition, some people are hypersensitive to milk products and show improvements in arthritis symptoms when these foods are removed from the diet.

Researchers at the University of Oslo in Norway placed patients on a fast followed by a vegetarian diet, while another group (the control group) fasted and then returned to normal dietary intakes. Within four weeks, the vegetarians showed significant improvements in the number of tender and swollen joints, pain, duration of morning stiffness, grip strength, and immune function.

*Glucosamine and Chondroitin:* These two components of cartilage are found in foods and can be made by the body. Researchers at the Boston University School of Medicine reviewed the literature on glucosamine and chondroitin supplementation and found that glucosamine had a moderate effect on reducing symptoms of osteoarthritis in at least half of all sufferers, and chondroitin effectively reduced pain in most people. Both supplements cause few side effects and take about two months of supplementation before benefits are noted. Most studies have used 1,500 mg a day of glucosamine and/or 1,200 mg of chondroitin.

## Arthritis: Diet Advice

The various forms of arthritis have different causes and symptoms, and require different types of treatment. Even one form of arthritis can vary from person to person, so treatment must be tailored to the individual.

Some rheumatoid arthritis symptoms might result from a food intolerance, allergies, or problems with digestion or absorption of foods, which might explain why symptoms lessen when women adopt vegetarian diets that remove the offending foods.

Elimination diets are effective for some people but must be carefully monitored by a physician and/or dietitian. With these diets, suspected aggravating foods, such as wheat or milk products, black walnuts, alfalfa, or nitrite-containing foods, are eliminated from the diet and gradually added back one at a time to monitor adverse reactions. Eliminating coffee, or at least limiting intake to three cups or less a day, might help curb symptoms, too. (See pages 328 to 332 for more information on food intolerance.)

Osteoarthritis and gout occur frequently in overweight people. Maintaining a desirable weight throughout life helps prevent these two forms of arthritis, while losing weight lowers the blood uric acid level in gout patients and helps in the treatment of osteoarthritis.

Until more is known about the causes and cures of arthritis, follow the guidelines of the Healthy Woman's Diet or the guidelines in chapter 2 for an optimal vegetarian diet. In addition,

- Boost intake of all antioxidants and consider supplementing with additional amounts of vitamins C and E.
- Include two or more servings of fish in the weekly diet.
- Avoid consuming too much iron from supplements, since this mineral might aggravate arthritis symptoms.
- Consider trying glucosamine and chondroitin supplements for osteoarthritis.
- Frequent, moderate exercise increases the blood flow, and therefore oxygen and nutrient supply, to all body tissues and can retard the aging processes of all tissues, including the bones and joints.

*Precautions:* Arthritis sufferers are susceptible to quackery, i.e., the quick, easy, secret, or special cure. Many fads, from copper bracelets to methylsulfonylmethane

(MSM) supplements, appear to work when in reality the disease disappeared on its own. Many fad diets for arthritis are not effective and might contribute to malnutrition and aggravation of arthritis symptoms. These diets include eliminating acid fruits and vegetables, eating only one type of food at each meal, altering the acid-base balance of the diet, low-protein diets, low-calorie diets (except for weight management), and low-carbohydrate diets.

The belief that overconsumption of calcium causes osteoarthritis also is unfounded. Optimal calcium intake improves bone density and strength, but has no effect on abnormal calcification of joints associated with osteoarthritis.

The fact that more than half of all cases of rheumatoid arthritis spontaneously cure themselves suggests the immune system often can overcome the disorder if supplied with the necessary nutritional ammunition to stage a full-scale war.

## Bowel Problems

Disorders of the bowel, including the small and large intestine, are numerous. The most common problems include flatulence (gas), constipation, diarrhea, irritable bowel syndrome (spastic colon), diverticular disease, and inflammatory bowel disease.

### Flatulence (Gas)

The average person generates one to three pints of gas each day, which is comprised of nitrogen, oxygen, hydrogen, and small amounts of methane. The causes of gas include swallowing air while eating or drinking, increased intestinal activity, and excessive bacterial fermentation of food components in the bowel. People with too much gas often produce the same amount as other people, but because of increased movement of food through the bowel, gas is not reabsorbed through the colon wall. Increasing the fiber content of the diet also can temporarily cause gas.

Carbohydrate-rich foods often are the worst offenders. Most gas results from sugars, starches, and fibers that reach the large intestine without being thoroughly digested and absorbed. Colonies of harmless bacteria in the colon eat the carbohydrates, giving off gases in some people. Gas production can be reduced or avoided by gradually replacing low-fiber foods with high-fiber foods and by cutting back on sweets.

A special type of sugar called raffinose is found in beans and, in smaller amounts, in some vegetables and grains. The human body lacks the enzyme—alpha-galactosidase—to digest this sugar so bacteria in the colon have a feast. The result is gas. Flatulence from beans can be prevented or reduced by:

- Soaking the beans overnight and discarding the water.
- Adding fresh water, cooking for half an hour, and again throwing away the water. Add nine cups of water for every cup of beans.
- Cooking beans thoroughly to avoid raw starch granules that also produce gas.
- Discarding the liquid from canned beans; it also is loaded with raffinose.

---

## TABLE 16. I    Vegetables and Fruits That Cause Gas

**VEGETABLES:**

| | |
|---|---|
| Beans: kidney, lima, navy, garbanzo, black, pinto | Peas, split or black-eyed |
| Broccoli | Peppers, green |
| Brussels sprouts | Pimentos |
| Cabbage | Radishes |
| Cauliflower | Rutabagas |
| Corn | Sauerkraut |
| Cucumber | Scallions |
| Kohlrabi | Shallots |
| Leeks | Soybeans |
| Lentils | Turnips |
| Onions | |

**FRUITS:**

| | |
|---|---|
| Apples, raw | Honeydew melon |
| Apple juice | Prune juice |
| Avocados | Raisins |
| Cantaloupe | Watermelon |

A product on the market called Beano contains the digestive enzyme alpha-galactosidase. A few drops added to a bowl of beans stops the gas-producing bacteria in the colon and reduces the bloating and distension that trouble many gas-sufferers.

Other tips for reducing gas include:

- Eat slowly.
- Chew with your mouth closed.
- Don't gulp food.

Also avoid gas-forming foods and then add back those foods that are well tolerated. People vary in their reactions to foods, so don't assume that what is gassy for one person will be gassy for another.

Excessive gas could be a sign of lactose intolerance (inability to digest milk sugar) or a deficiency of another intestinal enzyme. As a trial, omit milk and milk products from the diet, including ice cream, yogurt, milk, cheese, puddings, and custard, and observe any improvements in symptoms.

## Constipation

Constipation is a very subjective complaint. Ideally, a person should have a bowel movement each day; however, constipation is defined as less than three stools per week while eating a high-fiber diet, or when three or more days go by without a bowel movement. The causes of constipation are numerous and include lack of exercise, side effects of medication, disease, crash dieting, obesity, dehydration, and a low-fiber diet.

The first step is to increase the fiber content of your diet by eating more fresh fruits and vegetables, whole-grain breads and cereals, and more cooked dried beans and peas. The diet should contain at least five, and preferably eight to ten, servings of fruits and vegetables, six servings of whole grains, and one serving of cooked beans.

Avoid highly refined foods, such as white rice and bread, cream of wheat, pastries, pies, cakes, enriched noodles, and commercial snack foods. Prunes and prune juice are high in fiber and also stimulate intestinal movement. In addition,

- Drink at least eight to ten glasses of water daily.
- Avoid excessive intake of iron or calcium carbonate supplements.

- Avoid using large amounts of bran cereals as a source of fiber. Excessive amounts of this processed fiber can be irritating to the intestinal tract and can cause flatulence or intestinal blockage.
- The regular use of laxatives, including flaxseed meal, is discouraged, since this practice causes dependence on the laxative and possibly spastic constipation.
- Regular aerobic exercise improves bowel function and often cures constipation.

## Diarrhea

Diarrhea is a symptom, not a disease. Food passes rapidly through the intestine, resulting in potential nutrient deficiencies if the condition persists. Diarrhea should be differentiated from more serious conditions, such as dysentery, and is caused by a variety of conditions, including lactose intolerance or other intestinal disorders, bacterial and viral infections, laxatives such as castor oil, ulcerative colitis, and Crohn's disease. Coffee or caffeine consumption, even in moderate amounts of one to two cups each day, can cause diarrhea in sensitive people. Iron and/or calcium supplements also can cause diarrhea in some individuals.

The primary nutritional goal in the treatment of diarrhea is to remove the cause. A low-fiber diet often is used temporarily to reduce the undigestible bulk in the intestine. This diet consists of potatoes without the skin, enriched white bread and rice, strained fruit juices, plain crackers without seeds, milk (unless the person is lactose intolerant), creamed or broth-based soups, fish or chicken, and enriched pastas.

In contrast to the treatment of constipation, fiber-rich foods are avoided in the treatment of diarrhea. Drink daily at least ten glasses of water to replace fluids. Pectin in applesauce provides some therapeutic benefits, but never use concentrated canning pectin as a source of this fiber. Fiber foods are gradually reintroduced when the diarrhea subsides and the person can tolerate food. Chronic diarrhea may require vitamin and mineral supplementation to avoid deficiencies from poor food absorption.

## Irritable Bowel Syndrome

Irritable bowel syndrome (IBS), also called spastic colitis or spastic colon, probably results from disturbances in intestinal activity, stress, and dietary deficiencies or intolerances. Overstimulation of the nerves that trigger bowel activity results in excessive bowel contractions, abdominal pain, diarrhea or constipation, and nausea. Contributing causes vary, but often include use of laxatives, tobacco, caffeine, alcohol, antibiotic therapy, digestive tract infections, or irregularities in sleep, fluid intake, and bowel movements. People with IBS frequently are tense, underweight, and chronically upset. Because of past experiences, they are afraid to eat because of anticipated pain.

The goal of nutritional therapy is to relieve the condition, regain optimal nutritional status, and increase body weight. A low-fat, nutrient-dense, high-fiber diet helps relieve constricting pressure in the bowel and promotes normal bowel activity. Avoid large supplemental doses of vitamins and minerals that might irritate the intestinal tract. Relaxation and stress management also are essential in the long-term management of this bowel problem.

### Diverticular Disease

Diverticula are pouches in the weakened intestinal wall. The condition might go unnoticed or a person can experience discomfort, cramping, painful bowel movements, diarrhea or constipation, or nausea.

Diverticulitis is inflammation and infection of the pouches that result from accumulation of fecal matter in these pockets. The incidence of diverticular disease increases with age, possibly because of reduced strength of the intestinal wall or a lifetime of eating a low-fiber diet and not exercising.

The first line of nutritional defense is to increase the fiber content of the diet, which

1. reduces the pressure within the intestines that is thought to cause the pockets,
2. decreases the pain, and
3. speeds the movement of foodstuff through the bowel.

Even two teaspoons of bran three times a day relieve the symptoms of diverticular disease in most people. The high-fiber diet might produce temporary gas, which subsides within a few weeks.

## Inflammatory Bowel Disease

Inflammatory bowel disease (IBD) is classified according to the section of the bowel that is affected. Inflammation of the small intestine is usually called Crohn's disease, while inflammation of the rectum and right portions of the colon is called ulcerative colitis. Symptoms include diarrhea, bleeding, abdominal pain, fever, and weight loss. Viral infections, suppressed immunity, and nutrient deficiencies have been implicated in the development and progression of inflammatory bowel diseases; however, the exact cause(s) is unknown.

Nutrient deficiencies are common in people with IBD. Fever and infection increase nutrient requirements, while the pain and inflammatory processes reduce food intake and absorption. Impaired taste, reduced appetite, and suppressed immunity are common symptoms of IBD that might result from zinc deficiency and sometimes respond favorably to zinc supplementation.

Vitamin A is essential for the development and maintenance of the intestinal lining; however, there is no evidence linking this vitamin in the prevention or treatment of bowel disease. Dietary management of Crohn's disease and ulcerative colitis requires counseling and monitoring by a physician and dietitian.

# *Carpal Tunnel Syndrome*

A major nerve that carries signals from the brain to the hands passes through a narrow tunnel in the wrists formed by small bones called the carpals. The tunnel is rigid, so anything that causes swelling or inflammation of the encased tissues results in pressure and pinching on that nerve. The condition is called carpal tunnel syndrome (CTS) and it can affect one or both hands at the same time.

Symptoms of CTS include intermittent numbness, pain that shoots up the arm from the wrist, and a sensation of tingling or burning in the hands and fingers. Symptoms might increase throughout the day, might be severe enough to cause sleeplessness, and can become worse over time.

CTS is fairly common in women engaged in sports, such as volleyball or racquetball, or in jobs that place stress on the wrists. Minor injuries, such as falling backward on your hand, also might cause the tendons to swell. A change in the balance of hormones during pregnancy and menopause can result in an accumulation of fluid and subsequent swelling of the wrists, which might explain the increased prevalence of CTS in pregnant and menopausal women.

In some cases, CTS clears up without treatment. In others, a splint worn on the wrist at night helps relieve the pain. The usual treatment is anti-inflammatory or diuretic medications or cortisone injections to reduce swelling. Conditions unresponsive to medication require surgery to cut through the tough membrane and create a larger space for the encased nerve.

### Nutrition and CTS

Vitamin $B_6$ has been linked to the development and treatment of CTS. The issue is not a matter of poor dietary intake, but rather the possible benefits of pharmacological doses of the vitamin. The symptoms of CTS sometimes are reduced or relieved when vitamin $B_6$ intake is increased. Several case studies have reported that vitamin $B_6$ supplementation eliminated the need for surgery, although it might take up to twelve weeks before symptoms improve. Other studies have found no effect of vitamin $B_6$ supplementation.

If vitamin $B_6$ affects the development of CTS, the reasons are poorly understood. The vitamin is involved in the development and maintenance of healthy nerve tissue, while too little of the vitamin might cause inflammation of the nerve tissue resembling that seen in CTS. Sometimes vitamin $B_6$ therapy is effective despite normal blood levels of the vitamin. In these cases, it is conceivable that reduced blood flow in the cartilage and bone tissue involved in CTS results in a localized deficiency of vitamin $B_6$, whereas other tissues with increased circulation have an adequate supply of the vitamin.

### CTS: Diet Advice

If the muscles of the hands have begun to atrophy and weaken, then surgery is probably necessary. However, in most cases, a CTS patient might benefit from a three- to four-month trial of vitamin $B_6$ supplementation. Most studies reporting success have used daily supplements containing 50 mg to 200 mg of vitamin $B_6$. The daily dose can drop to 25 mg after several months if the symptoms respond to this therapy.

If the symptoms are not relieved, do not increase the dosage thinking more is better. Large doses of vitamin $B_6$ can cause numbness and tingling in the hands, a condition called peripheral neuropathy, and poor coordination. Megadose vitamin $B_6$ therapy also has caused permanent nerve damage. The threshold above which toxic symptoms occur appears to be above 250 mg of vitamin $B_6$ per day. However, a physician always should monitor the use of large supplemental doses of vitamin $B_6$ for the treatment of CTS. Other treatments that might help in the management of CTS include yoga and acupuncture.

# Cervical Dysplasia

Cervical dysplasia is an abnormal growth of tissue in the cervix. Most cases are harmless; however, in some cases the abnormal cells progress to cancer. Cervical cancer is largely preventable if this precancerous tissue is detected and treated at an early stage.

Although the causes of cervical dysplasia are poorly understood, this condition is associated with a sexually transmitted viral infection called the human papillomavirus (HPV). This virus also is found in healthy women, which implies something makes one woman more susceptible to infection than another. Several factors have been identified as possibly increasing the chances of developing dysplasia, including sexual and reproductive history, socioeconomic status, cigarette smoking, lowered immunity, and nutrition.

## Nutrition and Cervical Dysplasia

Vitamin deficiencies, especially folic acid and the antioxidants, are linked to increased risk for developing cervical dysplasia. These links are particularly interesting since deficiencies of these nutrients also are associated with other risk factors for cervical dysplasia, including oral contraceptive use, pregnancy, and cigarette smoking.

*Folic Acid:* Low levels of folic acid in cervical tissue are associated with an increased risk for developing cervical dysplasia. Marginal folic acid deficiency might make the cervical cells' genetic material more vulnerable to attack by the HPV, while normal to optimal folic acid intake might help genetic material within the cells resist viral attack. Another link is with homocysteine, a compound in the blood that increases when folic acid intake is inadequate. Elevated homocysteine might escalate risk for cervical dysplasia, according to a study from the University of Alabama.

Unfortunately, not all studies have shown a therapeutic effect. Some evidence suggests that too little folic acid predisposes a woman to cervical dysplasia, but trying to make up for lost time by supplementing won't reverse preexisting problems. It may be that folic acid is only beneficial in the prevention of cervical dysplasia, but has no effect once the condition is established.

Interestingly, some women with cervical dysplasia have normal blood folic acid levels, yet their cervical tissues are low in folic acid. Traditionally, nutrient requirements have been considered in terms of the whole person and are measured by blood levels. It now appears likely that localized nutrient deficiencies also can occur, sometimes triggered by medication (i.e., oral contraceptives) or other causes. In these cases, the blood levels of a vitamin such as folic acid are normal, while specific tissues remain deficient. These tissues appear to respond when greater than normal amounts of a nutrient are consumed.

*The Antioxidants:* The antioxidant nutrients, including vitamins C and E and beta carotene, show promise in preventing cervical dysplasia. Vitamin C intake is lower among women with cervical dysplasia compared to healthy women, and is related to as much as a tenfold higher risk for developing dysplasia. The risk for developing cervical dysplasia also increases as blood or cervical tissue levels of both vitamin E and beta carotene decrease.

It is hard to decipher the effects of these antioxidants alone, since they often are found in the same foods as folic acid. Beta carotene also might be a marker for other health-enhancing compounds in fruits and vegetables that prevent disease. Consequently, a deficiency of one is likely to result in deficiencies of other vitamins and phytochemicals. In addition, dietary intake and blood levels of both vitamin C and beta carotene are low in people who smoke, which is another risk factor for cervical dysplasia.

## Cervical Dysplasia: Diet Advice

The Healthy Woman's Diet is the foundation for the prevention of cervical dysplasia. Make sure to include two to three folic acid–rich foods, such as dark green leafy vegetables, legumes, or orange juice, in the daily menu. Choose very fresh produce (i.e., crispy dark green leafy vegetables), avoid long-term storage, and eat vegetables raw or only slightly cooked.

Make sure vitamin C and beta-carotene intakes are optimal by consuming additional citrus fruits and dark orange vegetables along with the folic acid–rich foods. A supplement that supplies moderate levels of vitamins C and E and folic acid also provides nutritional insurance.

Finally, and most importantly, schedule routine Pap smears and have your physician closely monitor any abnormal cell growth.

## *Chronic Fatigue Syndrome*

Chronic fatigue syndrome (CFS) is a collection of symptoms that includes muscle fatigue, sore throat, depression, insomnia, and poor concentration. A woman is exhausted, experiences head and joint aches, and has trouble remembering things. Upper respiratory infections, swollen lymph nodes, low blood pressure, and night sweats may develop. The symptoms are not dramatic; what makes this disorder unique is that symptoms linger for months and sometimes never resolve, but merely come and go. It also has been called the "yuppie disease," since most of the people who develop symptoms are white, educated professionals in their twenties and thirties. Women with CFS outnumber men two to one.

One theory is that the symptoms result from a viral infection, in particular the Epstein-Barr virus. Consequently, chronic fatigue syndrome also has been called chronic Epstein-Barr virus or CEBV. However, like chicken pox, the Epstein-Barr virus is very common. As many as 95 percent of all people have been exposed to this virus, but only a few develop CFS. Chronic fatigue sufferers often have high levels of antibodies to the Epstein-Barr virus, but that does not signify infection; antibodies also are high in energetic people with no symptoms. Consequently, the link between CFS and this virus remains controversial.

Accumulating evidence shows CFS should be classified into at least three categories:

- People with a previous history of psychological problems.
- People with other underlying disorders that exhibit similar symptoms to CFS.
- People with no history of emotional problems but who exhibit all the symptoms of CFS. This latter group might be suffering from a compromised immune system.

Since antibodies to the Epstein-Barr virus are found in both healthy and fatigued subjects, it is most likely that an abnormal immune system has led to infection, not just exposure to the virus. Several studies show CFS patients have lower numbers of white blood cells, such as T lymphocytes, and these immune cells are less active than those found in healthy individuals. At this time, it is not known whether the possible suppressed immunity is a cause or a result of CFS.

Interestingly, the integral link between mood, stress, and immunity is exemplified in CFS. Researchers report that depression is common in people with CFS, while antidepressant medications and sleep therapy are two treatments that appear to produce favorable results for CFS patients.

## Chronic Fatigue Syndrome: Diet Advice

Until more is known about the causes of CFS, the best dietary advice is to consume ample amounts of all the nutrients associated with a strong immune system. This would include a low-fat, nutrient-dense diet, as outlined in the Healthy Woman's Diet, comprised primarily of fresh fruits and vegetables, whole-grain breads and cereals, cooked dried beans and peas, with small amounts of nonfat milk or yogurt and fish or chicken. (See more on the immune system in chapter 15.) Amounts greater than recommended levels for the antioxidant nutrients, such as vitamin E, vitamin C, and beta carotene, might be required.

A few studies report that people suffering from CFS have low blood levels of magnesium and respond favorably to magnesium supplementation. How magnesium might exert its effects is poorly understood. Improvements in energy levels and mood reported in this study correspond with findings of other investigators who used magnesium at recommended levels to treat anxiety, insomnia, and organic mental disorders. Another study found that people with CFS have low blood levels of vitamin $B_6$. Whether or not increased intake of vitamin $B_6$ would aid in the treatment of CFS is unknown.

Bad habits, such as smoking, crash dieting, a sedentary lifestyle, and alcohol abuse, aggravate the symptoms of CFS, while regular exercise is good medicine for CFS. In athletes, overtraining or restrictive diets also are linked to an increased risk for CFS. In addition, it is likely a psychological component contributes to the condition. Professional women are at highest risk for CFS, which implies that the added stresses of career and maintaining a fit, not just thin, body combined with the age-old stress of maintaining a healthy marriage and raising well-adjusted children give women more to be sick and tired about.

Women spend four to eight hours a day on housework in addition to time spent on the job. In contrast, a typical husband spends less than two hours on domestic tasks. In another study, the average working mother spent forty hours at work and thirty-seven hours doing housework each week. In order to accomplish this schedule, women typically give up personal time, sleep, and play time. It is likely that this race to "do it all" contributes to the increased risk for developing CFS. If this is the case, then delegating responsibilities or letting go of the "super-woman" complex might be the best treatment for CFS.

# *The Common Cold*

The common cold is actually a group of minor infections lasting a few days that are caused by any one of almost two hundred different viruses. Symptoms usually are limited to congestion in the nose and a sore throat, but some viruses also affect the larynx (causing laryngitis) and the lungs (causing bronchitis). Sometimes a viral infection is followed by a more serious bacterial infection of the throat, lungs, or ears. Although colds are most common in infancy and early childhood when the immune system is still maturing, anyone at any time can catch a cold.

## Nutrition and the Common Cold

The link between nutrition and the common cold was made famous when the Nobel Laureate Linus Pauling theorized that megadoses of vitamin C would prevent or cure the common cold. Since that time, research on nutrition and the immune system has uncovered a wealth of evidence linking most vitamins and minerals to prevention of the common cold, the flu, other infections, and disease. In fact, all nutrients associated with strengthening the immune system, including beta carotene, vitamin E, the B vitamins, vitamin C, selenium, zinc, iron, and other minerals, are important for both the prevention and treatment of the common cold or any infection. (See chapter 14 for more information on nutrition and immunity.) Specific research on the common cold is limited to vitamin C, zinc, and a handful of herbs.

*Vitamin C:* Since Dr. Pauling's claims in the 1970s, a large number of studies have shown that vitamin C might not always prevent the common cold, but it is effective at reducing the duration and severity of its symptoms. In six out of eight studies investigating the effects of vitamin C on the common cold, doses of one to six grams taken daily decreased the duration or severity of the common cold by more than 20 percent in adults.

Vitamin C possibly stimulates the immune system, thus reducing the symptoms of the common cold. The vitamin is found in immune cells, such as phagocytes and lymphocytes, in concentrations up to a hundred times higher than in blood and other tissues, which suggests that it has an important physiological role in immunity. Vitamin C strengthens the immune system possibly by increasing the production or activity of interferon and white blood cells, which are responsible for destroying foreign invaders such as viruses and bacteria. There is a reduction in white blood cell formation and impaired wound healing when vitamin C is deficient in the diet, and the body's resistance to infection and disease improves with increased vitamin C intake.

*Zinc:* This trace mineral plays a fundamental role in maintaining a healthy immune system. Zinc deficiency impairs many aspects of immunity, while optimal intake enhances immune function even in healthy people. Zinc also has a direct effect on limiting the growth of microorganisms, such as bacteria and possibly viruses. For example, certain viruses cannot survive in a zinc-rich environment. This antiviral effect was the basis for zinc lozenges that dissolve in the mouth and coat the lining of the throat.

One study of forty-nine cold sufferers found that zinc gluconate lozenges reduced cold symptoms, including coughing, headaches, runny noses, and sore throats, within four days. Further research is needed before recommendations for the optimal dose of zinc in the treatment of the common cold can be made, especially since zinc is an example of more not necessarily being better.

*Herbs:* Extracts of echinacea (a member of the daisy family) are an age-old remedy for the common cold. A few studies show echinacea temporarily increases the body's resistance to upper respiratory infections. The liquid extract might work better than capsules. Other herbs that show some promise in helping reduce symptoms of the common cold include ginger, goldenseal, tiger balm, astragalus, peppermint tea, and mullein. Elderberry extract also might help fight the flu.

*Garlic:* Taking garlic at the first sign of a cold might help curb symptoms and shorten the duration of the illness. Allicin, a sulfur compound in garlic, has antibiotic effects and other compounds in garlic have antiviral and antibacterial properties.

### The Common Cold: Diet Advice

The Healthy Woman's Diet is the foundation for preventing and managing the common cold. In addition, make sure the diet contains optimal amounts of the vitamins and minerals essential for maintaining a strong immune system. Also consider the following:

- Extra nutritional insurance in the form of a moderate-dose vitamin C supplement might help prevent or curb the severity and/or duration of the common cold. For maximum effectiveness, take a low-dose vitamin C supplement (or better yet drink a glass of orange juice) every two hours beginning at the first sign of a cold and throughout the duration of the infection. Orange juice, oranges, and other citrus fruits high in vitamin C have an added advantage in that they also contain compounds called bioflavonoids that might help stimulate the immune system, providing additional health benefits in the fight against the common cold.
- Take zinc lozenges at the first sign of a cold. Take one lozenge every two to four hours (up to six a day) until symptoms subside. Allow the lozenges to dissolve in your mouth, don't chew them. Don't take lozenges for more than a week, since excessive zinc intake can produce a copper deficiency or even suppress the immune system. You also should eat something when you take them, since they can cause nausea on an empty stomach.
- Sip on chicken soup. Chicken contains an amino acid called cystine that is chemically similar to a drug prescribed for respiratory infections. The soup helps clear nasal congestion and eases breathing.
- Munch on garlic. Two cloves a day could keep the doctor away.

Other health habits that help prevent the common cold and aid in a speedy recovery include relaxation, seven or more hours of sleep each night, eight glasses of water daily, staying warm, increasing the moisture in the air with a vaporizer or humidifier, and possibly taking an aspirin at night to relieve aches and pains.

Consult a physician if the cold lasts more than ten days, if symptoms show the infection has spread beyond the nose and throat, or if you are susceptible to bronchitis or ear infections. Earaches, pain in the face or forehead, a temperature exceeding 102 degrees Fahrenheit, persistent hoarseness or sore throat, shortness of breath and wheeziness, and/or a dry painful cough are symptoms that require immediate medical attention.

# Cuts, Scratches, Bruises, and Burns

The healing of a cut, scrape, or wound requires a complex interplay of many body systems, including the immune system, the circulatory system, and cellular mechanisms responsible for the repair of damaged tissue and the growth of new tissue. Nutrition plays a fundamental role in each of these processes.

## Nutrition and Wounds

The nutritional needs for healing minor cuts and bruises are no different from those needed for maintaining health. However, even marginal deficiencies of some nutrients, such as vitamin C and zinc, can interfere with optimal recovery from everyday tissue damage, including athletic injuries, minor burns and cuts, or even sunburns. Nutrient needs before and following surgery increase to meet the demands of stress and wound healing. For example, poor healing of skin ulcers is associated with low blood levels of several trace minerals, such as zinc.

In general, all nutrients related to immune function (see chapter 14), the antioxidant system, and circulation, including protein, iron, the B vitamins, vitamin C, vitamin E, calcium, copper, and zinc, are needed in moderate amounts for optimal healing of cuts, burns, and bruises. Several of these nutrients also function directly in the healing process.

*Protein:* When tissues are damaged, the body rallies several systems to repair and build new tissue. Since skin and underlying tissues are composed primarily of protein, optimal dietary intake of this nutrient is essential for quick and complete healing of cuts, scrapes, burns, and other injuries. In addition, trauma and disease increase protein requirements above normal needs. Consumption of high-quality protein from nonfat milk, extra-lean meat, fish, chicken, or a combination of whole grains and legumes ensures production of specific tissue proteins during healing and recovery from surgery or minor wounds.

*Vitamin A:* The most well-defined role of vitamin A (and its building block beta carotene in fruits and vegetables) is to maintain healthy epithelial tissues of the skin, eyes, lungs, stomach, and other internal and external body surfaces. For years, vitamin A was called the "anti-infection" vitamin because it promotes the healing of infected tissues, such as the skin. More importantly, vitamin A maintains healthy skin so that it is less susceptible to infection and damage.

*The Antioxidants:* Limited evidence shows that vitamin E might be important in wound healing. Vitamin E reduces free radical damage to tissues, including skin grafts, and is helpful in the recovery from burns and other wounds.

Skin, blood vessel walls, and all body tissues are glued together by connective tissue, of which collagen is a major component. Repairing tissues includes producing and laying down new connective tissue and collagen. Vitamin C is a critical factor in collagen formation. In fact, most symptoms of scurvy, the classic deficiency syndrome associated with vitamin C, relate to the vitamin's role in collagen production. Small, dotlike bruises under the skin, swollen and bleeding gums, slow wound healing and poorly formed scars that break open, scaly skin, and tender joints are symptoms of vitamin C deficiency.

*Zinc:* A common symptom of zinc deficiency is poor wound healing, probably caused by defective production of collagen. In addition, trauma such as burns or surgery increases zinc loss in the urine, thus increasing the risk for poor wound healing and recovery. Marginal zinc intake even during healthy times has been reported in children, teenagers, pregnant women, seniors, vegetarians, athletes, and people following low-calorie diets. Zinc deficiency also is common during sickness and hospitalization.

Although increased intake of zinc either through dietary or supplemental sources is recommended for helping improve healing and recovery from injury, caution should be used in overdosing with this trace mineral. Intakes in excess of 50 mg could result in secondary deficiencies of other trace minerals, such as copper, or possibly could reduce immune function.

*Other Dietary Factors:* Many other substances help in wound healing. For example, compounds in garlic have antifungal and antibacterial properties that help combat infection. Several compounds in the aloe vera plant, when applied topically, also are effective in speeding the healing of cuts, burns, and other minor injuries.

## Cuts and Scrapes: Diet Advice

Dietary treatment of severe burns, surgical incisions, and other major wounds requires medical management, including supervision by a dietitian and physician. Minor cuts, burns, and bruises are most likely to heal quickly and completely when a woman follows the Healthy Woman's Diet. Make sure to consume daily:

- Two to three servings daily of high-quality protein. The typical American diet supplies two to three times normal dietary needs for protein and would be more than adequate to meet the extra tempo-rary demands during recovery and repair of damaged tissues. There is no need for protein supplements.

- Two to three servings daily of vitamin C–rich foods and of dark green leafy vegetables; beta carotene–rich foods, such as orange veg-etables; and vitamin E–rich foods, such as wheat germ.
- Several servings daily of zinc-rich foods. A supplement containing zinc in doses less than 30 mg might be necessary if dietary intake falls short of recommended amounts. Although zinc is best absorbed from lean meat, supplemental zinc also is well absorbed.

Other lifestyle habits that encourage optimal immune and circulatory func-tion, such as effective stress management, regular sleep patterns, daily exercise, avoidance of tobacco, and limited intake of alcohol, also help in the healing process.

## *Diabetes*

Diabetes is on the rise:

- 16 million people in the United States have diabetes, with only 10 million of those cases diagnosed; 8.1 million of those cases are women.
- 800,000 new cases of diabetes are diagnosed each year.
- Between 1990 and 1998, the incidence of diabetes increased: 70 per-cent in people thirty to thirty-nine years old; 40 percent in people forty to forty-nine years old; 31 percent in people fifty to fifty-nine years old.

### Defining Diabetes

Diabetes is classified into two separate types: Type I, also called insulin dependent (IDDM) or juvenile-onset diabetes and Type II, also called noninsulin dependent (NIDDM) or adult-onset diabetes. IDDM usually begins in childhood and starts suddenly. Severe symptoms develop soon after onset, and control of the disorder requires insulin. In contrast, NIDDM begins in the adult years, progression of the disease is slow, and symptoms are mild at first. It often progresses undetected, and is usually prevented and controlled with weight loss and lifestyle modification, or medication.

Diabetics are unable to use and metabolize dietary carbohydrates. Consequently, blood sugar levels are elevated (a condition called hyperglycemia) and there is an abnormal amount of sugar in the urine. In the diabetic, blood sugar cannot enter the cells at the normal rate. Cells are starved for energy, while blood sugar levels reach abnormally high levels and sugar spills into the urine through the kidneys. Diabetics are at increased risk for other life-threatening diseases, including heart disease, nerve damage, kidney failure, blindness, stroke, and gangrene.

## Diet and Diabetes

Diet is essential in the prevention, treatment, and control of diabetes. Eating well improves overall health and maintains a desirable body weight. It also helps stabilize blood sugar levels, and prevent or delay the development of cardiovascular disease, kidney disease, and eye or nerve disorders. The diet plan is designed to control the intake and percentage of carbohydrate, protein, and fat. Maintaining a desirable weight on the high-fiber, low-fat Healthy Woman's Diet reduces the need for medication and the risk for secondary diseases in patients with either NIDDM or IDDM. Vitamins and minerals, including the antioxidants, chromium, magnesium, zinc, and vitamin D, also contribute to the prevention and treatment of the disease and provide a second line of defense.

*Body Weight:* Excess body fat is a primary contributor to the development of NIDDM. Most women with NIDDM are overweight. Gaining as little as eleven pounds over a decade increases the risk for diabetes. In most cases, blood sugar stabilizes or returns to normal when a woman loses weight.

*Carbohydrates and Protein:* High-complex carbohydrate diets that include whole-grain breads and cereals, vegetables, cooked dried beans and peas, and other unrefined starches, with moderate amounts of protein and a low amount of fat are the mainstay in controlling diabetes, contrary to fad diets that blame carbohydrates as the cause of diabetes.

Replacing refined grains with whole grains lowers diabetes risk, state researchers at the Harvard University School of Medicine in Boston. Dietary intakes were taken for 75,521 women between the ages of thirty-eight years old and sixty-three years old and with no history of diabetes or heart disease. During the ten-year follow-up, 1,879 cases of diabetes were noted. Those women who consumed the most whole grains showed a 38 percent *reduction* in risk for diabetes, while women who consumed more refined grains showed a 31 percent *increase* in risk. The findings were most apparent in women who were overweight and the reduction in risk was caused by something more than just the increased content of fiber, magnesium, and vitamin E in the whole grains.

*The Glycemic Index:* Starchy foods produce different blood sugar responses. This effect is called the glycemic index of food. The index was developed by comparing the rise in blood sugar after a specific food was eaten. Pure sugar received a score of 100 and other sugary or starchy foods are compared to that. Cooked dried beans and peas produced some of the lowest scores (i.e., produced the smallest rise in blood sugar).

The glycemic index implies that dietary intake is more complicated than just simple versus complex carbohydrates. However, people seldom consume one food at a time, but rather eat meals comprised of a variety of foods, so the usefulness of the glycemic index has been questioned. Probably, most important to dia-

---

**TABLE 16.2    A Partial List of the Glycemic Index**

A high score on the glycemic index reflects a rapid rise in blood sugar when a food is consumed compared to a low score that reflects a modest rise in blood sugar.

| PERCENT | FOOD |
|---|---|
| 100 | Sugar |
| 80 to 90 | Carrots, cornflakes, honey, parsnips, potatoes |
| 70 to 79 | Whole-wheat bread, white rice |
| 60 to 69 | Bananas, white bread, raisins, brown rice |
| 50 to 59 | Oatmeal muffins, frozen peas, spaghetti, corn, yams, potato chips |
| 40 to 49 | Navy beans, oranges, orange juice, dried peas |
| 30 to 39 | Apples, chickpeas, milk, tomato soup, yogurt, ice cream |
| 20 to 29 | Kidney beans, lentils, fructose |
| 10 to 19 | Soybeans, peanuts |

betic control is consuming a variety of high-quality carbohydrate foods in conjunction with some protein and fat.

*Fiber:* Certain forms of fiber slow the rise in blood sugar after a meal, aid in the maintenance of normal blood sugar levels, and reduce the amount of sugar excreted in the urine. Oat bran, the fiber in cooked dried beans and peas, guar gum, and pectin in fruits are especially effective in the control of blood sugar levels; however, consumption of all fiber foods, including the fiber in whole-grain breads and cereals and vegetables, also lowers a woman's risk for diabetes.

*Fish Oils:* Fish oils and monounsaturated fats, such as olive oil, might be two types of fat that help prevent or control diabetes. Fish oils increase the concentration of these fats in the pancreas, blood, and muscles; help regulate blood sugar levels; and reduce the risk for developing heart disease and high blood pressure. Within one month of replacing meat and fatty dairy foods (saturated fats) with monounsaturated fats, diabetics at Texas Southwestern Medical Center in Dallas showed increased HDL-cholesterol levels, lower blood sugar levels, reduced insulin requirements, and decreased triglyceride levels.

*The Antioxidants:* Free radicals might damage cell membranes and impair insulin activity in diabetes, while optimal intake of antioxidants, including vitamins C and E and the carotenoids, helps prevent this damage. Adequate intake of vitamin C might help regulate blood sugar levels and aid in the prevention of diabetes. Diabetics show altered vitamin C metabolism and low tissue levels of the vitamin. This might partially explain why some immune functions are suppressed in diabetics. Caution must be used when diabetics supplement with vitamin C, since vitamin C even in moderate daily doses of 250 mg might interfere with the urinary test for glucose.

Besides its antioxidant effects in the prevention of diabetes, limited evidence shows vitamin E also might improve blood sugar regulation, insulin action, and insulin response. Diabetics and people at risk for developing diabetes often have low blood vitamin E levels, which suggests that the disease alters how the body uses vitamin E. Limited evidence shows that the progression of atherosclerosis in diabetics might be slowed when vitamin E is increased in the diet.

*Chromium:* The trace mineral chromium is a component of glucose tolerance factor, a compound made in the body that works with the hormone insulin to move sugar out of the blood and into the body's cells. Chromium improves insulin binding to cells, insulin receptor numbers, and activates insulin receptor enzymes leading to increased insulin sensitivity. A chromium deficiency resembles diabetes, including elevated insulin in the blood, numbness in the toes and fingers, increased blood sugar, glucose intolerance, and reduced muscle strength and coordination. These symptoms disappear with chromium supplementation in some people.

Chromium improves insulin resistance and lowers the risk for developing diabetes, even in the presence of a high-fat diet, according to researchers at the U.S.D.A. Human Nutrition Research Center in Beltsville, Maryland. Rats fed high-fat, chromium-poor diets showed poor glucose clearing from the blood and increased insulin resistance, both factors associated with the development of diabetes. Adding chromium to the diet lowers blood triglyceride levels, hastens glucose clearance from the blood, and reduces the insulin response. The researchers concluded that "insulin resistance induced by feeding a high-fat . . . diet is improved with chromium."

Most people do just fine with 50 mcg to 200 mcg of chromium, but according to Dr. Richard Anderson and colleagues at the U.S.D.A. Beltsville Human Nutrition Research Center, some diabetics might need as much as five times this amount. Type II diabetics were daily given either placebos or chromium supplements totaling 200 mcg to 1,000 mcg of chromium picolinate while continuing their normal diets and medications. Within two months, the diabetics taking

**TABLE 16.3    Where Do You Get Chromium?**

| FOOD | CHROMIUM (MCG/SERVING) |
| --- | --- |
| Beef, extra-lean, 3 ounces | 38.0 |
| Sweet potato, 1 | 36.0 |
| Egg, 1 | 26.0 |
| All-bran cereal, 1 cup | 14.0 |
| Oatmeal, 1 cup | 12.9 |
| Orange juice, 1 cup | 9.6 |
| Molasses, 2 tbsp. | 4.4 |
| Whole-wheat cereal, 1 cup | 3.0 |
| Wheat germ, 2 tbsp. | 1.4 |
| Banana, 1 | 1.0 |

1,000 mcg of chromium showed significant improvement in glucose tolerance, while the diabetics taking 200 mcg showed some improvement within four months.

*Magnesium:* Magnesium metabolism is altered in diabetics and might contribute to the development and progression of the disease. Not only is magnesium deficiency one of the most common disturbances in mineral metabolism observed in diabetics, but low blood magnesium levels are associated with many complications of diabetes, including heart disease and high blood pressure.

Magnesium functions in more than three hundred processes related to carbohydrate, protein, and fat metabolism and is involved in the regulation of insulin and blood sugar regulation. Magnesium supplementation restores low blood and tissue levels, helps correct glucose intolerance, produces a protective effect against heart disease, and might aid in the prevention of eye disorders associated with diabetes and, possibly, even the progression of the disease.

*Other Minerals:* Even marginal deficiencies of copper, vanadium, manganese, and zinc might contribute to abnormal blood sugar regulation and the development or progression of diabetes and its health complications. In addition, deficiencies of these minerals have been identified in diabetics; urinary losses often are increased, while blood levels are low in uncontrolled diabetes. Zinc is a component of insulin and might aid in insulin regulation. A zinc deficiency also impairs immune function, which would contribute to increased infection, leg ulcers, and other problems in diabetics. Copper, vanadium, and manganese deficiencies are associated with abnormal blood sugar regulation, which is reversed when dietary or supplemental intake of these minerals is increased.

*Herbs:* Ginseng might help in the prevention of diabetes. At the University of Toronto in Ontario, ten nondiabetic people on twelve separate occasions randomly received either placebos or three, six, or nine grams of American ginseng before an oral glucose challenge test. Results showed that compared with placebos, ginseng reduced blood glucose levels after an oral dose of sugar. All doses of ginseng were effective at lowering blood sugar levels.

## Diabetes: Diet Advice

The primary goal in the dietary management of diabetes, both IDDM and NIDDM, is control of blood sugar levels with a fasting blood sugar no higher than 109 mg. A woman with diabetes should work closely with a physician and dietitian to establish a high-fiber, low-fat diet and exercise program that balances blood sugar and food intake with exercise and body weight. Losing even ten to twenty pounds for an overweight woman often prevents the need for medication. The Healthy Woman's Diet can form the foundation for this individualized nutrition program.

Vitamin and mineral deficiencies are common in NIDDM diabetics. If the calorie intake is below 2,000 calories, a moderate-dose multiple vitamin and mineral supplement that contains all the vitamins and most of the minerals, especially chromium, copper, magnesium, manganese, and zinc, should provide adequate intake of these nutrients. Women who take moderate-dose vitamin and mineral supplements might lower their risk for developing diabetes, according to a study from the Center for Disease Control and Prevention in Atlanta. Using dietary intake information from a national nutrition survey, the researchers compared people who later developed diabetes with those who remained diabetes-free during the following twenty years. Results showed that women who took supplements lowered their diabetes risk by 16 percent.

*The Exchange Lists:* The Diabetic Exchange Lists developed by the American Diabetes Association and the American Dietetic Association are the most widely used system for diabetic menu planning. These lists group foods according to calorie, protein, carbohydrate, and fat contents into seven lists. For example, fruits are primarily found in one exchange list, while vegetables are found in another, and fats/oils are found in another list.

The term "exchange" refers to a serving of food that can be exchanged for any other food within the same list. The total calorie content of the diet, based on the number of servings from each list, depends on a woman's preferences, metabolic needs, and physical activity. The glycemic index was not considered when these lists were developed; however, a woman can combine the exchange lists with the Glycemic Index and choose those foods within each list that have a score of 50 or less.

Using the lists, diabetics need about 10 to 20 percent of calories from protein, 30 percent or less from fat, and the remaining 50 to 60 percent of calories from high-quality carbohydrates and a few sweets. The lists are used to make food selections and plan menus. Meal and snack intake must coordinate with insulin administration to guarantee the optimal balance between insulin and blood sugar levels. Vegetarian diets also are effective in the treatment of diabetes and can be designed using the same dietary guidelines and exchange lists.

*Lifestyle:* Aerobic exercise, such as brisk walking, aerobic dance, jumping rope, swimming, jogging, or stationary or outdoor bicycling, performed three to

**TABLE 16.4    The Exchange Lists**

| LIST | CARBOHYDRATE (GRAMS) | PROTEIN (GRAMS) | FAT (GRAMS) | CALORIES |
|------|------------|---------|-----|----------|
| Milk, nonfat | 12 | 8 | Trace | 90 |
| low-fat | 12 | 8 | 5 | 120 |
| whole | 12 | 8 | 10 | 165 |
| Vegetable | 5 | 2 | 0 | 25 |
| Fruit | 15 | 0 | 0 | 60 |
| Bread/starch | 15 | 3 | Trace | 80 |
| Meat/protein | | | | |
| low-fat | 0 | 7 | 3 | 55 |
| medium-fat | 0 | 7 | 5 | 75 |
| high-fat | 0 | 7 | 8 | 100 |
| Fat | 0 | 0 | 5 | 45 |
| Free foods | 0 | 0 | 0 | 0 |

four times a week, for twenty minutes or more with the supervision of a physician and trained exercise physiologist lowers blood sugar, body weight, body fat, and reduces the diabetic's risk for developing heart disease.

## *Eyes and Vision*

What you eat throughout life and whether or not you supplement might determine whether or not you battle the main causes later in life of vision loss, cataracts, and age-related macular degeneration (ARMD).

The lens of the eye must remain clear to focus light on the retina. As a person ages, an opaque, cloudy area can occur on the lens. This opacification, or cataract, blocks or distorts light entering the eye and progressively reduces vision. The main symptom of cataracts is a slow deterioration of vision in the affected eye(s), with the lens becoming visibly opaque or white in the later stages.

## Diet and Cataracts

The primary cause of cataracts was thought to be old age, since the majority of people over seventy-five years old develop cataracts, and many age-related injuries/debilities are associated with damage and accumulation of proteins that cloud the lens. However, many young people also develop the condition. Interestingly, in lesser-developed nations, cataracts occur more frequently in younger segments of the population, suggesting factors other than age might play a critical role in the genesis and progression of cataracts.

*The Antioxidants:* The formation of cataracts probably involves a number of physiological factors. However, a high correlation between cataract incidence and solar radiation, as well as the known cataract-producing effects of oxygen, suggest that free radical exposure results in a cascade of toxic reactions leading to cataracts. (See chapter 14 for more information on free radicals and antioxidants.)

Exposure to free radicals causes many of the changes in the lens that accumulate throughout life. Proteins within the lens are damaged, probably by repeated exposure to ultraviolet (UV) light and oxygen. These modifications might lead to the formation of protein "clumps" that scatter light and contribute to the development of cataracts. The lens takes the brunt of this exposure, since one of its prime functions is to serve as an optical filter so that UV light to the retina is greatly minimized. However, this filtering process also subjects the lens to constant exposure to free radicals and potential free radical damage.

According to two studies, one from the Harvard School of Public Health and another from Tufts University, free radical damage to the eyes' lenses is a major contributor to the development of cataracts. The Harvard study found that this free radical damage contributes to both heart disease and cataract formation. The Tufts study found that the lowest risk for cataract formation was in people who consumed antioxidant-rich diets, especially diets high in vitamin C, vitamin E, and the carotenoids beta carotene, lutein, and zeaxanthin. Risk also decreased when people took daily multivitamin and mineral supplements and in women who took vitamin C supplements for at least ten years.

People with cataracts consume significantly less beta carotene, vitamin C, vitamin E, and/or less than four servings daily of fresh fruits and vegetables compared to healthy people. Up to a 70 percent reduction in risk for developing cataracts is reported when people consume diets rich in carotenoids (the beta carotene–like compounds in dark green and orange vegetables) and vitamins C and E.

Some of the highest concentrations of vitamin C in the body are found in various fluids and tissues of the eyes. In humans, the vitamin C content of the eye is twenty times greater than in the blood. Interestingly, nocturnal animals with little exposure to UV light have very low concentrations of vitamin C in eye tissue, while diurnal animals have up to thirty-five times the vitamin C in ocular tissues. This suggests that a high vitamin C concentration is an adaptation that protects the eyes against solar radiation.

Women with cataracts have lower levels of this antioxidant nutrient in eye tissue than do women who are cataract-free, and the severity of the cataracts increases as vitamin C levels decrease. In contrast, persons with higher vitamin C status, especially women who supplement their diets for years, have diminished risk of developing cataracts.

Supplementation with vitamin C also raises eye concentrations of the vitamin, but dietary intake of vitamin C might not be adequate to prevent cataract formation. In one study, women who supplemented with vitamin C for more than ten years had up to an 83 percent lower prevalence of cataracts, compared with women who did not supplement. Other antioxidants, such as vitamin E, also show promise in reducing cataract formation.

People with high blood levels of antioxidants are at reduced risk for developing cataracts compared with people whose diets are low in these nutrients. While cataract risk increases and vitamin E levels decrease, risk is reduced by more than 50 percent when people supplement their diets with vitamin E. It appears that vitamin E cannot prevent cataracts, but optimal intake of the vitamin might delay the onset and slow the progression of lens damage associated with cataracts.

## Diet and ARMD

Macular degeneration is a disease affecting the retina, the light-sensitive area at the back of the eye that transmits visual impressions from the lens to the brain. Older persons with light-colored eyes are particularly susceptible, as are people who smoke or are frequently exposed to harsh sunlight. However, anyone can develop macular degeneration.

*Fruits and Vegetables:* People with ARMD typically consume fewer fruits and vegetables than do people who maintain healthy eyesight throughout life. In contrast, people who consume diets rich in fruits and vegetables, such as tomatoes and dark green leafy vegetables like spinach, maintain higher blood levels of carotenoids, including lycopene, lutein, and zeaxanthin. They are also less likely to lose their sight and if they do, the disease is less likely to progress to advanced stages.

*The Antioxidants:* The antioxidant nutrients, such as vitamins C and E, and the carotenoids including lutein and selenium, might counteract some of the harmful processes associated with macular degeneration, thus helping prevent damage to the retina. People who supplement with vitamin E have a lower risk for ARMD. The eye has one of the richest stores of selenium. This trace mineral, along with zinc, maintains optimal eye function and protects the eyes from free radical damage.

*Fat:* High-fat diets increase a person's risk for developing ARMD, while fish might protect against this leading cause of vision loss, according to data from the Nurses' Health Study and the Health Professionals Follow-Up Study at Harvard Medical School in Boston. The study included 42,743 women older than fifty years with no history of ARMD who were followed for several years. Those who consumed the highest-fat diets were 54 percent more likely to develop ARMD than those who consumed the lowest-fat diets. The greatest risk was noted for vegetable oils, while women who consumed at least four servings of fish each week had a 35 percent lower risk of developing ARMD compared to women who ate three or fewer servings of fish. Atherosclerosis of the arteries supplying the eyes is one possible contributor to ARMD. Thus, dietary fats that raise heart-disease risk also might increase risk for ARMD. In addition, fats susceptible to free radical damage, such as linolenic acid in vegetable oils, might explain why these fats raise ARMD risk, since they would generate increased oxidative stress on eye tissues.

*Zinc:* This trace mineral helps prevent ARMD. A zinc-dependent enzyme that is necessary for normal eye function slows with age. People who consume zinc-rich diets have a 40 percent reduction in risk compared to people who consume zinc-poor diets, especially if the nutrient-rich diet was consumed throughout life. Zinc appears to be less effective in halting or reversing the disease in later stages of ARMD.

## Vision: Diet Advice

Prolonged exposure to free radicals, not aging per se, is likely to be a primary cause of cataracts. Although the research is in the early stages, optimal intake of zinc, the antioxidant nutrients vitamins C and E, and the carotenoids including lutein, and selenium, might help prevent or slow the progress of eye disorders, such as cataracts and macular degeneration.

A vitamin-rich diet composed of eight to ten servings daily of fresh fruits and vegetables is usually sufficient to reduce cataract risk. However, some studies show supplemental doses of vitamin C (500 mg to 1,000 mg) and vitamin E (200 IU to 400 IU) might be necessary to provide maximum protection. Selenium and zinc should be limited to no more than 200 mcg and 30 mg, respectively, unless monitored by a physician.

In addition to the antioxidant nutrients, optimal intake of the B vitamins and vitamin A, and several servings weekly of fish, combined with a low-fat diet might help in the prevention and/or treatment of some eye disorders. Avoiding exposure to free radicals in tobacco smoke, air pollution, and sunlight also are important in the prevention of cataracts.

# Fatigue

Fatigue, tiredness, and lethargy are common symptoms of numerous emotional, mental, and physical problems. Stress, poor sleeping habits, overwork, infection, and disease are only a few of the causes of fatigue. A woman also might feel "under the weather," "not up to par," "not as energetic as I used to feel," because of marginal nutrient deficiencies. (Also see Chronic Fatigue Syndrome on pages 301 to 303.)

## Diet and Fatigue

Inadequate intake of any nutrient can cause fatigue. Protein and/or calorie malnutrition results in a number of symptoms, including lethargy and apathy. This condition is rare in the United States, but is seen in women with eating disorders such as anorexia, hospitalized patients, and the elderly. A compromised immune system resulting from marginal deficiencies of one or more nutrients also lowers a woman's energy level and increases the risk for fatigue, infection, and disease. (See chapter 14 for more information on nutrition and immunity.)

Poor dietary choices, such as grabbing a candy bar for quick energy, can affect a woman's "get up and go." The jolt of energy from a high-sugar food is a temporary high, but within no time the elevated blood sugar levels are countered by insulin and often fall to below normal levels, leaving a woman feeling more tired than before the snack.

The combined effect of coffee and doughnuts (or any sugary food) escalates blood sugar problems, since caffeine also stimulates the flow of insulin. In contrast, alcohol has a numbing effect on the nervous system, causing drowsiness and apathy. Alcohol and caffeine also interfere with a good night's sleep, resulting in fatigue. Finally, mild dehydration can cause fatigue and weakness. By the time a woman is thirsty, she is already dehydrated and suffering from fatigue as a result.

*Iron:* Next time you reach for a cup of coffee to boost your energy level, think again. If you are a premenopausal woman, you might need iron, not coffee. In one study on 14,762 young women (ages eighteen to twenty-three years old) and 14,072 middle-age women (ages forty-five to fifty years old), those women with recent histories of iron deficiency scored lowest on tests for physical and mental energy as well as vitality. The women were not anemic, but had been diagnosed with iron deficiency, a preanemic stage, within the past two years. The researchers conclude that "iron deficiency is associated with decreased general health and well-being and increased fatigue."

Low intake of iron is a main reason for fatigue in women (see pages 246 to 254 for more on iron-deficiency anemia). Iron gives red blood cells their ability to transport oxygen to all the body's tissues, including the muscles, brain and nervous system, and organs. Inadequate iron intake results in reduced oxygen supply to the tissues, which causes fatigue, weakness, being out of breath after minor physical effort, and poor concentration.

*Other Minerals:* A deficiency of one or more minerals results in fatigue because a malnourished body has less energy to complete normal daily tasks and because of direct effects on metabolism and nerve function. A magnesium deficiency causes muscle weakness and fatigue, possibly because of the mineral's roles in converting carbohydrates, protein, and fats into energy; removing toxic substances such as ammonia from the body; nerve transmission; and muscle contraction and relaxation.

Overt magnesium deficiencies are rare in this country; however, many Americans consume less than Recommended Dietary Allowance (RDA) levels and are at risk for marginal deficiencies. Lifestyle factors, such as physical or emotional stress, that also are associated with fatigue increase urinary loss of magnesium and further increase the need for this mineral.

Inadequate intake of potassium, chloride, or manganese also causes fatigue and muscle weakness. Deficiencies of cobalt, copper, or selenium result in anemia, which is associated with fatigue, poor concentration, and general weakness. As a component of the thyroid hormones, iodine helps regulate metabolism. Inadequate intake of this mineral results in goiter, with symptoms of lethargy. Finally, zinc is an essential component of numerous enzymes and functions in the metabolism of protein and the conversion of calorie-containing nutrients to energy. Zinc helps regulate insulin metabolism and blood sugar levels, strengthen the immune system, and maintain normal red blood cell levels. A deficiency of this trace mineral results in anemia and general weakness. Excessive intake of several essential minerals, including selenium, and toxic metals, such as silver, aluminum, cadmium, or lead, also is associated with weakness and fatigue.

*The Vitamins:* Several vitamins affect a woman's energy level. Deficiencies of vitamins E, $B_2$, $B_6$, $B_{12}$, and C; folic acid; or biotin result in anemia with symptoms of fatigue, poor concentration, apathy, and being out of breath after minor exertion. Many of the B vitamins, such as vitamins $B_1$, $B_2$, $B_6$; pantothenic acid; and niacin, are vital to the production of energy in the body. It is not surprising that even a marginal deficiency of one or more of these nutrients results in general fatigue, muscle fatigue, and weakness.

## Fatigue: Diet Advice

The Healthy Woman's Diet is the best protection against diet-induced fatigue. In addition,

- Consume at least six to eight glasses of water daily, even when not thirsty. Since thirst is a poor indicator of water needs, a general guideline for water intake is to drink twice as much water as quenches thirst.
- Limit caffeine intake to two cups or less each day and do not drink caffeinated beverages after midday.
- Avoid alcohol and limit sugary foods.
- Divide the total food intake into four or more small meals throughout the day to maintain normal blood sugar levels.
- Eat breakfast. Skipping the morning meal can result in reduced blood sugar levels (and fatigue) that do not return to normal even after eating later in the day.
- Avoid large or high-fat meals that can leave you drowsy.
- Include moderate daily aerobic exercise (i.e, brisk walking, jogging, swimming, or aerobic dance), relaxation, and stress management in the daily routine. Often people who complain of low energy find energy levels improve when they exercise.

Poor dietary habits are one of many causes of fatigue. If the fatigue lingers despite improvements in diet, exercise, and stress management, consult a physician to rule out other causes of chronic tiredness. (Also see sections on Hypoglycemia and Insomnia.)

## *Fibrocystic Breast Disease*

Fibrocystic breast disease (FBD) is characterized by painful, lumpy breasts. FBD is the most frequent disorder of the breast experienced by premenopausal women. More than one in every two women has obvious signs of FBD; 90 percent have at least the cellular changes associated with the condition. Women in their forties are at greatest risk.

FBD progresses through three stages. In the first stage, which usually develops between the late teens and early thirties, a few lumps are present and the breasts are tender and full for approximately one week prior to menstruation. In the second stage, which usually develops in the mid-thirties to early forties, the pain intensifies and continues longer. The breasts also might develop a granular or nodular consistency. Often a woman at this stage consults a physician for fear the lumps might be cancer. In the third stage, which develops during the late forties and fifties, the discomfort is more diffuse and pain often develops suddenly. Lumps can cluster and even the slightest touch is painful.

More than twenty-seven names are used for FBD, including benign breast disease, mammary dysplasia, and cystic mastalgia. FBD actually is an umbrella term for any condition characterized by cyclical changes in the breasts accompanied by lumps, cysts, and pain. Specific names for the condition are based on the type of breast tissue involved, such as the milk duct, the glands, or other tissue. FBD is such a vague diagnosis, with consequences ranging from none to breast cancer, that the American Cancer Society's National Task Force on Breast Cancer Control discourages the word "disease" and recommends the terms "fibrocystic changes" or "fibrocystic condition."

The cause of FBD is unknown, although an association with the ovarian hormones is suspected. This theory is supported by findings that oral contraceptives relieve the symptoms of FBD in as many as 85 percent of women. It is unknown, however, whether the association between hormones and FBD is caused by abnormal production of hormones or by exaggerated responses in breast tissue to the hormones. The pain experienced is probably caused by nerve irritation secondary to fluid accumulation (edema). Nerve pinching, the accumulation of tough fibrous tissue (fibrosis), and an associated inflammatory response to the fibrocystic changes also could produce pain and tenderness.

## FBD and Breast Cancer: Is There a Link?

There might be a link between FBD and breast cancer. Both diseases are associated with abnormal hormone metabolism, especially estrogen and progesterone. In addition, frequently the two coexist, which supports a relationship. This link is dependent on the woman's family history of breast disease and the type of cysts, their content, and possibly the number and frequency of development.

FBD typically precedes the development of breast cancer by about 10 to 15 years and only one in every eleven women with FBD develops breast cancer. However, a woman with the right type of FBD has as much as a five to nine times greater risk than does a woman with other types of FBD.

The Cancer Committee of the College of American Pathologists states the type of fibrocystic changes must be specified by a biopsy. Women with tissue changes called atypical hyperplasia with borderline lesions (that is, cancerlike cells are observed under a microscope but there are not enough to make a diagnosis of cancer) have a five times greater risk of developing breast cancer. Women with tissue changes called hyperplasia (increased numbers of cells) derived from a specialized cell type in the breast called epithelial cells, especially if those cells are located in the milk ducts, are up to two times more likely to develop breast cancer. (A family history of breast cancer raises the risk even higher.) All other types of cysts have little or no association with breast cancer.

## Diet and FBD

How, and even if, diet affects FBD is vague. Other lifestyle factors, such as lean body weight, high socioeconomic status, and advanced education, show a slight positive correlation with risk for developing FBD. These lifestyle factors also are related to increased consumption of saturated fats and other harmful dietary substances; however, a direct association between diet and FBD has not been found.

*Caffeine:* In early studies, as many as 65 percent of women experienced total disappearance of FBD symptoms when they eliminated coffee, tea, chocolate, and other caffeine-containing substances from their diets. However, this research was poorly designed and has not been widely accepted. More recent research shows little or no association between caffeine consumption and FBD.

*The Antioxidants:* Early studies on vitamin E and FBD produced promising results. However, subsequent studies, which were better designed, found no consistent association between vitamin E intake and the alleviation of FBD symptoms. Some women apparently do respond favorably to supplemental doses of vitamin E, with improvements in pain, congestion, and tenderness. Interestingly, women in these studies who take placebos (inactive pills thought by the person to be vitamin E) also report improvement in symptoms, suggesting a possible mind-over-matter component to the disorder.

*Dietary Fat:* A reduction in dietary fat might help prevent or treat FBD. Risk increases with high-fat diets; however, saturated fats show the strongest association with risk. When dietary fat is reduced to 20 percent of total calories, some women report a reduction in breast pain, while blood levels of the female hormones estrogen and prolactin decrease. Although a reduction in these hormones is associated with a reduced risk for developing cancer, the link to FBD remains unclear.

Evening primrose oil has received some attention as an FBD treatment. One study on two hundred women found a slightly lower incidence of cyst formation in the group given evening primrose oil. However, more studies are needed before recommendations can be made.

## FBD: Diet Advice

To be safe, every woman experiencing a solid mass in her breast after her menstrual cycle, regardless of what a mammogram shows, should have the tissue biopsied. As many as 15 percent of all palpable breast cancers are not evident on a mammogram, so a biopsy is the only way to detect a harmless lump from a lump or cyst that is associated with breast cancer.

Hormone and medication therapy is the most common treatment. In addition, a well-padded, supportive bra can reduce the strain on the ligaments. Stress also worsens symptoms, so effective stress management is advised.

It is wise to consume a low-fat, nutrient-dense diet, such as the Healthy Woman's Diet, that includes fresh fruits and vegetables, cooked dried beans and peas, and whole-grain breads and cereals, with a moderate intake of nonfat milk and milk products, fish, and poultry. Avoid or limit saturated fat to no more than 10 percent of calories, and consume alcohol in moderation, if at all.

Some women respond favorably to increasing vitamin E intake and eliminating methylxanthine-containing foods, such as coffee, cola drinks, and tea, from the diet. Since there is no harm in testing these dietary changes, a four- to six-month trial might be useful.

# *Fibromyalgia*

As many as six million Americans, most of them women, wake up every morning feeling terrible, and the pain doesn't let up all day. They have fibromyalgia, a musculoskeletal disorder with symptoms including pain in the muscles and soft tissues, unrelenting fatigue, headaches, bowel problems, anxiety, depression, and insomnia. If that wasn't enough, fibromyalgia is very difficult to diagnose. The symptoms ebb and flow and often overlap with other disorders, such as lupus, hypothyroidism, arthritis, or chronic fatigue syndrome. Often the only way to identify this problem is to press on eighteen points on the body that typically are tender in the fibromyalgic patient. If at least eleven of these points are painfully sensitive and the patient has had widespread pain for several months, a rheumatologist will probably rule out other disorders and settle on a diagnosis of fibromyalgia.

There is no known cause for fibromyalgia. Sufferers have higher levels of a compound called substance P, a chemical involved in pain transmission. They also have lower levels of the nerve chemical serotonin, which otherwise aids in sleep and pain tolerance. People with fibromyalgia have abnormal brain waves during deep sleep, a phase of sleep when the body usually makes growth hormone. Levels of this hormone, which help keep muscles and other soft tissues healthy, also are lower in people with fibromyalgia. Yet, what causes these imbalances remains a mystery.

No medication can cure fibromyalgia, but a combination of medications sometimes is helpful in relieving symptoms. Antidepressants aid mood and sleep problems and tranquilizers are used as muscle relaxants to promote sleep. Nonsteroidal anti-inflammatory medications, such as ibuprofen, have not proven very effective. Many people with fibromyalgia who find no relief from typical medical avenues, turn to unconventional therapies with varying success. Diet, exercise, supplements, acupuncture, massage, and herbs have helped some people.

## Fibromyalgia: Diet Advice

People with fibromyalgia find different dietary habits more or less effective in treating the symptoms of their disorders. While none of these dietary practices has been studied, it is worth trying some, such as eliminating all yeast-producing foods, in an effort to alleviate pain. The disorder is associated with low levels of some nutrients, such as selenium and vitamin D, but it is unknown whether increasing intake of foods rich in these nutrients will help curb symptoms. Symptoms of fibromyalgia were reduced when people consumed vegan diets rich in lactobacteria (from yogurt) in a study from the University of Kuopia, Finland. Eliminating foods that contain the additive MSG also might help reduce symptoms. Supplements of a green alga called *Chlorella pyrenoidosa* improved symptoms in some fibromyalgia patients in another study.

Other possible treatments include:

- Supplements of magnesium and malic acid, as well as the herbs boswellia extract and ashwagandha, help curb symptoms in some patients.
- Eliminate alcohol, since it typically aggravates symptoms.
- Exercise provides more symptom relief than many medications. Walking, swimming, cycling, and stretching rank highest in relieving pain.
- Whirlpools, warm baths, hot tubs, and massage might help.

Until more is known, your best bet is to consume the Healthy Woman's Diet, which provides all the building blocks your body needs to rally its own defenses against disorders like fibromyalgia.

# Fluid Retention

Fluid retention, more commonly called bloating, can result from simple temporary fluctuations in hormones such as is observed in premenstrual syndrome (PMS), or from excessive intake of salty foods, malnutrition, or serious disorders such as congestive heart failure or kidney disease.

## Nutrition and Fluid Retention

Edema, the technical term for fluid retention, is a consequence of several severe nutrient deficiencies, including protein and vitamin C. For example, a vitamin C–deficient diet reduces production and maintenance of the connective tissue that holds all cells and tissues together. The blood vessels, cell membranes, and other barriers that hold fluids in their appropriate spaces become porous, allowing fluids to leak into surrounding tissues and causing swelling. In contrast, excessive intake of some nutrients, such as vitamin A, also causes fluid retention in some people.

*Salt:* Do you wake up with puffy eyes in the morning? Do your shoes fit too tightly at certain times of the day? Is it well past noon before your rings are loose enough to remove? If so, your water retention probably stems from eating too many salty foods.

When the diet is high in salt, the body retains fluids in an effort to maintain a constant ratio of water to sodium. Once the sodium dilution reaches normal, then the kidneys excrete the accumulated water along with the sodium. Consequently, the best way to prevent salt-induced bloating is to eat a low-salt diet. The best way to treat this condition is to drink more water, which flushes out the sodium.

*Vitamin $B_6$ and GLA:* Bloating is a common problem in premenstrual syndrome (PMS). Some women report improvement in PMS-induced bloating with supplements of vitamin $B_6$ or evening primrose oil (a source of the fatty acid gamma linolenic acid or GLA). In addition, nutrients related to converting GLA to its metabolically active form include magnesium, vitamin $B_6$, zinc, niacin, and vitamin C. However, there is no evidence to show that these nutrients decrease fluid retention.

## Fluid Retention: Diet Advice

Temporary fluid retention most likely results from excessive salt intake. Eliminate or limit your intake of salty foods, remove the salt shaker from the table, reduce the amount of salt in recipes, and monitor other sources of sodium-containing foods and additives and you probably will remedy this form of fluid retention.

Drink six to eight glasses of water each day. Caffeinated beverages and alcohol are mild diuretics that interfere with normal sodium excretion. Drink them sparingly and don't consider them part of your total fluid intake.

More serious fluid retention, or edema, results from protein malnutrition. This condition is rare in the United States where most people eat too much, rather than not enough, protein. Women on very low calorie diets or poorly planned vegetarian diets, hospital patients, and the elderly are at potential risk for protein malnutrition, and are at increased risk for developing a variety of diet-related disorders.

# *Food Intolerance and Allergies*

One in every three people avoids a food for one reason or another. Considering the millions of known and unknown compounds in foods, both natural and added during processing and packaging, it is amazing that more people are not affected by food intolerances. It is likely that many symptoms are mild and go unnoticed or the reaction is vague or delayed and is not associated with a particular food. Reactions to a food are classified into a variety of disorders, including allergies, sensitivities, intolerance, pseudo-intolerance, and idiosyncrasies.

*Food Allergy:* Food allergies are rare and result from an immune system response to a food component. Reactions occur within minutes to several hours after consumption of the offending food or may take up to five days to develop. In either case, the symptoms reflect a release of histamine or other physiologically active compounds in the body. Symptoms of food allergies are restricted to the respiratory tract, the digestive tract, and the skin. Symptoms can be mild to severe, ranging from mild skin redness to anaphylactic reactions. The diagnosis is complicated and requires a diet history, a complete review of a person's medical and symptoms history, and multiple tests conducted by a trained health professional. Self-tests and tests conducted by a nonmedical person, including cytotoxic tests, sublingual tests, hair analysis, and symptom-provocation tests, are not reliable.

*Food Sensitivities:* These types of allergic response occur within six to twenty-four hours following ingestion of a food. An example of food sensitivity, such as the reaction to foods containing sulfiting agents, includes sweating, faintness, nausea, rapid pulse rate, low blood pressure, confusion, and/or loss of consciousness.

*Food Intolerance:* More commonly, people misdiagnose a food intolerance as being a food allergy. An intolerance to a food results from a genetic defect in a digestive enzyme or other metabolic process that interferes with the digestion or use of a food component. For example, people with inadequate amounts of the enzyme lactase cannot digest milk sugar, lactose, and are called lactose intolerant. The intestinal gas, bloating, diarrhea, or digestive discomfort that results from drinking milk is not an allergic reaction, but the result of undigested sugars that are fermented by intestinal bacteria to form gas. Celiac disease results when a person is unable to digest a protein in wheat flour called gluten. Sensitivities to gluten also are associated with skin problems and lung disorders.

**TABLE 16. 5    Symptoms of Food Allergy**

| RESPIRATORY TRACT | SKIN |
|---|---|
| Asthma | Hives |
| Rhinitis | Eczema or dermatitis |

| GASTROINTESTINAL TRACT | OTHER CONTROVERSIAL SYMPTOMS |
|---|---|
| Swelling or sores of the lips, mouth, tongue | Anaphylaxis |
| Swelling of the throat | Behavioral disorders |
| Nausea | Epilepsy |
| Cramping and pain | Arthritis |
| Abdominal discomfort | Ear infections |
| Vomiting | |
| Diarrhea | |
| Blood loss in the stool | |

*Pseudo-Intolerance:* A pseudo-intolerance or idiosyncracy is when a food "does not agree" with a person, but no physiological reason can be found. A person might complain that a food makes her tired or cranky, but these types of food reactions are usually more in her head than in her stomach.

## Diet and Food Intolerance and Allergies

Any food can cause allergic or adverse reactions; however, the most common causes of food allergies are milk, wheat, corn, and eggs. Other common foods include citrus fruits, tomato-based products, shellfish, nuts, fish, and chocolate. Salicylates found in a variety of foods, including grapes, oranges, peanuts, melons, tomatoes, pineapple, apples, pears, other nuts, and apricots, also produce allergic-like responses in some people.

*Additives:* Most food additives do not cause food allergies, intolerances, or sensitivities. A few additives, such as the sulfiting agents sodium or potassium metasulfite, monosodium glutamate (MSG), and yellow azo food dyes, produce symptoms in some people. Headaches associated with food sensitivities are significantly reduced when some women eliminate foods containing MSG, yellow dye, yeasts, nitrites, and salicylates from the diet.

Sulfites or whitening agents have been banned by the U.S. Food and Drug Administration (FDA) for use on fruits and vegetables, and food labels must contain a notice if even "detectable amounts" of this additive are present in the food. Some wine, beer, frozen and dried potatoes, vinegar, cider, maraschino cherries, dried fruits and vegetables, canned seafood soups, baking mixes, seafood such as shrimp, fruit drinks, and colas still contain sulfites.

Tartazine or FD&C yellow dye No. 5 causes allergic reactions in some people. The coloring is difficult to avoid, since it is found in a variety of foods, including cake mixes, orange drinks, instant puddings, gelatin, macaroni and cheese dinners, cheese-flavored snacks, and lemon-flavored candy.

## Food Intolerance and Allergies: Diet Advice

Diagnosing food reactions is a complicated process. Allergies are diagnosed differently than are intolerances, and one food intolerance is identified by different tests than is another food intolerance. For example, lactose intolerance is usually diagnosed by giving a fasting person 50 grams of lactose and measuring blood glucose levels. Celiac disease is often diagnosed by intestinal biopsy and the results of elimination-challenge tests, where the gluten-containing foods are first removed from the diet and then are reinstated to observe any adverse effects.

*The Food Diary:* Keeping a food diary and a symptom diary is very important. Write down everything you eat and observe any symptoms that develop within the next hour, including tiredness, cramping, stuffy nose, irritability, nausea, sneezing, headaches, or frequent urination. Once the offending food has been identified, the simplest treatment is to avoid that food(s) and use substitute foods, such as fortified soy milk for milk products in lactose intolerance or gluten-free flour for wheat flour in celiac disease.

*Combination Foods:* Combination foods present another problem, since the offending ingredient is not always obvious. A person with lactose intolerance must read labels on any food that contains milk products, including breads, biscuits, bologna, some salad dressings, cream sauces and soups, and pancakes. A woman allergic to eggs must avoid cream pies, custards, puddings, egg noodles, French toast, and many convenience mixes such as pancakes and cookies, hol-

## TABLE 16.6    Food Intolerance Symptoms

| OFFENDING FOOD | SYMPTOMS |
| --- | --- |
| Chocolate, aged cheese, brewer's yeast, canned fish, red wine | Migraine headaches |
| Coffee, tea, cola | Nerve disorders |
| Fermented cheese or foods, pork sausage, sardines, canned tuna | Migraine headaches, skin rash, itching |
| Food additives | Asthma, headaches, digestive tract problems, itching |
| Legumes (peanuts, beans) | Flatulence, diarrhea |
| Monosodium glutamate (MSG) | Asthma, flushing, dizziness, headaches, restless sleep |
| Strawberries, shellfish, alcohol, pineapple, tomatoes | Eczema, itching, sores on the mouth or tongue |
| Sulfiting agents | Asthma, fluid retention, nasal congestion, itching |

landaise sauce, and dumplings. In addition, cross-reactivity also must be considered. For example, a person who is allergic to peanuts also might react to other legumes, such as soybeans.

Often the sensitivity is not severe and a person can tolerate small amounts of the offending food when eaten as part of a normal diet. For example, most (but not all) people with lactose intolerance can drink small amounts of milk with a meal. Often people with lactose intolerance can eat yogurt or fresh cheeses such as cottage cheese and mozzarella. Sometimes cooking deactivates the offending ingredient, so that raw strawberries produce symptoms but cooked strawberries do not. Finally, often food intolerances spontaneously disappear, so an offending food might be reintroduced into the diet at a later date without a problem.

*The Elimination Diet:* An avoidance or elimination diet is most effective in diagnosing and treating food intolerances and allergies. A woman consumes a restricted diet that excludes all suspected foods. After several days and in intervals, one food is reintroduced at a time while signs of adverse reactions are noted. Keep a diary of food intake and symptoms, monitoring for changes in energy level, bowel function, headaches, sneezing or watery eyes, gas or abdominal pain, or bloating. The final diet is based on all foods that do not cause a reaction.

Designing the diet for food intolerance and allergies is a very individualized process that requires the help of a physician and dietitian. In contrast, self-diagnosis and designing a restrictive diet are seldom accurate and usually result in unnecessary avoidance of nutritious foods.

## *Hair*

Hair, along with skin and nails, are outer reflections of inner health. Flexible, shiny, vibrant hair is a sign of a healthy, well-nourished body, while dry, dull, lifeless hair is a signal of poor nutrition and overall health.

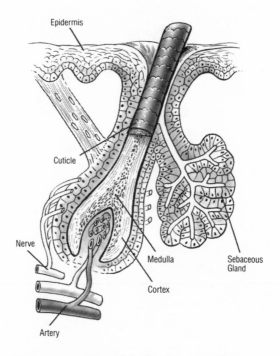

**FIGURE 16.1  The Hair Shaft and Follicle**

The hair shaft is composed of three layers: the outer cuticle; the middle, protein-rich cortex; and the inner medulla. Hair color depends on the pigments inside the cortex; an absence of pigments results in white hair. The hair shaft is embedded in a cavity called the follicle, which is surrounded by tiny blood vessels called capillaries that nourish the hair shaft and supply it with oxygen, water, and nutrients. Waste products, too, are removed via these blood vessels. Oil-secreting glands (called sebaceous glands) also attach to the follicle and secrete sebum, an oily substance that nourishes and moistens the hair shaft.

## Diet and Hair

Almost all of the more than fifty nutrients in the diet are associated with healthy hair, including protein, fat, vitamins, minerals, and water. Nutrients act directly on the growth and maintenance of healthy hair or function indirectly to build a healthy bloodstream that nourishes the hair shaft and follicle.

*Protein and Calories:* Inadequate intake of either protein or calories results in hair loss and dry, brittle hair. Hair loss has been observed in young women with anorexia or in dieters on very low calorie diets that supply insufficient protein or calories to meet minimal daily needs. Protein needs are easily met by following the dietary guidelines outlined in the Healthy Woman's Diet. In fact, Americans typically consume two to three times more protein than they need. Extra protein will not stop hair loss or speed the growth of hair. Instead, it is broken down and used either for energy or stored as body fat.

*Dietary Fat:* An essential dietary fat, called linoleic acid, is found in vegetable oils, such as safflower oil. Although very rare, a deficiency of this fat or consumption of a fat-free diet can result in reduced oil secretion from the sebaceous glands, causing dry, dull hair. Using oils externally on the hair will not compensate for the poor diet.

*Vitamin A and Beta Carotene:* Vitamin A is essential for healthy hair. This fat-soluble vitamin is necessary for normal oil production in the skin and scalp, and optimal intake of either vitamin A or beta carotene helps maintain healthy, shiny hair and scalp. In contrast, a deficiency results in a reddened and sore scalp and hair that is dry and bleached out. Hair loss and dandruff are common symptoms of vitamin A deficiency. However, vitamin A deficiency is only one of many potential causes of dandruff.

*The B Vitamins:* The B vitamins, especially vitamins $B_6$ and $B_{12}$, folic acid, pantothenic acid, and biotin, are needed for healthy hair. Certain forms of seborrhea (chronic inflammation of the sebaceous glands that causes overproduction of oil) respond well to vitamin $B_6$. This B vitamin, in addition to folic acid and vitamin $B_{12}$, is essential for red blood cell formation, thus maintaining the oxygen and nutrient supply to the hair. Folic acid and vitamin $B_{12}$ also are essential for the growth of new hair cells.

Pantothenic acid is important in the normal growth and color of hair. Limited evidence shows that a deficiency of this B vitamin might result in premature graying of hair. Biotin deficiency, although rare, results in hair loss and dry, dull hair. A protein in raw egg whites, called avidin, binds to biotin in the intestines and prevents its absorption. A person might develop a biotin deficiency if several raw eggs were consumed daily. Other causes of biotin or pantothenic acid deficiencies include chronic diarrhea, long-term use of antibiotics, or alcohol abuse.

*Vitamin C:* The oil-producing capability of the sebaceous glands depends on vitamin C. A diet low in this vitamin results in hair that easily breaks and splits. If the hair breaks just below the surface of the skin, the new hair will kink and either coil into an abnormal circular pattern or form imperfectly. These hairs are dry, kinky, tangled, and split.

*Minerals:* Several minerals are related to the maintenance of healthy hair, including calcium, copper, iron, magnesium, manganese, selenium, and zinc. A copper deficiency causes changes or loss of color from the hair. Iron is necessary for optimal blood and oxygen flow to the hair, while hair loss and baldness are signs of either a selenium or a zinc deficiency.

*Water:* The most commonly forgotten nutrient necessary for healthy hair is water. Water is the main component of perspiration, which is important in moisturizing skin and stimulating the sebaceous glands of the hair follicles to secrete oils that keep the hair moisturized.

## Hair: Diet Advice

Hair problems result from poor nutrition, although more often than not the most common problems, such as balding or graying, are caused by other factors such as genetics or the adverse side effects of medications.

In some cases, hair problems do stem from dietary deficiencies and respond quickly when these deficiencies are remedied. Follow the guidelines for the Healthy Woman's Diet. Make sure the diet contains at least one tablespoon of safflower oil (a source of linoleic acid) and several glasses of water daily. In addition,

- Limit the intake of coffee, tea, alcohol, and other fluids that increase water loss.
- Consume at least 1,600 to 2,000 calories of minimally processed foods.
- Exercise, effective stress management, and regular washing with a mild shampoo help reduce the risk of unnecessary hair problems.
- Save your money and skip those nutrient-fortified shampoos laced with protein, B vitamins, vitamins C and E, and more. Hair is only nourished from the inside before shampoos ever reach it, and is dead by the time you see the shaft on top of your head.
- Avoid long-term use of hair dyes, since limited evidence shows they might increase the risk for leukemia and non-Hodgkin's lymphoma.

# *Headaches*

Although some headaches are symptoms of other disorders, such as the flu, eyestrain, a sinus infection, or a hangover, most headaches are usually brought on by tension, depression, and stress that strains the muscular tissues or blood vessels in the head or neck. Lack of sleep, noisy or stuffy environments, or strenuous work also can cause temporary headaches.

Up to eighteen million Americans, most of them women, suffer from migraine headaches, which are severe, throbbing headaches often accompanied by nausea, vomiting, or disturbed vision. Migraines are disabling, intermittent, and last for a few hours to several days. Often bright lights are unbearable so the woman remains in a darkened room or in bed. Migraine headaches tend to occur within families, suggesting there might be a genetic factor to the disorder.

## Diet and Headaches

Both deficiencies and excesses of certain nutrients can cause headaches. Some food substances, as well as food intolerances or allergies, also trigger migraine headaches. The issue is complicated, since a suspected food might not always trigger an attack, depending on other circumstances and how much of the food is eaten. A headache also might not develop for several hours or even days after eating a trigger food.

*The B Vitamins:* Marginal deficiencies of many of the B vitamins, such as niacin, folic acid, and pantothenic acid, can produce headaches. A vitamin $B_1$ deficiency is associated with reduced tolerance to pain and heightened pain response. In one study, women suffering from stress-induced headaches consumed suboptimal amounts of vitamins $B_1$ and $B_2$ and folic acid as compared to headache-free women. Migraine sufferers might benefit from large doses of vitamin $B_2$, with symptoms improving in up to 70 percent of women in one study.

The use of vitamin $B_6$ in the treatment of migraines is based on the vitamin's role in producing the nerve chemical serotonin. If migraines are caused by depletion of serotonin, then vitamin $B_6$ supplementation would help raise serotonin levels and prevent or modify the pain of migraines. To date, vitamin $B_6$ has not proven consistently effective in causing, preventing, or treating migraines. However, vitamin $B_6$ is successful in treating headaches associated with premenstrual syndrome (PMS) in some cases. The treatment appears most effective if taken for five days prior to the onset of PMS. In addition, estrogen-related headaches that occur during the early stages of pregnancy, with the use of postmenopausal estrogen, or with the birth control pill, might be responsive to vitamin $B_6$ supplementation.

*Minerals:* Several minerals are suspected to aid in the management of headaches, including calcium and magnesium. Researchers at Mount Sinai Hospital in New York report two cases of vitamin D and calcium supplementation relieving migraine headaches. Two postmenopausal women suffering from migraine headaches (one following the initiation of hormone replacement therapy and the second following a stroke) reported reductions in the frequency and duration of headaches after taking 1,000 mg of elemental calcium each day and therapeutic weekly doses of vitamin D. One woman reported a reduction from eight to one attack per month as long as the supplement therapy was continued.

*Food Components:* Several substances in foods trigger headaches and migraines. For example,

- A compound called tyramine might produce migraines. Tyramine-containing foods include herring, organ meats, aged cheeses, peanuts and peanut butter, fermented sausages such as bologna and pepperoni, chocolate, sauerkraut, and alcoholic beverages.
- Tannins in apple juice, blackberries, tea, and red wine are suspected to trigger headaches. Other foods associated with headaches include milk/cheese, wheat, grapes or raisins, citrus fruits, and shellfish.
- Phenylethylamine, a compound in chocolate, affects the blood ves-

sels and might produce migraine headaches. Headache sufferers who eat chocolate are more likely to develop headaches than are headache sufferers who eat carob, a chocolate-like replacement.

- Some food additives, such as monosodium glutamate (MSG) used as a flavor enhancer in Chinese foods and many processed foods, also cause headaches in susceptible people.
- Nitrites found naturally in foods and used as preservatives in hot dogs and other processed meats have been reported to cause headaches.
- Some people report increased frequency of headaches when they consume the noncaloric sweetener aspartame (NutraSweet).

Coffee, wine, and possibly tea are linked to headaches. Some people develop allergic-like symptoms to coffee and tea, including irritability, heart irregularities, and headache. Coffee withdrawal results in headaches that might linger for several days. On the other hand, 100 mg to 200 mg of caffeine can relieve regular headaches, especially when combined with painkillers like ibuprofen.

*Fish Oils:* The omega-3 fats in fish and/or fish oil capsules might help prevent or treat migraine headaches. Several studies report improvements in headache symptoms, even in patients unresponsive to medication, when fish oils were included in the diet. Although poorly understood, researchers speculate fish oils reduce spasms of the cerebral arteries and possibly alter serotonin levels.

## Headaches: Diet Advice

Keep a daily journal of your diet, exercise, and sleep habits along with any headaches that develop. After a week, review your records for trends that might precipitate a headache. Also, develop a routine for diet, sleep, and exercise, and stick with it.

Eliminate tyramine-containing foods if you suffer from migraine headaches. If headaches persist after following a tyramine-free diet, then other foods thought to aggravate the condition should be eliminated one at a time to determine if symptoms respond. This type of elimination diet should be monitored closely by a physician and/or dietitian. In addition,

- Avoid caffeine-containing beverages, misuse of alcohol, and tobacco smoke.

- Eat frequent, small nutrient-packed meals rich in fruits, vegetables, whole grains, legumes, and other real foods. Avoid high fat and processed foods.
- Limit ice cream, since it can trigger migraines in some people. Migraine sufferers also should avoid drinking icy cold beverages, which stimulate the nerve center at the back of the palate that controls blood flow to the head.
- Fasting, or even allowing more than five hours to elapse between meals, can trigger a migraine attack.
- Get regular and adequate sleep.
- Mild headaches might respond to 125 mg of dried feverfew leaf standardized extract.

Effective coping skills also are helpful for reducing the stress associated with headaches. Make sure the diet contains at least recommended levels of all vitamins and minerals. Chronic trouble with headaches should be reviewed by a physician.

## *Hypertension*

In the United States alone, one in every five women has hypertension. This figure includes about 75 percent of women over the age of seventy-five. Many of these women don't know they have the disorder, and only a small percentage have their blood pressures under control through medication and/or diet.

A blood pressure reading contains two figures: the top and higher number (systolic blood pressure) reflects the maximum amount of blood pressure in the arteries when the heart contracts; the bottom and lower number (diastolic blood pressure) is the lowest amount of pressure in the arteries when the heart relaxes between beats. Although hypertension is not a disease, it is an indication of cardiovascular problems and is a major risk factor for the development of atherosclerosis, stroke, and other cardiovascular diseases, as well as kidney failure and hemorrhages in the eye.

### Diet and Hypertension

In most cases, blood pressure drops and even normalizes with improved diet, frequent exercise, and weight loss. In fact, the National Institutes of Health recom-

**TABLE 16.7     Blood Pressure Readings: What Do They Mean?**

|  | SYSTOLIC/DIASTOLIC |
|---|---|
| Normal | 120/80 or less |
| Hypertension | 140/90 to 160/95 |
| Hypertension that requires immediate treatment | 200/120 |

mend that physicians have their patients try a three- to six-month trial of dietary and behavioral change before they prescribe medications to control hypertension. Antihypertensive medications are a last resort, especially since many of their side effects, such as elevated blood fats and lowered magnesium levels, increase a woman's risk for developing heart disease.

*Weight Control:* Weight loss has one of the greatest effects on lowering blood pressure of any nonmedicine treatment. Even small amounts of weight loss (i.e., ten pounds) result in significant reductions in blood pressure. The benefits are directly proportional to the amount of weight lost, while blood pressure tends to increase as a woman gains weight.

*Sodium, Potassium, Calcium, and Magnesium:* At one time, the effect of diet on hypertension was thought to be a simple matter of restricting salt intake. Current understanding of the mechanisms that control blood pressure show that it is much more complex than previously thought, with several minerals (called electrolytes), including sodium, potassium, calcium, and magnesium, working as a team.

Populations where people consume salty diets, such as the Japanese and Americans, have a higher incidence of hypertension than do societies where salt intake is low. Approximately one-half of all hypertensives are "salt sensitive" and respond favorably when salt (i.e., sodium) is restricted.

The average American consumes ten to twenty times the recommended amount of sodium, which would be considered a "megadose" of any other nutrient. The kidneys cannot always keep up with the excessive influx of sodium, so the body tries to minimize the toxic salty excess by diluting it with water in the blood and cells of the body. A woman can accumulate five to ten pounds of excess fluid just to keep the accumulated salt diluted. The expanded blood volume places pressure on the cardiovascular system and hypertension develops. Diuretic medications force the kidneys to excrete water and sodium at a faster rate, thus reducing blood pressure in some people.

The ratio of potassium to sodium in the diet might be as, or more, important than sodium alone. The American diet is low in potassium relative to sodium. The body appears to retain sodium and water when potassium intake is low, while increased intake of potassium combined with salt restriction increases sodium excretion, reduces the risk for developing hypertension, lowers blood pressure, and reduces medication requirements.

Calcium also has an integral role in blood pressure, in part by interacting with sodium, potassium, and magnesium. Increased calcium intake, either from diet or supplements, can offset some of the hypertensive effects of sodium, possibly by increasing urinary excretion of sodium. In one study, calcium supplementation (i.e., 1,000 mg/day for twelve weeks) increased urinary excretion of sodium and consequently reduced both systolic and diastolic blood pressures in women over the age of forty. In contrast, a high-sodium diet increased urinary calcium loss and increased the risk for developing hypertension. Replacing table salt (sodium chloride) with potassium salt halts calcium loss and improves hypertension risk in women.

Calcium even lowers blood pressure in healthy women with normal blood pressures. Low-fat, calcium-rich foods and calcium supplements lower blood pressure, while fattier calcium sources, such as cheese, do not. In addition, studies on animals show that a pregnant mother who consumes ample calcium during pregnancy is less likely to give birth to babies who later in life suffer from hypertension. Potassium also might play a role in maintaining normal calcium balance in the body, further showing the interrelationship between these minerals.

Low magnesium intake, although not a cause of hypertension, contributes to its development by its direct effect on the blood vessels and by indirectly affecting potassium balance in the body. Approximately 30 percent of women with hypertension consume inadequate amounts of magnesium. In addition, many diuretic medications increase urinary loss of this essential mineral. In either case, low magnesium status results in low potassium levels, which in turn alters sodium and increases blood pressure. In contrast, consumption of magnesium-rich foods or magnesium supplementation often aids in the prevention and treatment of hypertension and other cardiovascular disorders.

*Vitamin C:* Both vitamin C–rich diets and vitamin C supplementation are associated with a reduced risk for developing hypertension. In contrast, the diet and blood levels in people with hypertension often are low in vitamin C as compared to healthy people. Vitamin C supplementation increases the flexibility and responsiveness of artery walls, showing that increased free radical damage to blood vessel walls might contribute to the disease.

*Fiber and Fat:* A low-fat, low-sugar, high-fiber diet also helps prevent and treat hypertension. A high-fat diet increases the risk for developing hypertension, while a reduction in saturated fat primarily from foods of animal sources and a moderate increase in polyunsaturated fats from vegetable oils, nuts, and seeds reduces blood pressure. Researchers speculate that the polyunsaturated fats are converted to hormonelike substances called prostaglandins in the body that help regulate blood pressure. For the same reasons, frequent inclusion of fish in the diet or supplementing with fish oils lowers blood pressure, especially when consumed in conjunction with a low-salt, high-calcium diet. Fiber helps lower blood pressure, especially when combined with a low-fat diet.

*Fruits and Vegetables:* While the salt shaker is the villain in the hypertension story, fruits and vegetables are the heroes. Researchers at Johns Hopkins University in Baltimore report that a low-fat diet loaded with fruits and vegetables and laced with low-fat milk products lowered systolic and diastolic blood pressures in a group of mildly hypertensive adults. In adults with higher blood pressures, the fruit- and vegetable-filled diet lowered systolic pressure even more. Even people with normal blood pressure benefit from eating more produce.

## Hypertension: Diet Advice

If fat is reduced to 25 percent or less of total calories, salt is restricted, and a desirable body weight is maintained, hypertension would be controlled or eliminated in 85 percent of all hypertensives without the use of medication.

To restrict salt intake, eliminate or curb the use of salt in cooking or at the table. Purchase low-salt foods and avoid processed foods high in salt. Gradually reduce salt in recipes to wean yourself from the salty taste. In addition,

- Boost intake of potassium, magnesium, calcium, vitamin C, and fiber preferably from dietary sources, such as fresh fruits and vegetables, whole-grain breads and cereals, cooked dried beans and peas, and low-fat or nonfat milk products.
- Consume small amounts of or eliminate red meat and the dark meat of poultry.

- Include two or more servings of fish in the weekly menu.
- If you don't consume daily the calcium equivalent of three glasses of nonfat milk and several servings of magnesium-rich soy, nuts, and whole grains, consider a supplement that supplies these two minerals in a ratio of 2 parts calcium for every 1 to 1.5 parts magnesium (e.g., 800 mg calcium and 400 mg to 500 mg magnesium).
- Drink coffee and tea in moderation, if at all. Tea and/or coffee might increase the risk for developing hypertension, possibly because these beverages increase urinary excretion of calcium or contain substances that directly affect blood pressure.

*Beyond Diet:* Other lifestyle habits associated with a reduced risk for developing hypertension include:

- reduce alcohol intake to five or fewer drinks a week,
- reduce stress and competitive behaviors,
- exercise aerobically (brisk walk, jog, swim) four to five days a week,
- avoid oral contraceptives, and
- do not smoke.

People with normal blood pressure at home might appear hypertensive at the doctor's office. So learn how to routinely take blood pressures at home or at work, or ask the physician to take several blood pressure readings at different times and average the results. Wearing an acupressure device on the ear is safe, but is no more effective at lowering blood pressure than a placebo, say researchers at Columbia University College of Physicians and Surgeons in New York. Finally, comply with medication and physician instructions if you have been diagnosed with hypertension.

# Hypoglycemia

Hypoglycemia or low blood sugar is not a disease but a symptom of abnormal blood sugar regulation. It is common in diabetes and in other conditions and is typically characterized by blood sugar levels below 50 mg per 100 deciliters of blood. Symptoms include pallor, fatigue, irritability, inability to concentrate, headaches, palpitations, perspiration, anxiety, hunger, and shakiness or internal trembling.

Traditionally, hypoglycemia was divided into two basic categories: reactive hypoglycemia, which develops within three to four hours of a meal, and fasting or organic hypoglycemia, which is characterized by symptoms developing eight hours or more following a meal. Reactive hypoglycemia results from the foods you choose, especially sugary foods in sensitive people. This condition is sometimes associated with an increased risk for developing diabetes and reflects a delay in the secretion of insulin, the hormone that regulates blood sugar levels. Fasting hypoglycemia is rare and usually results from other serious conditions, such as diabetes, a tumor on the pancreas (the organ that secretes insulin), liver damage, starvation, or cancer.

Many more people complain of hypoglycemic-like symptoms than actually show specific low blood sugar levels on a glucose tolerance test (GTT). In fact, hypoglycemia became a fad in the 1970s when popular books attributed everything from behavior problems and crime to heart disease and allergies to this condition. None of these associations have been verified by well-designed studies. Although many cases of hypoglycemia are more psychological than physiological, there is more to low blood sugar than was previously thought.

Low blood sugar syndromes develop on a continuum. On one end are very healthy people who occasionally experience a slight decrease in blood sugar with mild or no symptoms. At the other end, are the rare cases of fasting hypoglycemia. In between, there are as many variations on blood sugar levels and symptoms as there are people who complain of hypoglycemia.

The GTT should be the definitive test for monitoring blood sugar levels; however, it is inconclusive in the diagnosis of hypoglycemia. For this test, a person consumes a sugary drink on an empty stomach and blood sugar levels are monitored every half hour. The GTT can produce false positive results, since it creates an unrealistic situation—seldom do people consume only sugar.

Another test, the meal tolerance test (MTT), provides a more reliable estimate of blood sugar levels and reflects blood sugar response to normal dietary intake. However, even in the MTT, one person showing low blood sugar levels can exhibit no symptoms, while another person with normal blood sugar levels will report numerous symptoms.

Thus, the traditional definition of "normal" or "low" blood sugar is likely to be arbitrary, with low blood sugar levels affecting different people differently.

What is clear is that self-diagnosis or using inadequate procedures, such as questionnaires, to identify hypoglycemia is an unreliable diagnosis.

### Hypoglycemia: Diet Advice

The diet for hypoglycemics is similar to that for diabetics. (See pages 309 to 315.) A low-fat, high-fiber, nutrient-dense diet, such as the Healthy Woman's Diet, should be followed with no more than 30 percent fat calories, no more than 20 percent protein calories, and the rest from high-quality carbohydrates. Focus on low glycemic-index carbohydrates, such as whole-grain breads and cereals, starchy vegetables like sweet potatoes, fruits and vegetables, and cooked dried beans and peas. Avoid high glycemic-index foods, such as white bread, sweets, and potatoes.

The soluble fibers found in fruits, vegetables, cooked dried beans and peas, and oats, and in guar gum supplements are especially effective in regulating blood sugar levels. Avoid sugar, sugary foods, caffeine, and alcohol, and divide the diet into six or more minimeals and snacks throughout the day with each meal containing some protein, some starchy food, and fiber. This will slow the rate of absorption of carbohydrates and help regulate blood sugar levels.

Supplementation with 200 mcg of chromium has proved beneficial in some cases of hypoglycemia, since this trace mineral is essential in insulin metabolism and blood sugar regulation. Also consume chromium-rich foods, such as whole grains and legumes, and cook in stainless-steel cookware, which increases the chromium content of the meal because the mineral leaches from the pot into the food during preparation. Maintain a desirable body weight, exercise daily for at least twenty to forty minutes, and always bring foods with you so you are prepared for a bout of low blood sugar. Finally, eat a little, but not a lot, in response to hypoglycemic symptoms, since overeating only aggravates blood sugar irregularities.

## *Insomnia*

Insomnia, having difficulty falling or staying asleep or awakening too early, is the most common sleep disturbance. Sleep problems usually result from or accompany other life events, such as stress, depression, physical discomfort, perimenopause, or medication use. In some cases, nutrition might aggravate or cause insomnia.

### Diet and Insomnia

Many dietary habits can interfere with getting to sleep, staying asleep, or even how peacefully you doze. Several dietary habits—including consumption of coffee and alcohol, the size and spiciness of the evening meal, quick weight-loss dieting, and even some food additives—could keep you tossing and turning.

*Caffeine:* This stimulant, found in coffee, tea, colas, and chocolate, can linger in the body for up to fifteen hours, disrupting sleep and leaving you groggy and tired the next day. Coffee also is a diuretic, and the increased need to urinate can cause night awakenings.

*Alcohol:* Alcohol and other depressant medications suppress a phase of sleep called REM (Rapid Eye Movement), during which most of your dreaming occurs. Less REM is likely to mean more night awakenings and a restless sleep. A glass of wine at dinner probably won't affect your sleep; however, it's best to limit the amount to no more than two glasses and avoid drinking any alcohol within two hours of bedtime. You should start sleeping better within two weeks of being alcohol-free, if alcohol is a contributing factor in your sleep problems. Of course, *never* mix alcohol with sleeping pills!

*The Evening Meal:* Large dinners with fatty foods might make you drowsy, but you won't sleep soundly. Heavy meals keep the digestive tract busy, which means you'll be awake, too. Eat your biggest meal of the day at breakfast or lunch and keep the evening meal light. Include some chicken, extra-lean meat, or fish at dinner to help curb middle-of-the-night snack attacks.

*Spicy Foods:* Spicy or gas-forming foods can contribute to sleeping problems. Dishes seasoned with garlic, chilies, cayenne, or other hot spices can cause heartburn or indigestion. Foods seasoned with MSG (monosodium glutamate), a taste-enhancer often added to Chinese food, can cause sleep disturbances, vivid dreaming, and restless sleep in some people. The higher the dose, the greater the likelihood of a reaction. Eating gas-forming foods or eating too fast and swallowing air also can leave you bloated and uncomfortable, which in turn interferes with sound sleep.

*Carbohydrates:* Serotonin is the brain's sleep chemical. When levels of serotonin are high, people typically sleep like babies. You can self-regulate serotonin levels by eating all-carbohydrate snacks, which raise brain levels of the building block for serotonin, an amino acid called tryptophan.

In contrast, a high-protein bedtime snack, such as a slice of turkey or a glass of milk, is a great source of tryptophan, but also provides large quantities of other amino acids that compete with tryptophan for absorption and entry into the brain. Consequently, these snacks do not produce the serotonin rise and might even produce a drop in brain levels of serotonin, which could aggravate insomnia. (The warm milk still might help with sleep because the warm liquid soothes and relaxes and provides a feeling of satiety.)

*Vitamins:* Deficiencies and excesses of certain vitamins, including vitamins $B_6$ and $B_{12}$, might increase the risk for insomnia. Vitamin $B_6$ helps form the nerve chemical serotonin, which regulates sleep. Marginal dietary intake of this B vitamin might lead to insomnia, irritability, and depression. These symptoms disappear when vitamin $B_6$ intake increases. Vitamin $B_{12}$ aids in the wake-sleep cycle governed by melatonin. People who take vitamin $B_{12}$ supplements sometimes show a rise in melatonin and an improvement in sleep.

*Minerals:* Inadequate trace mineral intake also might increase the risk for insomnia. For example, poor copper intake is linked to difficulty falling asleep, longer total sleep time, and feeling less rested upon awakening. Low iron intake might contribute to increased nighttime awakenings and longer total sleep time, possibly because of iron's role in serotonin metabolism. Optimal magnesium intake and avoidance of aluminum-containing foods were associated with high-quality sleep time and few nighttime awakenings in one study on women with sleep disorders. Poor dietary intake of calcium can cause muscle cramping, abnormal nerve function, and changes in deep-sleep eye movements that, theoretically, might affect sleep patterns.

*Melatonin:* Sleep disturbances are a common complaint among seniors. Now there might be a simple solution to this age-old problem. Seniors who suffer from sleep disturbances and who have low melatonin production during the night were given 2 mg of controlled-release melatonin or a placebo. After three weeks, sleep quality, as measured by wrist actigraphy, was significantly improved and wake time was reduced with melatonin compared to the placebo. The only adverse side effect reported was in two patients who developed pruritus (itching).

## Insomnia: Diet Advice

What you eat could be affecting how you sleep. If you suffer from insomnia and drink more than two cups of coffee during the day or drink coffee after 1 P.M., try eliminating caffeine from your diet. If you feel and sleep better after two weeks of being caffeine-free, then avoid caffeine permanently. Some people experience withdrawal symptoms, including depression, irritability, headaches, fatigue, or even tearfulness, within a few hours of going off coffee. These symptoms might last up to four days, after which energy level and mood should improve, leaving you feeling better than ever. In addition,

- Avoid spicy foods at dinnertime.
- Limit your intake of gas-forming or spicy foods to the morning hours, eat slowly to chew food thoroughly, and avoid gulping air. Avoid foods with the additive MSG in the evening.
- Keep your evening meal light.
- Forget those quick-fix diets. Women following very low-calorie diets sometimes complain of sleep disorders.
- Have a light all-carb snack just before bedtime, such as air-popped popcorn, half a whole-wheat English muffin with honey or jam, or two cookies, which helps raise serotonin levels.
- Limit alcohol to no more than two small drinks in the evening.
- Herbs, such as kava, chamomile, catnip, hops, lemon balm, passionflower, Saint-John's-wort, and valerian, have helped some people with mild insomnia.

The Healthy Woman's Diet will ensure adequate intake of all vitamins and minerals. Effective stress management and daily exercise also help prevent and treat sleep disorders. Physical activity helps a person cope with daily stress, produces a surge in sleep hormones, and tires the body so it is ready to sleep at night. Prolonged insomnia should be treated by a physician and might require medication or psychological counseling.

## *Memory and Mind*

Memory begins to fade in our fifties, just about the time that reaction times begin to slow, affecting how quickly we learn new skills or remember the dog's name. Mental slumps, poor concentration, slowed reaction times, forgetfulness, and loss of creative thinking aren't limited to the middle years; they can hit us at any age. Much of this mental decline has more to do with being tired, stressed, depressed, lonely, or just plain not taking good care of your health than it does aging. There is much you can do to slow and even stop memory loss and boost thinking ability.

## Diet, Memory, and Mind

What you eat affects how you think, how much you remember, and even your intelligence level. Our brain cells (all 100 billion of them!) require the right mix of brain-boosting nutrients to function optimally. Miss even one nutrient and you can experience memory loss, reduced ability to think clearly and quickly, poor concentration, acceleration of the age-related changes in brain tissue, reduced ability to learn and reason leading to lowered IQ scores, and a dwindling desire to learn.

On the other hand, choosing the right mix of foods and nutrients could help you think quickly and remember well throughout life. In one study, cognitive performance went up as dietary intakes improved. Women who consumed the most vitamins E, A, $B_6$, and $B_{12}$ also had better recall memory and performed better on abstract thought problems. High intakes of vitamins $B_1$, $B_2$, niacin, folic acid, and vitamin C also boosted test scores, while adequate protein intake improved memory. But don't take feeling good as a sign of thinking good! Impaired mental function always precedes physical problems, so look to your diet first before blaming age or heredity for lapses in memory, thinking, or concentration.

*Breakfast:* Women who eat breakfast think better and faster, remember more, react quicker, and are mentally sharper than breakfast skippers. They also miss

---

**TABLE 16.8    Food and Mind**

What you eat affects:

1. The level of nerve chemicals in the brain that regulate all mental processes.
2. The development and maintenance of brain-cell function and structure.
3. The insulating sheath surrounding nerve cells that speeds the transport of messages from one neuron to the next.
4. The level of enzymes and their activity, which enhances brain functions.
5. The amount of oxygen that reaches the brain.
6. The rate of accumulation and removal of cell waste products.
7. The ability of brain cells to transmit electrical messages.
8. The efficiency of brain-cell membranes to transport nutrients into, and debris out of, the cell.

---

fewer days of school and work. Just about every measure of thinking ability improves after eating a good breakfast—from math scores and creative thinking to speed and efficiency in solving problems, concentration, recall, and accuracy in work performance. Compared to breakfast skippers, people who eat breakfast communicate more effectively, make fewer mistakes, get the job done more quickly, and have better ideas throughout the day.

The trick to thinking clearly and avoiding mental fatigue is to eat breakfast, but stick with low-fat choices. Eating a high-fat breakfast will leave you feeling less vigorous, imaginative, and alert, and more feeble and fatigued, according to researchers at the University of Sheffield in the United Kingdom. Instead, have a bowl of whole-grain cereal with nonfat milk or soy milk, a piece of fruit, and orange juice.

*Lunch Rules:* A high-fat or high-sugar meal at lunch will make you drowsy and less mentally alert. Researchers at Harvard University in Cambridge, Massachusetts, report that mental alertness and ability to concentrate decrease after a midday meal of carbohydrate-rich foods, especially sugary foods. Keep lunch light and combine a little protein with more whole-grain foods, such as a turkey sandwich on whole-grain bread with mustard, a piece of fruit, and juice or a salad (oil-free dressing).

*Skip the Fad Diets:* Crash diets don't work. In fact, they might make you dumb. Research from the Institute of Food Research in the United Kingdom found that women following fad diets processed information slowly, took longer to react, and had more trouble remembering sequences compared to nondieting women. While dieting might make you mentally dull, losing weight the good old-fashioned way—that is a gradual weight loss of no more than two pounds a week—allows you to lose the right kind of weight (fat weight), keep it off, and stay clearheaded in the process.

*Dietary Fat:* Most people know that gobbling the typical high-fat American diet will put on the pounds and increase the risk for heart disease. But did you know it also slows the thinking process? Researchers at Baycrest Center for Geriatric Care in Toronto fed young rats high-fat diets (from either animal or vegetable fats) or regular diets and put them through a series of tests for memory and problem-solving. Rats on either high-fat diet did poorly compared to leaner rats fed standard diets. "High-fat diets impair performance on virtually all our measures," says Gordon Winocur, a lead researcher in the study. "It's remarkable how impaired these animals are."

*Fish Oils:* The omega-3 fats in fish protect the brain from damage associated with memory loss. Researchers at the National Institute of Public Health and the Environment in the Netherlands found that people who eat fish regularly show less cognitive decline as they age compared to people who consume more vegetable oils. The diets of people between the ages of sixty-nine and eighty-nine years were compared with cognitive ability during a four-year period. The results showed that a high linoleic-acid intake (a fat found in vegetable oils) impaired thinking, while the omega-3 fatty acids in fish improved thinking ability. More research is needed before specific recommendations can be made. In the meantime, your best bet is to cut back on red meat consumption to no more than three servings of extra-lean (no more than 7 percent fat by weight) a week and substitute fish, especially omega-3-rich fish such as salmon. Then grill, bake, or sauté your fish in oil-less marinades. Or add flaxseed meal to your daily diet, since it is one of the few vegetable sources of the omega-3 fatty acids.

*Coffee:* You'll notice a mental boost within minutes of drinking a cup of coffee. The caffeine in coffee (or tea, cola, and chocolate) revs up the nervous system so you think more clearly, are more alert, have a faster reaction time, and can concentrate better. You also perform tasks, such as typing, faster and more accurately. While some is good, more is not necessarily better. Caffeine lingers in the system for four to fifteen hours and keeps you up at night, interfering with mental function the next day. Caffeine also is effective only up to your jitter threshold; add more coffee after this and you're too buzzed to think clearly. Finally, coffee and tea contain compounds called tannins that reduce other brain-boosting nutrients, such as iron, by up to 75 percent. Limit caffeinated beverages to two to three servings a day and drink them between meals.

*The Antioxidants:* The antioxidants protect delicate brain tissue from free radical damage, which accumulates over years and is associated with age-related memory loss. Maintain antioxidant levels in brain tissue throughout life and you might keep a more youthful brain power. You also will offset the damage from stress that otherwise leads to age-related memory loss.

A study from Erasmus University Medical School in the Netherlands found that thinking ability remained high throughout life when people consumed lots of antioxidant-rich foods. Healthy centenarians with great memories and concentration also have the highest antioxidant levels and consume the most antioxidant-rich fruits and vegetables. In a study from the University of Sydney in Australia, men and women who consumed ample vitamin C performed the best on tests for attention, recall and memory, and calculation.

The antioxidants, especially vitamin E, also might help slow the progression of Alzheimer's disease, the major cause of dementia in older persons. A study from Columbia University College of Physicians and Surgeons in New York found that people with Alzheimer's disease who took vitamin E supplements were able to slow the progression of the disease. Other antioxidants that might help curb the symptoms of Alzheimer's include ginkgo biloba, lipoic acid, and compounds called flavonoids in fruits and vegetables.

To keep your antioxidant defenses strong, consume daily at least six to eight servings of fresh fruits and vegetables, such as orange juice, strawberries, carrots, sweet potatoes, spinach, broccoli, kiwi, and cantaloupe. Also take daily supplements of vitamin E supplement (400 IU) and vitamin C (250 mg to 1,000 mg).

*B Vitamins:* Inadequate intakes of several vitamins, including vitamin $B_1$, vitamin $B_2$, niacin, vitamin $B_6$, vitamin $B_{12}$, pantothenic acid, and folic acid, can lead to memory loss and mental decline. For example,

- Poor intake of vitamin $B_1$ leads to fatigue, mental confusion, reduced attention span, and memory loss.
- Even a mild deficiency of niacin produces symptoms that include depression, confusion and disorientation, anxiety, irritability, and short-term memory loss.
- Low intake of vitamin $B_6$, folic acid, or vitamin $B_{12}$ contributes to a variety of mental problems, including dementia, depression, poor concentration, moodiness, confusion, reduced learning ability, and even convulsions.
- Vitamin $B_6$ might also help soothe the mental distress experienced during times of grief.
- Up to 42 percent of older women are vitamin $B_{12}$ deficient, which increases their risk for memory loss and dementia. The good news is, their mental function improves when they supplement with this B vitamin.

*Iron:* Iron deficiency is the most common nutrient deficiency in the United States and could be a major contributor to shortened attention spans, lowered IQ scores and intelligence, lack of motivation, poor hand-eye coordination, lowered scores on vocabulary tests, inability to concentrate, limited educational achievement, and suboptimal work performance in children and adults. Women during their childbearing years, pregnant and breast-feeding women, and seniors are at particularly high risk for developing iron deficiency. Increasing iron intake in deficient people stimulates brain activity, especially in the left hemisphere of the brain, the region of the brain responsible for analytic thought and abstract thinking. Optimal iron intake also is linked to greater verbal skills and overall improved mental functioning.

Include several iron-rich foods, including spinach, extra-lean red meat, legumes, dried apricots, raisins, and lima beans, in the daily diet. Always combine a vitamin C–rich food, such as orange juice, with an iron-rich food to maximize iron absorption, and cook in cast-iron pots.

*Choline:* Choline is a building block for a special category of fats called phospholipids (fats containing the mineral phosphorus) found in cell membranes and the nerve chemical acetylcholine, which regulates memory. Although the body manufactures this B vitamin–like compound, boosting brain levels with supplements of choline might improve memory or slow age-related memory loss, although the evidence is not conclusive. The best dietary sources of choline are wheat germ, egg yolks, liver, peanuts and peanut butter, and brewer's yeast. Small amounts of choline are found in potatoes, tomatoes, whole-wheat bread, milk, oranges, cauliflower, and cucumbers.

*Aluminum:* Women with Alzheimer's disease show abnormal accumulation of aluminum in their brains. On the other hand, while aluminum levels are high in the brains of Alzheimer's patients, it has never been confirmed that dietary intake of this metal contributes to the disease. If it does, consuming more optimal amounts of calcium (at least three to four servings daily of calcium-rich, low-fat milk products) reduces aluminum absorption and, thus, might have an indirect effect on maintaining brain function.

*Phosphatidylserine:* A compound related to choline, called phosphatidylserine (PS), accumulates in the brain and might boost brain power. PS helps brain cells conduct nerve impulses, enhancing communication within the brain. A few studies show that PS supplements improve memory and learning in animals, depressed or Alzheimer's patients, healthy people, and seniors, and with no side effects. No specific effective dose has been identified, although some researchers speculate that 300 mg taken for the first few weeks followed by a 100 mg maintenance dose is safe. Be sure to purchase only standardized products from reputable manufacturers, since these products are not regulated by the U.S. Food and Drug Administration (FDA). You also boost PS levels by including more fish in your diet, since the omega-3 fatty acid DHA (see page 355) appears to boost the body's ability to make PS.

*Lipoic Acid:* This fat-soluble substance is found in liver and brewer's yeast and might protect the brain from free radical damage. Researchers at the University of California, Berkeley, report that this antioxidant easily crosses the blood-brain barrier, making it an ideal defense against free radical damage of nerve and brain cells.

## Memory and Mind: Diet Advice

The Healthy Woman's Diet forms the basis for the best nutrition for body and mind, today and in the future. In addition,

- Eat regularly, starting with breakfast.
- Keep the midafternoon meal light and low-fat.
- Forget fad diets. Lose weight sensibly, following the guidelines in chapters 7 and 8.
- Include two or three servings of fish in the weekly menu.
- Feast daily on eight to ten antioxidant-rich, deep-colored fruits and vegetables.
- Take a moderate-dose vitamin and mineral supplement that contains 100 percent of the Daily Value for all the B vitamins and iron (if you are a premenopausal woman).
- Limit caffeine to two to three beverages a day.
- Include more choline-rich wheat germ and brewer's (not baker's) yeast in your daily diet.
- Consume three calcium-rich foods a day to help block aluminum absorption.
- Consider taking supplemental phosphatidylserine.

Finally, physically active people stay mentally sharp longer than couch potatoes. So, stay active, engage in vigorous exercise throughout life, and enjoy every minute of it!

# *Mood and Emotions*

What you eat affects how you feel. Long before you develop osteoporosis from lack of calcium or heart disease from eating too much fat, you experience the emotional consequences of your food choices. In fact, what you eat or don't eat for breakfast will affect how you feel by midafternoon.

## Diet, Mood, and Emotions

Nerves communicate by releasing chemicals, called neurotransmitters. Some neurotransmitters, such as acetylcholine, stimulate nerves and are responsible for increased mental processes. Other neurotransmitters, such as serotonin, inhibit nerve function and result in relaxation and other calming mental processes. Diet affects the formation and activity of these neurotransmitters by regulating how much of what the body makes.

*Starches:* It is no coincidence that women turn to pasta, desserts, and other carbohydrate-rich foods when they feel down in the dumps. Carbohydrates increase concentrations of an amino acid called tryptophan. Tryptophan is the building block for the neurotransmitter serotonin. Consequently, increased tryptophan means higher levels of serotonin in the brain, which in turn relieves depression, insomnia, and irritability.

People with Seasonal Affective Disorder (SAD)—a condition characterized by depression, lethargy, and an inability to concentrate combined with episodic bouts of overeating and excessive weight gain—crave carbohydrates when they feel down in the dumps. Women battling premenstrual syndrome (PMS) also eat more carbohydrates the ten days before their periods. Like people with SAD and PMS, many women report increased desire to snack on sweets when they feel depressed or emotionally vulnerable. Even women with the eating disorder bulimia have lowered serotonin levels that respond to increased intake of carbohydrates. Often persons describe the "craving" for carbohydrates as "I just need something to calm myself." They feel more relaxed and clearheaded after the snack.

*Sugar:* Although a carbohydrate, sugar might affect mood and behavior for other reasons in addition to its effect on serotonin production. Sugar provides an energy boost followed by an energy lull as the hormone insulin reacts to elevated blood sugar levels and transfers the sugar from the blood into the cells. Consequently, a woman feels tired, depressed, confused, or hungry.

Using sugar to self-regulate mood is a temporary fix. In the long run, it could create a vicious cycle. A woman suffering from depression who turns to sugary foods might relieve the fatigue and feel better for a short while, but the depression and fatigue return. She then must either reach for another sugar fix or seek help elsewhere.

Sugar raises other brain chemicals, called endorphins, that are natural, morphinelike chemicals in the brain that ease stress and discomfort. The taste of sugar on the tongue appears to release these endorphins and result in a calming effect.

*Protein:* Protein-rich foods, such as milk or turkey, are good sources of tryptophan, but they do not boost serotonin levels. Only a carbohydrate-rich snack can do that. Protein does release other nerve chemicals, such as epinephrine, which increases alertness. You might consider eating a little protein with the noon meal to keep yourself energized throughout the afternoon hours. On the other hand, if you want to put your feet up and rest during the afternoon, choose a carbohydrate-rich meal for lunch.

*Fat:* While fatty meals can make you sluggish, the fats in fish improve mood. Cultures where people regularly eat fish have low incidences of depression, while depression and suicide rates increase as fish consumption decreases. Researchers at the National Institute on Alcohol Abuse and Alcoholism state there is a link between the omega-3 fatty acids—the fats most commonly found in fish—and a person's risk for depression, impulsive violence, and suicide. These harmful behaviors are strongly associated with low levels of serotonin breakdown products called 5-hydroxyindoleacetic acid, or 5-HIAA, in cerebral spinal fluid. Since it is difficult to measure serotonin levels in the brain, 5-HIAA in cerebral spinal fluid (CSF-5HIAA) is an excellent and readily accessible marker for this neurotransmitter. In this study, blood levels of omega-3 fatty acids, especially docosahexaenoic acid (DHA), were directly related to CSF-5HIAA; as blood DHA increased, so did CSF-5HIAA and both decreased at similar rates. In addition, significant differences in blood DHA levels were noted between the healthy controls and alcoholic patients.

*Meal Size:* The size of a meal also affects mood. A big lunch supplying 1,000 calories or more interferes with mental alertness, especially if a woman is not accustomed to eating a large midday meal. In contrast, small, low-fat midday meals and snacks improve mental alertness and work performance.

*Coffee and Caffeine:* Caffeinated beverages, including coffee, tea, and colas, are central nervous system stimulants that affect mood. One to two cups of coffee increase alertness, combat fatigue, and improve performance on work tasks that require detailed attention. Higher doses result in agitation, headaches, nervousness, and decreased ability to concentrate.

In women who do not regularly consume caffeine, even a small dose of coffee results in irritability, nervousness, and insomnia. In contrast, regular coffee drinkers develop similar symptoms when they are deprived of coffee. Some individuals who suffer from depression and other distress symptoms respond favorably to removing caffeine (and sugar) from the diet.

*Vitamins:* B vitamin deficiencies, including vitamins $B_1$, $B_2$, $B_6$, $B_{12}$, and niacin, as well as vitamin C deficiencies are often found in psychiatric patients. Other vitamins that might improve mood include vitamins D and E. In some cases, these deficiencies result from poor dietary habits. However, vitamin deficiencies often result in a cycle of depression, disinterest in food or poor eating habits, progressive malnutrition, and increasing mental or emotional disorders, which respond best to a combination of diet and moderate supplementation. Vitamin deficiencies seldom occur alone and almost always are accompanied by inadequate intake of other vitamins, protein, iron, and/or trace minerals.

Even marginal deficiencies of vitamins $B_1$, $B_2$, $B_6$, and niacin are associated with irritability, nervousness, fatigue, mental confusion, depression, memory loss, or emotional instability. Other symptoms include personality changes, dramatic mood changes, insomnia, abnormal EEG readings, or aggressiveness. These deficiencies are common in people suffering from depression and negative mood patterns. For example, people battling depression often are low in folic acid. Their mood improves when they increase their intake of this B vitamin.

Vitamin $B_{12}$ is essential for the formation and maintenance of the insulation around nerve cells. A long-term deficiency of this B vitamin results in moodiness, confusion, agitation, delusions, dizziness, disorientation, and, in severe cases, permanent nerve damage. A folic acid deficiency is also directly linked to depression and mood changes. Mental illness in the elderly is often attributed not to aging, but to poor dietary intake or absorption of one or both of these B vitamins.

In addition, vitamin $B_{12}$ and folic acid are essential for the formation of all body cells, including red blood cells that carry oxygen to the brain and nervous system. A deficiency of folic acid or vitamin $B_{12}$ results in anemia, lethargy, depression, and fatigue, which is treatable with improved diet.

Mental changes associated with vitamin C deficiency include depression and lethargy. Vitamin C is involved in the production of several essential nerve chemicals, which might explain the vitamin's role in mood and behavior.

*Folic Acid:* Of all the nutrients linked to neuropsychiatric disorders, folic acid appears most closely tied to depression. Depression is the most common neurological disorder associated with folic acid deficiency. Low folate levels are noted in up to 38 percent of women suffering from depression; the severity of depression is directly related to the degree of deficiency. Patients with low blood levels of folic acid are less likely to respond to antidepressant medications; consequently, folic

**TABLE 16.9     What Foods Have Folic Acid?**

| FOOD | AMOUNT | FOLIC ACID (MCG) |
|---|---|---|
| Lentils | I cup cooked | 358 |
| Beans: kidney, garbanzo, black | I cup cooked | 229–282 |
| Spinach | I cup cooked | 262 |
| Wheat germ | ½ cup | 199 |
| Orange juice | I cup | 109 |
| Green peas | I cup cooked | 101 |
| Meat, chicken, fish | 3 ounces | Less than 20 |
| Milk | I cup | Less than 15 |
| Whole-wheat bread | I slice | 16 |
| White bread | I slice | 10 |

acid status might predict whether a patient will improve on some forms of antidepressant therapy.

Depressed patients who are low in folic acid show improvement in mood with folic acid supplementation. In one study, psychiatric patients treated with folic acid spent less time in the hospital and showed significant mood improvement and better social functioning than did those with low folic acid levels who did not receive supplements. In patients with bipolar and unipolar mood disorders, daily supplemental doses of 200 mcg of folic acid are sufficient to produce improvement in mood. In other cases, up to 15 mg of folic acid have been used to obtain mood improvement in patients who receive ongoing treatment with standard antidepressant medications.

How folic acid affects brain chemistry is only partially understood. Folic acid is essential in the metabolism of many neurotransmitters, the formation of membrane phospholipids, and the synthesis and repair of nucleic acids. A defect in any of these processes could underlie some psychotic and mood disorders.

*Minerals:* Both calcium and magnesium are essential for normal nerve function and in neurotransmitter production. Although no association between calcium and behavior has been noted, even marginal magnesium deficiency results in confusion, personality changes, depression, lack of coordination, weakness, and poor concentration. Low zinc also has been linked to depression.

Poor dietary intake of iron causes anemia and altered brain and nervous system chemistry, which results in mood disorders, lethargy, depression, poor concentration, impaired reasoning and judgment skills, irritability, decreased attention span, apathy, personality changes, and reduced desire to learn. Iron-deficient children and university students have reduced verbal ability, perform poorly on intelligence tests, and exhibit impaired concentration and memory skills. Even iron-deficient infants who later consume adequate amounts of iron score lower on mental and physical tests than do children with optimal iron intakes. These findings are consistent with studies on adults, which show that work performance, mood, and memory are impaired when iron intake is poor.

In a study conducted at the University College in Wales, people taking selenium supplements (100 mcg per day) showed improved mood and reduced anxiety, fatigue, and depression compared to people taking placebos. As dietary intake of selenium was reduced, reports of anxiety, depression, and fatigue increased. How selenium might affect the brain and nervous system is unknown.

While some dietary minerals and metals might play a beneficial role in maintaining healthy emotions and attitudes, other minerals consumed in excess are harmful. For example, excess copper and manganese impair brain function. Lead or mercury poisoning also have profound effects on the nervous system.

*Herbs:* Several herbs show promise in improving mood, including Saint-John's-wort for depression and ginkgo biloba for dementia, tryptophan and phenylalanine as adjuncts to enhance conventional antidepressants. S-adenosylmethionine (SAM) combined with the omega-3 fatty acids also show promise in stabilizing mood, according to researchers at George Washington University School of Medicine in Washington, D.C.

## Mood and Emotions: Diet Advice

Depression and other mood disorders are common symptoms of many physical, emotional, and situational problems unrelated to diet or nutritional status. However, in some cases, improving dietary habits or choosing a well-balanced vitamin/mineral supplement might improve, or even cure, a troublesome condition.

Any drastic change in normal eating patterns can alter brain chemistry. Severe dieting, bingeing on sweets, skipping meals such as breakfast, or other abnormal eating habits affect neurotransmitter levels and, consequently, mood and behavior.

The Healthy Woman's Diet is the basis for managing your moods. In addition,

- Consume several small meals/snacks throughout the day, rather than two to three big meals to avoid wide fluctuations in blood sugar and neurotransmitter levels.
- Carbohydrate cravers cannot "will away" their cravings, so they should work with them instead. Make sure every meal contains some complex carbohydrate. In addition, plan a carbohydrate-rich snack during that time of the day when you are most vulnerable to snack attacks, and choose whole-grain breads and cereals, rather than sugary foods.
- Include two to three servings of fish, such as salmon, in the weekly menu.
- Consider a well-balanced vitamin/mineral supplement. (See chapter 6 for more information on choosing a supplement.)
- Limit caffeinated beverages to one or two servings a day.

Include regular exercise, coping skills, and a strong social support system in your daily life. Limit or avoid alcohol, cigarettes, and medications that compound emotional problems. Finally, consult a physician if emotional problems persist or interfere long-term with the quality of life and health.

## *Muscle Cramps*

A cramp is an involuntary, violent, and painful spasm of a muscle. Women, especially during pregnancy or with intense exercise, are most likely to experience cramps in calf muscles, but the hamstrings, quadriceps, small muscles of the feet and hands, or any voluntary muscles are also common targets.

Figuring out the type of cramp provides the first clue to the underlying causes and most effective treatment. A true cramp, or "charley horse," is most common. These cramps are most frequent in people with well-developed muscles. Heat cramps develop when a woman performs intense muscular work in a hot environment and perspires profusely. During heat exposure, electrolytes (i.e., sodium, potassium, chloride, and other minerals) are lost in perspiration. Muscle pain and spasms, especially in the calves, occur if these electrolytes are not replaced. Intermittent, painful spasms of the muscles, called tetany, are usually attributed to low calcium levels. However, low blood magnesium levels also can result in tremor and seizures and low potassium levels produce tetany-like symptoms in some people.

Researchers suspect cramps result from overactivity of the nerves sending messages to specific muscle groups. In addition, changes in the fluid outside the cells, such as occurs in dehydration and electrolyte imbalances, or alteration of intracellular metabolites, such as enzymes, can initiate and terminate muscle cramps.

### Diet and Muscle Cramps

Alterations in tissue mineral levels are linked to all forms of muscle cramps. The minerals and electrolytes most likely to affect the muscles include calcium, magnesium, potassium, and some trace minerals. These nutrients work as a team. For example, low blood magnesium levels often develop when a person is deficient in potassium and/or calcium. Vitamin E shows moderate usefulness in the treatment and prevention of muscle fatigue and cramping, and even vitamin D might help prevent muscle weakness.

*Calcium:* This mineral helps regulate muscle contractions and is stored within the muscle cells. Low calcium levels increase the irritability of the nerves and result in muscle spasms, such as leg cramps. Increased calcium intake might help alleviate this form of leg cramps, although the research is inconclusive. Some studies show improvements in leg cramps with calcium supplementation, while other studies report no effect.

*Magnesium:* The balance between calcium and magnesium is critical to normal muscle function: calcium stimulates muscle contraction, while magnesium stimulates muscle relaxation. The two minerals also help regulate nerve transmission and the heartbeat. Inadequate magnesium intake affects all tissues, especially the muscles. Even marginal magnesium intake can result in tremors, spasms, and weakness of the muscles.

Strenuous exercise alters magnesium concentrations in the muscles and blood, which might affect muscle relaxation and contraction. Blood levels of magnesium are low after endurance exercise, and blood levels remain below preexercise values for as long as several months after a strenuous exercise session. Levels of hormones, such as norepinephrine and epinephrine (adrenaline), rise in response to strenuous exercise and these hormones also increase urinary loss of magnesium. In addition, muscle concentrations of magnesium can be low despite normal blood concentrations of the mineral. Low blood levels reflect potentially serious loss of magnesium from the tissues.

Dietary surveys show that self-selected diets often contain less than recommended amounts of magnesium. In addition, the recommended amount might not be optimal for women who exercise. The physical stress of sports training, exercising in the heat, and even the psychological stress of competition increase magnesium losses.

Dr. Mildred Seelig, at the American College of Nutrition, recommends that optimal magnesium intake might be as much as 500 mg per day for a 135-pound woman. An intake that ranges between 350 mg and 450 mg is probably adequate for nonexercising women.

*Potassium:* Potassium is the main electrolyte inside the muscle cells. It maintains nerve and muscle function and normal contraction of the muscles and heart. Muscle spasms, tremors, tetany, heart arrhythmias, and muscle weakness are caused by increased nerve excitability associated with inadequate intake of potassium. Chronic low intake of potassium combined with frequent exercise or work in hot climates could increase a woman's need for potassium.

*Zinc:* Several cellular components associated with muscle cramping could be susceptible to the harmful effects of free radicals. Free radical activity is higher in zinc-depleted tissues than in tissues with adequate levels of this trace mineral, which places these tissues at risk for damage, cramps, and generalized weakness. Zinc intake often is low, while the physiological demands of both exercise and pregnancy increase the risk for poor zinc status.

*Vitamin $B_6$:* Nocturnal leg cramps are common in up to 70 percent of older persons and might be prevented by taking a B vitamin supplement, according to a study from Taipei Wan Fang Hospital in Taiwan. In this study, twenty-eight older patients suffering from leg cramps were given either placebos or vitamin B complex supplements that contained 50 mg of vitamin $B_1$, 250 mcg of vitamin $B_{12}$, 30 mg of vitamin $B_6$, and 5 mg of vitamin $B_2$. After three months, 86 percent of the patients taking supplements reported remission of leg cramps, while no significant reductions in leg cramps were noted in the placebo group. The supplements significantly reduced the frequency, duration, and intensity of the cramps.

*Carnitine:* Carnitine supplementation improves muscle aches, cramps, and muscular exhaustion, according to a study from Nagoya University in Japan.

Patients were given 500 mg of carnitine daily. After twelve weeks, two-thirds of the patients reported improvement in muscular symptoms. The researchers speculate that carnitine improves muscle problems by restoring tissue levels of carnitine and removing metabolic waste products that cause muscle fatigue and cramping.

### Muscle Cramps: Diet Advice

Although the exact cause of muscle cramps is unknown, it is likely that cramps result from a variety of factors working independently or in combination. Regardless of the type of muscle cramp, several minerals, including calcium, magnesium, potassium, and zinc, apparently perform combined roles in the prevention of muscle injury and cramps. Include several servings daily of foods rich in these minerals.

General recommendations for preventing muscle cramps include the following:

- Drink plenty of water and fluids.
- Eat a high-carbohydrate, nutrient-packed diet.
- Maintain optimal mineral and electrolyte intake.
- Frequently and gently stretch the troublesome muscles and/or warm up and cool down before and after exercise.

## Premenstrual Syndrome

Premenstrual syndrome (PMS) is the troublesome period before your period. For one to fourteen days prior to the onset of menstruation, many women experience a physical and emotional roller coaster that includes such symptoms as bloating and breast tenderness, headaches, nausea, backache, moodiness, increased cravings, and irritability. Symptoms vary from woman to woman and even from month to month.

Up to 90 percent of women experience PMS, with the greatest percentage occurring during the thirties and forties. It is likely that PMS results from a complex of factors, including hormone imbalances, fluid and sodium retention, alterations in neurotransmitters and prostaglandins (hormonelike substances that affect the nervous system and numerous metabolic functions), low blood sugar, and nutritional inadequacies or excesses.

## Diet and PMS

Numerous dietary factors might contribute to the development or severity of symptoms in PMS. These include calories, fat, sugar, fiber, and salt intake; food cravings; several vitamins, such as vitamin B$_6$ and vitamin E; and minerals such as calcium and magnesium.

For example, studies show that women with PMS, as compared to other women, consume less fluids, B vitamins, zinc, iron, calcium, magnesium, and manganese, and more fatty dairy products, salt, sugar, protein, and saturated fat. Some women respond to vitamin/mineral supplementation despite normal blood levels of these nutrients.

*Calories:* Many women with PMS say they are hungrier during the premenstrual phase, which explains why calorie intake can increase by up to 87 percent during this time of the month. Changes in hormones and nerve chemical coincide with the increased appetite and might be partially responsible. For example, estrogen and progesterone levels are highest at the times when women experience the greatest increase in hunger.

Serotonin levels might also dip during this time, increasing cravings for sweets. Women with PMS add as much as twenty teaspoons of additional sugar to their daily diets. PMS-induced depression is linked to fluid retention and increased cravings for sweets and chocolate, while women who do not suffer from depression are also less likely to crave sweets. A high-carbohydrate, low-sugar, low-protein diet during the premenstrual phase sometimes improves symptoms of depression, anxiety, anger, fatigue, and confusion, while increasing alertness and tranquility, possibly by elevating levels of the neurotransmitter, serotonin.

*Fiber, Protein, and Fat:* Elevated estrogen levels might contribute to some symptoms of PMS. Dietary fiber helps remove excess estrogen from the body and might help alleviate some of these symptoms.

Reduced consumption of meat and protein is recommended for some symptoms of PMS. Vegetarian diets are associated with improved estrogen and progesterone levels during the premenstrual phase and, therefore, might be helpful in reducing symptoms of PMS. Soy foods, such as tofu or soy milk, show promise in reducing PMS symptoms. (See chapter 2 for information on how to plan a vegetarian diet.)

Some research shows that limiting animal fats and emphasizing vegetable oils might aid in the regulation of PMS symptoms. Animal fat directly influences blood estrogen levels, and since excess blood estrogen might contribute to PMS symptoms, avoiding these fats could help. Evening primrose oil, which contains vitamin E and a fatty acid called gamma linolenic acid (GLA), might help regulate the production of hormonelike compounds called prostaglandins that affect PMS symptoms, such as breast tenderness, irritability, and depression.

*Fish Oils:* Women who suffer monthly from menstrual cramps and bloating might consider taking fish oil capsules. Researchers at Aarhus University in Denmark gave young women who typically suffered from menstrual cramps five fish oil capsules daily, fish oil plus vitamin $B_{12}$, seal oil, or placebos for three to four months. By the third month, the women taking fish oils reported a significant reduction in menstrual symptoms. The most dramatic reduction in symptoms came from the group supplemented with both fish oils and vitamin $B_{12}$.

*Vitamin $B_6$:* Some women respond favorably to vitamin $B_6$ supplementation during the premenstrual phase, including reduced depression, irritability, dizziness, vomiting, headaches, swelling, acne, and fatigue. Other women experience no improvements while, in some cases, 70 percent of the women taking placebos also report improvements in symptoms. This suggests a possible psychosomatic component to some women's PMS symptoms that is responsive to any type of therapy the woman believes will work.

How vitamin $B_6$ might help treat PMS is controversial. Some researchers theorize that pharmacological doses of this vitamin (200 mg to 800 mg) reduce blood estrogen levels and increase progesterone levels, thus improving the balance between these two female hormones. Other researchers speculate that the vitamin aids in the manufacture and release of the neurotransmitter serotonin, which in turn regulates appetite, pain, sleep, and mood. Another theory is that a suboptimal level of vitamin $B_6$ produces a domino effect on the body's hormones—it decreases the release of dopamine, which increases levels of a hormone called prolactin, which triggers PMS symptoms. In short, disagreement prevails over if, why, or how vitamin $B_6$ is useful in the treatment of PMS.

*Calcium:* Calcium and vitamin D help curb many of the symptoms of PMS. Alterations in calcium metabolism during a woman's cycle are associated with many of the emotional symptoms characteristic of PMS, including depression, anxiety, and irritability. In fact, the symptoms of low calcium status and PMS are remarkably similar. Clinical trials on women with PMS found that calcium supplementation effectively reduced many mood and emotional symptoms. Researchers at Columbia University report: "PMS represents the clinical manifestation of a calcium deficiency state that is unmasked following the rise of ovarian steroid hormone concentrations during the menstrual cycle." Since the average woman consumes approximately half her recommended intake for calcium, it is not surprising that lack of this mineral could be a major player in PMS symptoms.

*Magnesium:* Red blood cell concentrations of magnesium are low in women with PMS, although other blood indices of magnesium are normal. Symptoms of magnesium deficiency resemble those of PMS, including muscle spasms, appetite changes, nausea, personality changes, and apathy. Women who increase their intake of magnesium-rich foods report improvements in water retention, including weight gain, swelling of the extremities, breast tenderness, and abdominal bloating. Some researchers speculate that stress promotes magnesium excretion, which in turn leads to fluid and sodium retention.

*Herbs:* Vitex agnus castus (VAC) is an herb native to the Mediterranean area and Asia that has been used to treat premenstrual symptoms since antiquity. In one study, women who took VAC capsules experienced a reduction in PMS symptoms, such as breast tenderness, edema, tension, headaches, constipation, and depression. Minor side effects were reported, including gastrointestinal discomfort and headaches. VAC contains essential and fatty oils and flavonoids, which might contribute to its effectiveness. Compounds in this herb might alter metabolism in the hypothalamus and pituitary glands, which secrete luteinizing hormone (LD) and help regulate prostaglandins, both contributors to PMS symptoms.

## PMS: Diet Advice

Premenstrual syndrome is definitely linked to diet. During these ten days to two weeks before a woman's period, intake of sweets, fats, and calories skyrockets, according to researchers at the University of Adelaide. That's the bad news. The good news is there are a few diet tips that could curb PMS symptoms. Begin by following the Healthy Woman's Diet. In addition:

- Calcium supplementation, at a dose of 1,000 mg to 1,200 mg a day, decreases many of the symptoms of PMS, including pain, food cravings, and water retention.
- Magnesium supplements, at doses of 200 mg to 400 mg a day, might relieve some symptoms, including water retention, headaches, and moodiness. However, the link here is sketchy.
- Frequent inclusion of soy foods, such as fortified soy milk or tofu, in the weekly diet might help curb PMS symptoms.

- Limit sugar to 10 percent of calories and focus on whole grains.
- Drinking eight or more glasses of water daily and limiting salty foods help reduce bloating and breast tenderness.
- Supplements of vitamins $B_6$ and E have produced conflicting results.
- Herbal supplements, such as dong quai, Saint-John's-wort, and kava, might interact with prescription medications and are considered unsafe for women who might become pregnant. Vitex agnus castus (VAC) might be useful, but has some side effects.
- Include one to two tablespoons of safflower oil in the daily diet.
- Include physical activity in the daily routine.

A physician should be consulted if symptoms intensify or persist, since hormone and/or drug therapy might be indicated.

## Sexually Transmitted Diseases (STDs)

Sexually transmitted diseases, also called venereal diseases, are infections transmitted from one person to another person through sexual contact. Examples of STDs include gonorrhea, nonspecific urethritis (NSU), syphilis, herpes genitalis, and genital warts. The vaginal infections trichomoniasis and yeast infection can be transmitted through sexual conduct but are more frequently contracted through nonsexual means.

### Diet and STDs

The literature is sketchy on how diet affects a woman's risk for contracting an STD. Since maintaining a strong immune system is a primary defense against all forms of infection and disease, it is wise to consume a diet high in the nutrients known to aid in immunity, including the antioxidant nutrients (vitamin C, vitamin E, beta carotene, and selenium), the B vitamins, and the minerals iron, magnesium, and zinc.

One study from the Centers for Disease Control in Atlanta reports that vitamin C inactivates the herpes virus within days of exposure. This study concluded that vitamin C might be an effective antiviral agent in the treatment of both oral and genital herpes. (See chapter 14 for more information on nutrition and immunity.)

*Lysine and Herpes:* In the 1970s, researchers reported that supplemental doses of the amino acid lysine were effective in reducing the severity and frequency of herpes infections; however, lysine had no effect on preventing the infection. Some people report the pain subsides within hours and the herpes sores do not spread when supplements containing between 800 mg and 2 grams of lysine are consumed. Healing normally takes six to fifteen days, but with lysine as many as 83 percent of patients report lesions healed in five days or less. Some studies report that if the maintenance dose is too small (i.e., less than 750 mg per day) or is discontinued, herpes lesions reappear within one to four weeks.

L-lysine is thought to be the only effective form of lysine. Failures with lysine therapy might result from an inadequate dose of the amino acid or using D-lysine, which has no effect on viral growth. Normal dietary intake of lysine is not sufficient to produce the beneficial effects observed in some patients taking supplements.

The theory is that the herpes virus cannot grow in a lysine-rich environment, while another amino acid, arginine, triggers the growth of this virus. Consequently, an arginine-poor diet combined with lysine supplements is recommended for the treatment of herpes infections. Some studies show improvements in herpes symptoms in both the lysine-supplemented and the placebo groups, suggesting that a psychological factor exists and a person might be able to "will away" some infections.

## STDs: Diet Advice

The only dietary advice for the prevention and treatment of STDs is to consume a low-fat, nutrient-dense diet, such as the Healthy Woman's Diet. This diet supplies ample amounts of all the nutrients known to strengthen the immune system. In addition, supplementation with L-lysine (in doses of 750 mg or higher) combined with avoidance of arginine-containing foods, such as nuts, seeds, and chocolate, might reduce the frequency or severity of recurrent infections in some people.

Good sleeping habits, relaxation, and effective stress management are important, since physical and emotional stress suppress the immune system, which in turn increases a person's susceptibility to infection. Other stressors that should be avoided include tobacco smoke, alcohol, and caffeinated beverages.

The use of condoms is one way to reduce the risk of contracting an STD (other than abstinence). Inspecting the partner's genitals, routine medical evaluations, as well as the use of birth control foams, jellies, or creams also might reduce

STD risk. In addition, the more sexual partners a woman has, the higher her risk for contracting an STD.

In all cases, diet plays a minor role in the prevention and treatment of STDs. More importantly, a physician should be consulted at the first suspicion of infection and diagnostic tests and medical treatment should be initiated immediately.

## *Skin*

The skin's cells have a short life span and are replaced every few days; consequently, signs of nutritional deficiencies develop quickly. In contrast, clear, moist, glowing skin is a sign of internal health and optimal nutritional status.

The skin is comprised of three layers. The subcutaneous layer is the deepest layer and is primarily fat and a protein called collagen. The corium, or middle layer, shields underlying layers from injury and repairs surrounding layers when they are damaged. The upper portion of this layer has an abundant supply of blood

**FIGURE 16.2  The Layers of the Skin**

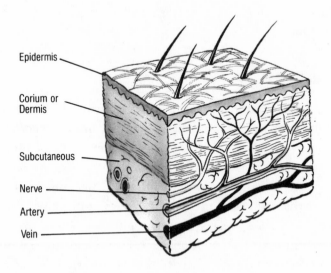

The skin consists of three layers: the subcutaneous, the corium (middle layer), and the epidermis (outer layer).

vessels and nerve endings; it is here that wrinkles originate. The epidermis, or top layer, is the thinnest layer of skin. The nails and hair grow from the epidermis. Covering all the layers of the skin is a layer of dead "keratinized" cells that swell in response to moisture and are shed daily.

## Diet and Skin

You skin is an outer reflection of your inner health. If you don't believe me, check out people's grocery carts. We look just like the food we buy. Carts filled with white bread, doughnuts, soft drinks, and potato chips are most likely pushed by people with pasty complexions, lifeless hair, and a glazed look in their eyes. The lady with the cart loaded with fresh spinach and strawberries, fat-free milk, whole-wheat bread, fresh salmon, and beans has a rosy glow to her cheeks, her hair is shiny, and she's downright perky.

OK, maybe I'm exaggerating . . . just a little, but what you eat *does* have a profound effect on how you look, both today and down the road. I'm not talking about severe deficiencies; you needn't be so drained of vitamin C that you bruise easily (a sign of scurvy) or so lacking in vitamin $B_2$ that you have cracks at the corners of your mouth. Even slight shortfalls from an optimal diet leave subtle effects on your looks.

The good news is that the nutrients needed for a healthy glow also revitalize your whole body, since every cell needs the same arsenal of vitamins and minerals to stay well tuned. Vanity might just be your best vice!

All nutrients, including calories, protein, fat, vitamins, minerals, and water, play important roles in maintaining healthy skin and in treating many skin disorders. For example, inadequate intake of any nutrient or calories results in reduced blood and oxygen flow to the skin, altered oil secretions within the skin, diminished maintenance and repair of injured tissue, dry skin, alterations in skin color, and limited ability to fight off infections.

*Vitamin A:* This fat-soluble vitamin is essential for the maintenance of epithelial tissues, with skin being the largest epithelial tissue you've got. Skimp on this vitamin and your skin might be dry, scaly, and rough. Excessive intake of vitamin A can cause skin itching, hair loss, and cracked lips. Your best source for this vitamin is nonfat milk fortified with vitamin A. The body can convert beta carotene found in orange and dark green vegetables into vitamin A. This conversion is carefully regulated so it's impossible to overdo it on produce.

*B Vitamins:* Poor intake of almost any B vitamin, including vitamin $B_2$, niacin, vitamin $B_6$, vitamin $B_{12}$, pantothenic acid, or biotin, can cause dermatitis-like symptoms, such as dry or scaly skin, itching, or a burning sensation. Vitamins $B_2$ and $B_6$ also are important in maintaining the oil-producing glands (the sebaceous glands), which keep the skin moist and smooth. For vitamin $B_2$, include in your diet several servings of nonfat milk, asparagus, and mushrooms. For more niacin, eat chicken, peanut butter, and green peas. Vitamin $B_6$ can be found in red meat, fish, and bananas, and good sources of vitamin $B_{12}$ include red meat, nonfat milk, and tempeh.

*Zinc:* This trace mineral helps maintain collagen and elastin fibers that give skin its firmness and help prevent sagging and wrinkles. Zinc is important in healing cuts and scrapes, while a deficiency causes dry, rough skin. Limited evidence suggests zinc also helps treat acne. Zinc-rich foods include oysters, turkey, pork, and wheat germ.

*Low-Fat Diets:* Adopting a diet that supplies 20 percent fat or less, rather than the typical American diet with almost twice the fat, lowers your risk for skin cancer, according to studies from Baylor College of Medicine in Houston. In a two-year study where people consumed typical-fat or low-fat diets, researchers found that the high-fat diets increased skin-cancer risk fourfold. "The benefits were noted only after sixteen months on the low-fat diet," says John Wolf, M.D., chairman of the department of dermatology where these studies were conducted. That means you must make a commitment to low-fat and stick with it for life. "The sooner you start the better," says Dr. Wolf, "since it's better to eat healthy before you develop precancerous skin lesions." However, Dr. Wolf adds that it's never too late to reap the benefits, no matter what your age.

*Linoleic Acid:* This essential fat is important for healthy, moist skin. A deficiency causes dry, rough, itchy, or blotchy skin. Make sure you include a couple of servings of nuts, wheat germ, or safflower and sunflower oils in the daily diet.

*Fish Oils:* In general, a high-fat diet increases your risk for skin cancer, while cutting back on fat reduces risk. The omega-3 fats in fish, such as salmon, herring, and mackerel, are exceptions; they lower skin-cancer risk, at least in animals, says Dr. Wolf.

*The Antioxidants:* The number one enemy of skin is the sun. Ultraviolet (UV) rays in sunlight generate oxygen fragments called free radicals. These highly reactive compounds pierce delicate cell membranes and attack the genetic code within skin cells, damaging underlying structures such as collagen and elastic fibers. UVA light penetrates the outer layers of the skin, causing sunburn, sun spots, rough texture, and skin cancer. UVB light penetrates deeper skin layers, resulting in wrinkles. Don't think you're off the hook because it's winter! Those UV rays can get you on the ski slopes and through cloud cover just as easily as they can reach you on the beach on a sunny day.

Fortunately, the skin has an anti–free radical system comprised of antioxidants that protect the skin from free radical damage. Frequent sun exposure and smog deplete the skin's antioxidants, such as beta carotene and vitamins C and E. It also takes up to three months to accumulate antioxidants in skin. "Along with sunscreen and a hat, people should boost their intake of antioxidant-rich foods now to get additional protection from sunburn later on," recommends Ronald Watson, Ph.D., professor of Public Health Research at Arizona Health Sciences Center in Tucson. Also, these antioxidants work as a team, so a combination is better than focusing on only one.

Vitamin C is an important antioxidant defender of the skin. Sun exposure (as well as stress) drains C from the skin for up to seventy-two hours, leaving skin vulnerable to damage. The combination of vitamins E and C is especially effective in reducing sunburn damage. (Don't get carried away and think you can leave the house without sunscreen!) Vitamin C in citrus fruits, kiwi, and other fruits and vegetables also helps maintain collagen, the underlying supporting structure of skin.

Sun exposure depletes vitamin E from the skin (by up to 50 percent!), while boosting intake of this antioxidant, alone or in combination with other antioxidants like beta carotene, helps lower skin-cancer risk. Vitamin E in nuts, seeds, wheat germ, and avocados also slows the aging of skin cells, by reducing the production of an enzyme called collagenase that otherwise breaks down collagen, causing the skin to sag and wrinkle. To get enough of this vitamin, consider taking a supplement. Natural vitamin E (d-alpha tocopherol) is best (100 IU to 400 IU daily).

As little as one-half cup of cooked carrots every day provides enough beta carotene to reduce the redness and skin inflammation of sunburn, a sign of accelerated aging and cancer of the skin. "Beta carotene accumulates in the skin providing twenty-four-hour protection against sun damage," says Dr. Watson. He adds that the more carotene-rich produce you eat, the more skin protection you get. Caution: Eating too many carotene-rich foods, such as sweet potatoes, carrots, and mangoes, can turn skin yellowish, but don't worry, this fades when you cut back on carrots and doesn't show up at all with a light tan.

Selenium, an antioxidant found in seafood, whole grains, and legumes, protects against the damaging effects of UV light, reducing your risk for sunburn and skin cancer. Low blood levels of selenium increase skin-cancer risk.

*Tea:* Tea contains antioxidant compounds called polyphenols that reduce sun damage to the skin associated with wrinkling and cancer. Tea also reduces the inflammation and redness associated with sunburn. While green tea is the best source of polyphenols, black tea also contains these helpful compounds.

*Phytochemicals:* Carotenoids (cousins to beta carotene) combine with vitamin E to reduce redness associated with sunburn and to reduce skin sensitivity to sunlight. "There appears to be substantial protection against sun damage from dietary antioxidants, including vitamin E and carotenoids like lutein," says Jeffrey Blumberg, Ph.D., professor in the School of Nutrition Science and Policy at Tufts University in Boston. He adds that the antioxidant alpha-lipoic acid, found especially in spinach, also shows promise in reducing the risk of skin injury from sun exposure. Phytoestrogens in soy products, such as soy milk and tofu, also might lower skin-cancer risk. Dr. Watson's work with pycnogenol (an antioxidant-rich extract of pine tree bark) has found similar benefits to beta carotene in reducing skin damage.

*Glutathione:* Glutathione is a proteinlike antioxidant made in the body that protects tissues, including the skin, from free radical damage. Levels of this compound drop when skin is exposed to sunlight, a sign that glutathione helps defend skin from damage. Sources of glutathione include fruit and raw vegetables, such as peaches, asparagus, cabbage, and cauliflower. The building blocks for glutathione, including the amino acids cysteine and methionine, are found in extra-lean meat, chicken, fish, and milk.

## Skin: Diet Advice

The Healthy Woman's Diet forms the basis for healthy skin. Make sure to include at least eight to ten servings daily of dark-colored fruits and vegetables and focus on whole grains and other minimally processed foods. In addition,

- Consider taking a vitamin E supplement.
- Drink tea instead of coffee.
- Drink plenty of water; at least eight glasses a day, more if you exercise.
- Always use sunscreen with number 15 SPF or higher, wear a hat in the sun, and use other protection against the sun's damaging rays.
- Keep skin clean and well moisturized.

## TABLE 16.10    New Skin Nutrients

The antioxidants from that carrot you munched at lunch are mostly stored in the deeper subcutaneous layer of the skin, thus leaving the outer epidermis only partially protected. A wealth of research is accumulating to show that rubbing some nutrients or phytonutrients (plant nutrients) on the top of your skin helps nourish from the outside in. Look for these ingredients in future skin-care products.

*Aloe Vera:* The gel extracted from this plant soothes sunburned skin, reducing inflammation, according to a study from the University of Texas Medical Branch in Galveston.

*Vitamin K:* Considering laser treatment to erase those fine lines? You might consider topical vitamin K, too. A study from Cornell Medical Center in Ithaca found that the redness associated with facial lasering healed faster when a topical cream containing vitamin K and retinol (a vitamin A derivative) was applied after surgery, under physician supervision of course!

*Vitamin C:* The skin receives only 8 percent of the vitamin C absorbed from a glass of orange juice. But the outer skin layers need more than that for protection against sun-generated free radicals that break down delicate cell membranes, resulting in wrinkling and sagging of skin, as well as skin cancer. Accumulating evidence suggests you get the maximum protection with a combination of vitamin C and vitamin E. Topical vitamin C also might speed healing after laser resurfacing, but discuss this with your physician, since only water-based vitamin C solutions worked in one study, while creams were ineffective.

*Vitamin D:* Topical application of vitamin D reduces symptoms of a type of dermatitis called prurigo, characterized by itching and hivelike bumps on the skin.

*Selenium:* A 0.02 percent solution of this antioxidant mineral reduces sun damage to skin, including risk for skin cancer.

*Melatonin:* Look for this hormonelike compound in future skin creams, since preliminary evidence suggests it works to curb sun damage when applied topically with vitamins E and C.

*Green Tea:* Polyphenolic compounds in tea curb sun damage whether you drink them or rub them on your skin. Applied topically, green tea appears to reduce skin-cancer risk, inflammation from sunburn, and skin aging.

# *Urinary Tract Infections*

Urinary tract infections (UTI) or bladder infections are the most common kidney-related disorder in women. Bladder infections can be caused by congenital obstruction, kidney stones, injury to the urinary tract, or chronic inflammation by bacteria. In the latter, bacteria migrate from the outside of the body up the urethra into the bladder. They also can travel to the kidneys from another part of the body through the bloodstream. Once in the urinary tract, the bacteria multiply and spread, which disrupts normal function and causes inflammation and swelling. If untreated, bladder infections can lead to chronic pyelonephritis, a condition where the kidneys become increasingly damaged by repeated infections.

Symptoms of a bladder infection include pain when urinating, frequent need to urinate, and sometimes blood in the urine. Urethritis is inflammation of the urethra (the tube that leads from the bladder to the outside of the body). The symptoms are similar to a bladder infection, but urethritis usually occurs in women as a result of bruising during sexual intercourse.

## Bladder Infections: Diet Advice

The common nutritional therapy for bladder infections is to force fluids—consume three to four quarts of water daily—and an "acid-ash" diet, which consists of high-protein foods, such as meats, fish, eggs, and gelatin products; cranberries, plums, and prunes; and vitamin C supplements. This produces an acidic urine that helps limit bacterial growth.

Cranberries contain a group of phytochemicals called tannins that block the binding of germs to cells in the lining of the urinary bladder, thus helping to flush these bugs out of the body and prevent or treat bladder infections. (Blueberries also contain these compounds.) A Harvard study found that women who drank ten ounces of cranberry juice daily reduced their risk for developing urinary tract infections over a six-month period. A word of warning: Cranberry juice is a help, not a substitute for medical treatment. Check labels, since most cranberry beverages contain anywhere from 10 to 33 percent cranberry juice, and some are sweetened with highly processed pear or apple juice so that the label reads 100 percent juice. New versions on the market are fortified with vitamin C, which also might reduce the growth of bacteria in the urinary tract.

Although vitamin A is essential for the development and maintenance of a healthy urinary tract, there is no evidence that this vitamin is effective in the prevention or treatment of bladder infections.

Always seek immediate medical advice for the treatment of bladder infections and always comply with medication use. To prevent bladder infections, wear cotton underwear, urinate regularly, empty the urinary bladder after intercourse, avoid bath salts or bubble bath, and wipe front to back.

# *Yeast Infections*

*Candida albicans* is a common organism found on the skin and in the mouth, digestive tract, or vagina. Under normal conditions, this fungus causes no problems; the numbers are small and are kept in check by harmless bacteria. The fungus proliferates and symptoms develop when conditions change to favor their growth. The result is a yeast infection that causes numerous problems, including vaginitis.

For example, antibiotic medications or feminine hygiene sprays destroy helpful bacteria and allow uncontrolled growth of *Candida* in the vagina. Pregnancy, diabetes, douching, sexual activity, or taking birth control pills also alter the vaginal environment and favor the growth of yeast, as does a compromised immune system.

Symptoms of *Candida albicans* growth include itching, a thick white discharge, irritation of the vagina, and swelling or redness of the vulva. Pain or soreness during intercourse and a need to urinate more frequently also might develop. *Candida* also might trigger nonspecific allergic reactions, including histamine release.

## Diet and Yeast Infection

The role of diet in the development and progression of yeast infections is unclear.

*Sugar:* One theory is that diets high in sweets or alcohol increase urinary loss of sugar and elevate the risk for vaginal *Candida* infection. According to this theory, reducing sugar intake, which means cutting back on table sugar, honey, and dairy products such as milk that contain milk sugar or lactose, might reduce the loss of sugar in the urine, and result in fewer complaints of yeast infection. No well-designed studies have proven that sugar has any influence on yeast infections. Yet, since most women consume too much sugar, cutting back on these useless calories is safe and possibly helpful in the treatment of yeast infections.

*Fish Oils:* Preliminary research also shows a possible association between fish oils and *Candida albicans* infection. A fatty acid in fish oils called EPA (eicosapentaenoic acid) reduces inflammation, while enhancing the body's immune response to counteract the growth of *Candida* infection.

*Yogurt:* The home remedy of using yogurt to treat *Candida* infections might have merit. One study found a threefold decrease in *Candida* infections and a significant reduction in the amount of *Candida albicans* numbers in the vagina of women who consumed daily one cup of yogurt containing *Lacto-bacillus acidophilus*. This culture does not kill the infection, but changes the microbial environment of the vagina to encourage the growth of normal, healthy bacteria. In addition, consuming live, active cultures found in yogurt enhances specific immune processes and might have a secondary benefit in strengthening a woman's defense against future infections.

*Yeast-Containing Foods:* Limited research also shows a possible connection between dietary intake of yeast-containing foods and *Candida albicans* infection. Women already at risk for developing an infection, i.e., people on long-term antibiotic therapy, have unusually high antibodies to yeasts found in baker's and brewer's yeasts. This hypersensitivity to dietary yeast products might contribute to the development of *Candida albicans* infections. In some cases, recurrent yeast infections have been successfully managed with medication and by reducing the intake of yeast-containing foods.

*Garlic:* Garlic might help prevent or treat *Candida albicans* infections. A component in garlic called allicin is a potent fighter against yeast, such as *Candida*. Garlic supplements must contain allicin to provide a protective effect. An optimal dose is unknown, although daily inclusion of a clove or two in the normal diet is safe, tolerable, and potentially useful.

*Vitamins:* Vaginal yeast infections are associated with impaired immunity. The number and activity of specialized immune cells, called monocytes, is reduced in women susceptible to repeated infections of *Candida albicans,* which might be caused by fluctuations in female hormones, especially progesterone, or other factors that suppress the immune system, including marginal nutrient intake.

Limited research shows a connection between vitamin status and risk for *Candida* infections. Vitamin A helps maintain the lining of the vagina and stimulates immune responses that defend against infection. Vitamin A deficiency has been noted in some women with recurrent vaginitis; however, the evidence is inconclusive whether a deficiency causes or is a result of the infection. Other vitamins that might help include vitamins $B_6$, $B_2$, and C, beta carotene, and biotin.

*Minerals:* Magnesium deficiency is sometimes noted in women with yeast infections. How magnesium might affect the development and progression of infection is unknown. A magnesium deficiency might reduce resistance to *Candida* infection or stimulate the release of histamine, which suppresses the immune system. A magnesium deficiency also might be secondary to marginal intake of vitamin $B_6$. Mild zinc deficiency also might increase a woman's susceptibility to, or contribute to, the development and progression of yeast infections.

## Yeast Infections: Diet Advice

Until more is known about how diet affects the risk and development of this type of infection, it is best to consume a low-fat, nutrient-dense diet, such as the Healthy Woman's Diet, that supplies ample amounts of all the nutrients associated with a strong immune system. In addition,

- Limit sugar, including table sugar, honey, "raw" sugar, or corn syrup.
- Consume fiber-rich foods, such as fruits and vegetables, cooked dried beans and peas, whole-grain cereals, and nuts.

Include one or more servings daily of yogurt that contains the *Lacto-bacillus acidophilus* bacteria. Not all yogurt contains *Lacto-bacillus acidophilus,* while many commercial yogurts include cultures of *L. bulgarius, L. lactis,* or *S. thermophilus.* These bacteria do not establish residency in the intestine or migrate as well into the vagina and do not show the same beneficial effects of *Lacto-bacillus acidophilus.* Some commercial yogurts claim to have *Lacto-bacillus acidophilus* but actually contain little or none. The effectiveness of *Lacto-bacillus acidophilus* tablets is controversial; some women report they are effective, while other women must rely on yogurt or bottled refrigerated *Lacto-bacillus acidophilus* liquid. You should research the content of any commercial yogurt to make sure it contains the advertised *Lacto-bacillus acidophilus.* Finally, whether it is consumed from dietary or supplemental sources, moderation remains the rule. More is not necessarily better.

If the above dietary recommendations combined with medication therapy are not effective, try avoiding yeast-containing foods, such as yeasted breads, brewer's yeast, and pastries made with yeast. There is no need to continue this dietary change if no improvements are noted within a few months.

In addition to dietary changes, avoid wearing nylon underwear or panty hose; long hours in tight-fitting clothes such as leotards, bathing suits, or garments made from fabrics that do not breathe naturally; or fabrics that irritate. Instead,

- Wear cotton underwear and polypropylene workout clothes.
- Use a hair dryer on a cool setting to dry the pubic area after a workout or shower.
- Sleep in cotton pajamas to allow air to circulate at night.
- Do not use feminine hygiene sprays or powders, or douche the vaginal area more than once a week.

Over-the-counter antifungal medications are now available to treat yeast infection; however, always consult a physician if you are not sure whether the condition is a yeast infection. Boric acid suppositories also might help prevent or treat the condition. Women who smoke, are overweight, became sexually active at an early age, or have had several sexual partners also are at increased risk of developing yeast infections.

# *Glossary*

**Acetylcholine:** A neurotransmitter associated with the regulation of numerous body processes, including memory.

**Achlorhydria:** Lack of stomach acid. A condition that increases in frequency as women age and can interfere with nutrient absorption.

**Additive:** A chemical substance added to food, either intentionally or unintentionally.

**Aerobic:** In the presence of oxygen. Aerobic exercise is any slow, steady exercise, such as bicycling, jogging, swimming, or walking, that requires constant long-term use of large muscle groups. Aerobic fitness refers to increased ability to transport oxygen to the tissues and is associated with cardiovascular fitness.

**Allicin:** A sulfur-containing compound in garlic that has antibiotic effects.

**Amenorrhea:** Cessation of the menstrual cycle.

**Amino Acid:** A building block or precursor of protein. More than twenty-one amino acids are used by the body to manufacture different proteins in hair, skin, blood, and other tissues.

**Anabolic:** Building tissue.

**Androgens:** Male hormones, such as testosterone.

**Anemia:** A reduction in the size, number, or color of red blood cells that results in reduced oxygen-carrying capacity of the blood.

**Anorexia:** The lack or loss of appetite for food, associated with weight loss and muscle wastage. Anorexia nervosa is a condition characterized by self-induced starvation.

**Antibody:** A substance in body fluids that is a component of the immune system and protects the body against disease and infection.

**Antioxidant:** A compound produced in the body or a nutrient supplied in the diet that neutralizes harmful substances called free radicals. Examples of antioxidants include vitamin C, vitamin E, beta carotene, and selenium.

**Arginine:** An amino acid.

**Artery:** A blood vessel that supplies blood, oxygen, and nutrients to the tissues.

**Ascorbic Acid:** Vitamin C.

**Aspartame:** A sugar substitute sold as NutraSweet or Equal.

**Atherosclerosis:** The accumulation of fat in the artery wall. It is the underlying cause of cardiovascular disease.

**Balanced Diet:** A diet where all vitamins, minerals, protein, essential fats, fiber, and other nutrients are supplied in optimal amounts. The typical balanced diet supplies a variety of foods from fruits and vegetables, breads and cereals, low-fat milk products, and extra-lean meats, chicken, fish, and cooked dried beans and peas.

**Beta Carotene:** A building block for vitamin A found in dark green or orange fruits and vegetables. Beta carotene also functions as an antioxidant independent of its vitamin A activity.

**Biotin:** A B vitamin important in the breakdown of fats, proteins, and carbohydrates for energy.

**Blood Cholesterol Levels:** Blood cholesterol levels are the best indicators of whether a person will have or has developed heart disease. A total blood cholesterol level greater than 200 mg/dl of blood is indicative of elevated risk.

**BMI:** Body Mass Index. A measurement using height and weight to identify body fat.

**Bulimia:** An eating disorder characterized by excessive food intake followed by vomiting, laxative use, or fasting.

**Caloric Density:** Refers to the amount of calories in a food relative to its nutrient content. A calorie-dense food supplies few nutrients for its calorie cost.

**Calorie:** A measurement of energy in food. Dietary calories are really kilocalories or kcalories and are one thousand times as large as the physicist's calorie. A kcalorie is the amount of heat energy necessary to raise the temperature of 1,000 grams of water 1 degree Centigrade. ("Calor" means heat and "kilo" means one thousand.) In foods, protein and carbohydrates supply 4 calories per gram, fat supplies 9 calories per gram, and alcohol supplies 7 calories per gram.

**Candidiasis:** An infection by a fungus called *Candida*. The infection can occur in the lungs, heart, vagina, gastrointestinal tract, skin, nails, or other tissues. Also called a yeast infection.

**Carbohydrate:** The starches and sugars in the diet.

**Carcinogen:** A cancer-causing substance.

**Cardiovascular Disease:** A disease of the heart and blood vessels often caused by the accumulation of cholesterol in the lining of the blood vessels.

**Cataract:** A milky film that forms over the eye and is one of the most common reasons for loss of eyesight.

**Celiac Disease:** A digestive tract disease caused by a sensitivity to a protein in wheat called gluten. Other terms for this condition include gluten-sensitive enteropathy, nontropical sprue, and idiopathic steatorrhea.

**Cell Membrane:** The outer covering of each cell composed of fats and proteins.

**Cervix:** The neck or opening to the uterus.

**Cholesterol:** A type of fat that supplies no calories and is found only in foods of animal origin, such as eggs, organ meats, meat, chicken, fish, dairy products, or processed foods made with these ingredients, such as egg noodles or pie crust made with lard. Increased dietary intake of cholesterol-rich foods is associated with elevated blood levels of cholesterol and an increased risk for developing heart disease.

Cholesterol is an essential component in the body and is needed for the manufacture of certain hormones, bile, and other compounds. However, the body manufactures all it needs, so intake of this fat only contributes to excesses, not to health.

**Cholesterol Oxides:** Cholesterol damaged by free radicals.

**Choline:** A B vitamin–like compound obtained from the diet and manufactured by the body. Whether or not choline is an essential nutrient remains controversial.

**Collagen:** A protein in connective tissues and the organ substance in teeth and bones.

**Complementary Protein:** Two or more proteins whose amino acid compositions complement each other so that the essential amino acids missing from one are supplied by the other. An example would be whole-wheat bread and cooked split peas.

**Complex Carbohydrate:** The starches in the diet comprised of ten to more than a thousand glucose units linked much like pearls on a string.

**Connective Tissue:** A weblike tissue located in every organ that holds together and supports the various tissues within the organ.

**Corium:** The middle layer of the skin.

**Coronary Arteries:** The arteries that supply the heart.

**Cortisol:** A hormone secreted by the adrenal glands that acts much like cortisone in stimulating the body to manufacture more glucose for energy.

**Cruciferous Vegetables:** Vegetables in the cabbage family, including broccoli, asparagus, Brussels sprouts, kohlrabi, and cabbage, that contain compounds called "indoles," which are protective against cancer.

**Daily Value:** Based on the Recommended Dietary Allowances, these values appear on labels to provide information on the nutritional quality of a supplement or processed food.

**Diastolic Blood Pressure:** The lower of two readings that make up a blood pressure test. Diastolic blood pressure corresponds to the least amount of pressure in the cardiovascular system at any one time and reflects the pressure inherent in the heart and blood vessels when the heart relaxes between beats (contractions).

**Docosahexaenoic Acid (DHA):** An omega-3 fatty acid in fish oils.

**Dysplasia:** Abnormal cell growth.

**Eclampsia:** See *Toxemia.*

**Eicosapentaenoic Acid (EPA):** An omega-3 fatty acid in fish oils.

**Electrolyte:** A substance or salt that dissolves into positive- or negative-charged particles and conducts an electrical charge. Sodium, potassium, and chloride are examples of electrolytes.

**Endometrium:** Lining of the uterus.

**Endorphins:** A group of neurotransmitter-like substances that produce a calming effect on the brain much like morphine.

**Energy:** The fuel that powers all body processes. Equivalent to calories. The nutrients that supply energy or calories include protein (4 calories/gram), carbohydrates (4 calories/gram), fat (9 calories/gram), and alcohol (7+ calories/gram). The body stores energy as fat tissue, and to a limited amount as glycogen (sugar) in the muscles and liver.

**Enriched:** The addition to processed foods of a few nutrients to bring the level back to the original vitamin or mineral content. Only four nutrients are added back in the enrichment process, while many more nutrients are lost.

**Enzyme:** A compound that acts as a catalyst in starting chemical reactions in the body.

**Epidermis:** The outer layer of the skin.

**Epinephrine:** A hormone and nerve chemical. Also called adrenaline.

**Epithelial:** The tissues that line the internal and external surfaces of the body, including the skin, lining of the blood vessels, uterus, urinary bladder, and outer surface of the eye.

**Esophagus:** The passageway or tube from the throat to the stomach.

**Essential Fatty Acid:** A polyunsaturated fat that cannot be manufactured by the body, i.e., linoleic acid.

**Essential Nutrient:** A necessary substance that cannot be manufactured in sufficient amounts in the body and must be obtained regularly from the diet.

**Estrogen:** A family of female hormones that regulates menstruation and possibly protects against heart disease and osteoporosis.

**Extracellular:** Outside the cells. Extracellular fluid includes blood, lymph, and fluid between the cells (interstitial fluid).

**Fat Calories:** The amount of calories supplied by fat in the diet. This percentage is calculated by multiplying the total grams of fat in a food or menu by 9 (fat supplies 9 calories per gram), dividing by the total calories in the food or menu, and multiplying by 100.

**Fatty Acid:** A fat-soluble molecule that consists of a long chain of carbon atoms with hydrogen attached. Three fatty acids combined to a glycerol molecule comprise a triglyceride. Eicosapentaenoic acid (EPA) and linoleic acid are examples of fatty acids.

**Ferritin:** A form of iron in the blood. The serum ferritin test measures iron status, in particular iron deficiency prior to the onset of anemia.

**Ferrous:** Iron.

**Fiber:** The indigestible residue of food, composed of the carbohydrates cellulose, pectin, and hemicellulose; vegetable gums; and the noncarbohydrate lignin.

**Flavonoids:** More than two hundred phytochemicals, including rutin, hesperidin, and quercetin, found in fruits and vegetables that enhance vitamin C activity and exert antioxidant capabilities.

**Folacin:** Folic acid or folate, a B vitamin.

**Follicle Stimulating Hormone (FSH):** A hormone secreted by the pituitary that stimulates the growth and maturation of follicles in the ovaries.

**Food and Drug Administration (FDA):** An agency of the United States government responsible for monitoring the safety and effectiveness of food, drugs, and cosmetics sold in the United States.

**Food Intolerance:** Inability to digest a food as a result of individual chemical idiosyncrasies, food contamination, psychological factors, or digestive enzyme deficiencies. Lactose intolerance is a food intolerance resulting from inadequate amounts of the digestive enzyme lactase.

**Fortified:** The addition of vitamins or minerals to a processed food to levels higher than naturally found. Milk is fortified with vitamin D.

**Free Radical:** Highly reactive substances found in air pollution, tobacco smoke, foods, pesticides, ultraviolet sunlight, and manufactured during normal body processes that damage cell components and contribute to disease and aging.

**Fructose:** A simple sugar or carbohydrate sometimes known as fruit sugar. High fructose corn syrup (HFCS) used in soft drinks contains between 40 to 90 percent fructose. Honey is approximately 50 percent fructose.

**Functional Food:** A food or food component that provides a health benefit beyond the traditional nutrients it contains. Calcium-fortified orange juice is an example.

**Gamma Liolenic Acid (GLA):** An omega-3 fatty acid in plants.

**Gastritis:** Inflammation of the stomach lining.

**Gastrointestinal Tract:** The digestive tract, including the stomach and intestines.

**Genetics:** The branch of biology that studies heredity and biological variation.

**Glucose:** Sugar, blood sugar, the building blocks of starch.

**Glucose Tolerance Factor (GTF):** A compound containing chromium that aids the hormone insulin in regulating blood sugar levels.

**Glucose Tolerance Test (GTT):** A test that measures blood sugar regulation, in particular the presence of hyperglycemia or diabetes and hypoglycemia. Oral administration of a glucose solution on an empty stomach with monitoring of blood sugar levels for up to four hours.

**Glutathione (Gla):** A nonessential substance in the diet that has antioxidant capabilities.

**Glycogen:** The storage form of glucose in the body. Glycogen is formed and stored in the liver and muscles and is converted to glucose when energy is needed.

**Gram:** A unit of weight. Twenty-eight grams equal one ounce.

**HDL Cholesterol:** Cholesterol packaged in high-density lipoproteins. HDL is comprised of fats and protein and serves as a transport for fats in the blood. A high level of HDL is associated with a reduced risk for developing cardiovascular disease.

**Hematocrit:** A test for iron-deficiency anemia. The volume percent of red blood cells in blood.

**Heme Iron:** Iron associated with hemoglobin in red blood cells. This form of iron, found in meat, chicken, and fish, is well absorbed, i.e., 30 percent is absorbed compared to only 2 to 7 percent absorption in nonheme iron foods, such as vegetables, grains, and fruit.

**Hemoglobin:** The oxygen-carrying protein in red blood cells. Each molecule of hemoglobin contains four atoms of iron. The hemoglobin test is a measure of iron status, in particular iron-deficiency anemia.

**Hemolytic Anemia:** Destruction of red blood cells, typically caused by vitamin E deficiency.

**Homocysteine:** An amino acid found in the blood. When levels are high, a condition called hyperhomocysteinemia, a woman is at increased risk for heart disease.

**Hormone:** A substance, produced by an organ called an endocrine gland, that is released into the blood and transported to another organ or tissue, where it performs a specific action. Examples of hormones include adrenaline and estrogen.

**Hot Flashes:** A common symptom of menopause, possibly caused by fluctuations in hormones. Visible redness in the face, neck, and throat, followed by profuse sweating and lasting for a few minutes.

**Hyperglycemia:** High blood sugar levels, often associated with diabetes or risk for developing diabetes.

**Hyperplasia:** An increase in the number of cells in a tissue. Can be a precursor for cancer.

**Hypertension:** High blood pressure.

**Hypoglycemia:** Low blood sugar levels.

**Immune System:** A complex system of substances, tissues, and organs that protects the body against disease and infection.

**Immunity:** The body's resistance to disease provided by a complex system of specialized cells, tissues, organs, and chemicals, such as antibodies and interferon.

**Indoles:** A group of phytochemicals in cruciferous vegetables (vegetables in the cabbage family) associated with a reduced risk for developing cancer.

**Insomnia:** Inability to sleep, to stay asleep, or to fall asleep.

**Insulin:** A hormone produced by the pancreas that regulates blood sugar levels.

**Interferon:** An immune system chemical produced in response to a virus that prevents the virus from multiplying.

**International Unit (IU):** An arbitrary measurement used for the fat-soluble vitamins A, D, and E. These units standardize the potency of the vitamin, rather than measure it by weight (i.e., grams or milligrams). IUs can be converted to weight measurements. For example, 3.33 IU of vitamin A are equivalent to 1 mcg.

**Intracellular:** Inside the cell.

**Intrinsic Factor:** A substance secreted in the digestive tract that is essential for vitamin $B_{12}$ absorption.

**Keratin:** A tough protein substance that gives hardness or structure to nails, hair, and the skin.

*Lacto-bacillus acidophilus:* A bacteria found in some yogurt that helps maintain a healthy environment in the digestive tract and vagina. Also called *L. acidophilus* or acidophilus.

**Lacto-Ovo Vegetarian Diet:** A diet that omits meat, chicken, and fish and is derived from fruit, vegetables, whole-grain breads and cereals, nuts, seeds, eggs, and dairy products.

**Lactose:** Milk sugar.

**LDL Cholesterol:** Low density lipoprotein. A molecule comprised of fats and protein that transports cholesterol in the blood. A high level of LDL is associated with an increased risk for developing cardiovascular disease.

**Lecithin:** A compound that has fat-soluble and water-soluble sides, thus making it a good emulsifier. Lecithin is a source of choline, is a constituent of cell membranes, is manufactured in the liver, and is found in food.

**Legume:** Dried beans and peas.

**Linoleic Acid:** An essential fatty acid found in safflower oil and to a lesser extent in other vegetable oils.

**Lipid:** Fat, including triglycerides, phospholipids, and cholesterol.

**Lipoprotein:** A compound comprised of fat and protein that carries fats, such as triglycerides and cholesterol, in the blood.

**Luteinizing Hormone:** A hormone produced in the pituitary gland that stimulates the secretion of sex hormones by the ovaries.

**Lymphocyte:** A specialized white blood cell that is a component of the immune system and aids in the protection of the body against disease and infection. There are B lymphocytes and T lymphocytes or B-cells and T-cells.

**Lysine:** One of the ten essential amino acids.

**Macrophage:** A large blood cell involved in the immune response and the body's resistance to infection and disease.

**Macula:** Macula lutea. A pigment area of the retina in the eye.

**Megadose:** Large intake of a nutrient; more than ten times the recommendation.

**Megaloblastic Anemia:** Anemia characterized by large, misshapen red blood cells that result from a deficiency of folic acid or vitamin $B_{12}$.

**Menopause:** The permanent cessation of the menstrual cycle.

**Menses:** Menstruation.

**Menstrual:** Pertaining to menstruation or the monthly discharge of blood and tissue from the uterus occurring between puberty and menopause.

**Menstruation:** The monthly discharge of blood and tissue from the uterus.

**Metabolism:** The sum of all the chemical processes that convert food and its components to fundamental chemicals the body uses for energy or for repair, maintenance, and growth of tissues.

**Microgram (mcg):** A metric unit of weight equivalent to one one-thousandth of a milligram or one-millionth of a gram.

**Microorganism:** Bacteria, viruses, and other minute life-forms that are visible only through a microscope.

**Milligram (mg):** A metric unit of weight equivalent to one one-thousandth of a gram.

**Mineral:** An inorganic, fundamental substance found naturally in the soil with specific chemical and structural properties.

**Monocytes:** A specialized white blood cell important in the immune response.

**Monounsaturated Fat:** A type of fat that has one site on the fatty acid for the addition of a hydrogen atom. An example of a monounsaturated fat is oleic acid in olive oil.

**Mucus:** A thick liquid secreted by the mucous glands.

**Myoglobin:** The iron-containing storage molecule for oxygen in the tissues, similar to hemoglobin in the blood.

**Neoplasia:** Abnormal, precancerous cell growth.

**Neural Tube Defects:** A congenital condition where the tube surrounding the spinal cord does not form correctly, such as spina bifida. A primary cause of birth defects.

**Neurotransmitter:** A chemical that serves as a communication link between nerve cells or between a nerve cell and a muscle or organ. Serotonin and acetylcholine are examples of neurotransmitters.

**Niacin:** A B vitamin important in breaking down carbohydrates, protein, and fat for energy. Also called nicotinic acid or niacinamide.

**Nutrient Density:** Refers to the amount of vitamins, minerals, and other nutrients in a food relative to its calorie content. A nutrient-dense food is one that supplies ample amounts of nutrients for few calories.

**Obesity:** Body fat weight more than 20 percent above ideal body weight. The body weight is excess fat, not muscle or lean tissue.

**Omega-3 Fatty Acid:** Fatty acids found in fish oils and gamma linolenic acid that reduce the risk for heart disease, cancer, arthritis, and other disorders, while strengthening the immune system.

**Oral:** Pertaining to the mouth.

**Ovary:** A glandular organ in the female reproductive system that produces the ovum (egg) and secretes the female hormones estrogen and progesterone.

**Ovulation:** The growth, maturation, and release of the egg (ovum) from the ovaries each month.

**Oxidative Stress or Oxidative Damage:** Free radical damage to tissues and molecules in the body associated with premature aging, disease, and suppressed immune function.

**Oxidized LDL Cholesterol:** LDL cholesterol that has been damaged by free radicals and is suspected to promote the development of atherosclerosis more than normal LDL cholesterol.

**Ozone:** A highly reactive modification of oxygen whereby the two atoms in oxygen $(O_2)$ are increased to three $(O_3)$.

**Pancreas:** The organ responsible for the production and secretion of numerous digestive enzymes and the hormone insulin.

**Perimenopause:** The period immediately prior to, and for one year following, the menopause with hormonal, chemical, and biological symptoms associated with the approach of the menopause.

**Pernicious Anemia:** Anemia caused by inadequate secretion of intrinsic factor, whereby vitamin $B_{12}$ is not absorbed and anemia develops.

**Peroxide:** One of a number of highly reactive free radicals.

**Phytochemical:** Thousands of health-enhancing compounds in fruits, vegetables, whole grains, legumes, tea, and other real foods. These compounds lower disease risk.

**Phytoestrogens:** Phytochemicals in soy that lower heart disease and possible cancer risk.

**Phytosterols:** Phytochemicals in legumes that slow the progression of and even prevent colon cancer.

**PKU:** Phenylketonuria. Excretion in the urine of excessive amounts of a breakdown product of the amino acid phenylalanine. It results from a genetically determined metabolic disorder and causes mental retardation unless foods containing phenylalanine are eliminated from the diet.

**Placebo:** A medicine or pill that has no pharmacologic effect, but is used to test the efficacy of a substance or drug. The "placebo effect" occurs when a health condition improves when the patient believes the treatment will work even if the patient is taking a placebo.

**Placenta:** An organ that develops during pregnancy and serves as the go-between for all nutrients and waste products for the mother and developing baby.

**Plaque:** The accumulation of fat, calcium, and other debris in the artery walls associated with the development of atherosclerosis.

**Platelets:** Blood cell fragments that aid in blood coagulation. Abnormal clumping of platelets is associated with atherosclerosis.

**Polyphenols:** Phytochemicals in tea and fruits that protect tissues from free radical damage. Tannins are polyphenols.

**Polyunsaturated Fat:** A triglyceride in which one or more of the three fatty acids is unsaturated, that is, it has room for more hydrogen atoms. Examples include the fats in vegetable oils and fish oils.

**Postmenopause:** After the menopause; determined after a period of twelve months of spontaneous amenorrhea has been observed.

**Prebiotics:** Compounds that favor the growth of probiotics.

**Precursor:** A substance used as a building block for another substance. Beta carotene is a precursor for vitamin A, and tryptophan is the precursor for serotonin and niacin.

**Preeclampsia:** Toxemia associated with the later stages of pregnancy, characterized by high blood pressure, edema, and protein in the urine.

**Pregnancy-Induced Hypertension (PIH):** See *toxemia.*

**Premenopausal:** Prior to the onset of menopause.

**Premenstrual Syndrome (PMS):** The ten days to two weeks before a woman's period when she experiences a variety of symptoms, including increased food cravings, bloating, moodiness, and weight gain.

**Probiotics:** Bacteria in foods, such as yogurt, that reduce disease risk by reducing harmful bacteria in the digestive tract and producing natural antibiotics.

**Procyanins:** Phytochemicals in chocolate that have antioxidant capabilities.

**Progesterone:** A female hormone that induces premenstrual changes of the uterus lining following ovulation and possibly inhibits contractions of the uterus during early pregnancy. Also called progestin.

**Prostaglandin:** A group of hormonelike substances formed from polyunsaturated fatty acids that have a profound effect on the body, including contraction of smooth muscle and dilation or contraction of blood vessels in the regulation of blood pressure.

**Pruritus:** Chronic itching of the skin.

**Recommended Dietary Allowances (RDAs):** Reference amounts of most vitamins and minerals necessary for health, based on a person's gender, age, and size.

**Refined:** The process whereby the coarse parts of plants are removed. For example, the refining of whole wheat into white wheat flour involves removing three of the four parts of the kernel, the chaff, the bran, and the germ, leaving only the endosperm or high-carbohydrate inner core.

**REM:** Rapid Eye Movement. A phase of sleep characterized by an increase in dreams.

**Retina:** The layer of light-sensitive cells lining the back of the inside of the eye.

**Retinol Equivalents (RE):** A unit of measurement for vitamin A; one RE is equivalent to 1 mcg or 3.33 IU of vitamin A as retinol.

**Saponins:** A group of phytochemicals in seeds and dried beans and peas that lower blood cholesterol levels.

**Saturated Fat:** A triglyceride with the maximum possible number of hydrogen atoms. Saturated fats are typically solid at room temperature and increase the risk for elevated blood triglyceride, heart disease, and some forms of cancer.

**Scurvy:** A disease caused by a deficiency of vitamin C and characterized by bleeding gums, loosened teeth, small hemorrhages below the skin, and weakness.

**Sebaceous Glands:** Glands in the skin that secrete a greasy lubricating substance called sebum.

**Secondary Deficiency:** A nutrient deficiency caused by something other than poor dietary intake, including excessive intake of one nutrient that interferes with absorption or utilization of other nutrients.

**Serotonin:** A neurotransmitter produced in the brain that regulates mood, sleep, pain, and numerous other body processes.

**Simple Carbohydrate:** Sugars in the diet, including sucrose (table sugar), glucose, fructose (in fruits and honey), and lactose (in milk).

**Sodium:** An electrolyte that combined with chloride makes table salt.

**Sphingolipids:** Compounds in milk that might lower colon cancer risk.

**Strict Vegetarian Diet:** A diet that contains only foods of plant origin, such as whole-grain breads and cereals, cooked dried beans and peas, fruits, vegetables, and nuts and seeds. Also called a vegan diet.

**Subcutaneous:** The deepest of three layers of the skin.

**Sucralose:** A sugar substitue sold under the name of Splenda.

**Systolic Blood Pressure:** The higher of the two readings that make up a blood pressure test. Systolic blood pressure represents the greatest amount of pressure in the cardiovascular system at any moment and corresponds to the pressure exerted by the heart during a heartbeat (contraction).

**Tannin:** Tannic acid. A phytochemical in tea with antioxidant capabilities. A form of polyphenols.

**Tetany:** Muscle twitching, cramps, and convulsions.

**Tocopherol:** Vitamin E.

**Total Iron Binding Capacity (TIBC):** A test to measure iron status, in particular iron deficiency prior to the onset of anemia.

**Toxemia:** A disorder that sometimes develops in the later portion of pregnancy characterized by high blood pressure, protein in the urine, edema, salt retention, convulsions, or sometimes coma. Also called eclampsia or pregnancy-induced hypertension (PIH).

**Trace Mineral:** An essential mineral found in the body in amounts less than 0.0005 percent of body weight.

**Trans Fatty Acids (TFAs):** Polyunsaturated fats formed during hydrogenation of vegetable oils to make margarine or shortening. The shape of these fats is different from other polyunsaturated fats and these fats are suspected to act more like saturated fats in the promotion of heart disease.

**Triglycerides:** The primary fats in food, in a person's fat tissue, and in the blood. Triglycerides can be saturated or unsaturated, and the unsaturated ones can be either monounsaturated or polyunsaturated. All triglycerides supply more than 250 calories per ounce and can contribute to weight gain and elevated body fat. Saturated triglycerides or fats are associated with numerous diseases, from heart disease to cancer.

**Tryptophan:** An amino acid essential for life and converted in the body to the B vitamin niacin.

**Unsaturated Fat:** A triglyceride that contains one or more fatty acids that could accept more hydrogen atoms. A polyunsaturated and monounsaturated fat. Examples of unsaturated fats include vegetable oils and fish oils.

**Urinary:** Pertaining to urine.

**Vegan:** A strict vegetarian who consumes no foods of animal origin.

**Virus:** Any of a large group of minute particles that are capable of infecting plants, animals, and humans.

**Vitamin:** An essential nutrient, which must be obtained from the diet, and is required by the body in minute amounts.

**Waist-to-Hip Ratio (WHR):** A measurement of regional distribution of body fat. A high WHR reflects excessive fat accumulation above the waist, which is associated with increased risks for heart disease, diabetes, cancer, and other disorders.

**Whole Grain:** An unrefined grain that retains its edible ouside layers (the bran) and the highly nutritious inner germ.

**Yo-Yo Dieting:** Repeated attempts to lose weight, followed by a regain of the lost weight. Also called weight cycling.

# Selected References

INTRODUCTION

Block G, Abrams B: Vitamin and mineral status of women of childbearing potential. *Ann NY Acad* 1993;678:244–254.

Braam L, Ocke M, Bueno-de-Mesquita H, et al: Determinants of obesity-related underreporting of energy intake. *Am J Epidem* 1998;147:1081–1086.

Flynn M, Sugrue D, Codd M, et al: Women's dietary fat and sugar intakes: Implications for food-based guidelines. *Eur J Cl N* 1996;50:713–719.

Frazao E (editor): U.S.D.A.'s *America's Eating Habits: Changes and Consequences*. Economic Research Report, Agriculture Information Bulletin Number 750. Washington, D.C., 1999, pp 77, 134.

Harrison G, Galal O, Ibrahim N, et al: Underreporting of food intake by dietary recall is not universal: A comparison of data from Egyptian and American women. *J Nutr* 2000;130:2049–2054.

Heitmann B, Lissner L, Osler M: Do we eat less fat, or just report so? *Int J Obes* 2000; 24:435–442.

Kennedy E, Ohls J, Carlson S, et al: The Healthy Eating Index: Design and applications. *J Am Diet A* 1995;95:1103–1108.

Krebs-Smith S, Cleveland L, Ballard-Barbash R, et al: Characterizing food intake patterns of American adults. *Am J Clin N* 1997;65(suppl):1264S–1268S.

Lichetman S, Pisarska K, Berma E, et al: Discrepancy between self-reported and actual caloric intake and exercise in obese women. *N Eng J Med* 1992;327:1893–1898.

Mertz W, Tsui J, Judd J, et al: What are people really eating? The relation between energy intake derived from estimated diet records and intake determined to maintain body weight. *Am J Clin N* 1991;54:291–295.

Pennington J: Intakes of minerals from diets and foods: Is there a need for concern? *J Nutr* 1996;126:2304–2308.

Putnam J: U.S. food supply providing more food and calories. *Food Review* 1999;Sept–Oct:2–12.

Putnam J, Kantor L, Allshouse J: Per capita food supply trends: Progress toward dietary guidelines. *Food Review* 2000;Sept–Oct:2–14.

Roberts R: Can self-reported data accurately describe the prevalence of overweight? *Publ Heal* 1995;109:275–284.

Subar A, Krebs-Smith S, Cook A, et al: Dietary sources of nutrients among U.S. adults, 1989–1991. *J Am Diet A* 1998;98:537–547.

Subar A, Ziegler R, Patterson B, et al: U.S. dietary patterns associated with fat intake: The 1987 National Health Interview Survey. *Am J Pub He* 1994;84:359–366.

Tippett K, Mickle S, Goldman J, et al: Food and nutrient intakes by individuals in the United States, 1 day, 1989–91. U.S.D.A. Agriculture Research Service, NFS Report No. 91–2, Sept 1995.

Zhang J, Temme E, Sasaki S, et al: Underreporting and overreporting of energy intake using urinary cations as biomarkers: Relation to body mass index. *Am J Epidem* 2000;152:453–462.

Zive M, Nicklas T, Busch E, et al: Marginal vitamin and mineral intakes of young adults: The Bogalusa Heart Study. *J Adoles H* 1996;19:39–47.

## CHAPTER 1: NUTRITION BASICS

Anderson J, Hanna T, Peng X, et al: Whole-grain foods and heart-disease risk. *J Am Col N* 2000;19:S291–S299.

Ascherio A, Katan M, Zook P, et al: Trans fatty acids and coronary heart disease. *N Eng J Med* 1999;340:1994–1998.

Ascherio A, Willett W: Health effects of trans fatty acids. *Am J Clin N* 1997;66:1006S–1010S.

Astrup A, Grunwald G, Melanson E, et al: The role of low-fat diets in body weight control: A meta-analysis of ad libitum dietary intervention studies. *Int J Obes* 2000;24:1545–1552.

Craig W: Phytochemicals: Guardians of our health. *J Am Diet A* 1997;97:S199–S204.

Denke M: Metabolic effects of high-protein, low-carbohydrate diets. *Am J Card* 2001;88:59–61.

Eckhardt R: Genetic research and nutritional individuality. *J Nutr* 2001;131:S336–S339.

Enig M: Trans fatty acids in diets and databases. *Cereal F W* 1996;41:58–63.

Goldman I, Kader A, Heintz C: Influence of production, handling, and storage on phytonutrient content of foods. *Nutr Rev* 1999;57:46S–52S.

Grundy S: What is the desirable ratio of saturated, polyunsaturated, and monounsaturated fatty acids in the diet? *Am J Clin N* 1997;66:988S–990S.

Hill J, Melanson E, Wyatt H: Dietary fat intake and regulation of energy balance: Implications for obesity. *J Nutr* 2000;130:S284–S288.

Howard B, Kritchevsky D: Phytochemicals and cardiovascular disease. *Circulation* 1997; 95:2591–2593.

Jacobs D, Pereira M, Meyer K, et al: Fiber from whole grains, but not refined grains, is inversely associated with all-cause mortality in older women: The Iowa Women's Health Study. *J Am Col N* 2000;19:S326–S330.

Liu S, Manson J, Stampfer M, et al: A prospective study of whole-grain intake and risk of type 2 diabetes mellitus in U.S. women. *Am J Pub He* 2000;90:1409–1415.

Louheranta A, Turpeinen A, Vidgren H, et al: A high trans fatty acid diet and insulin sensitivity in young healthy women. *Metabolism* 1999;48:870–875.

Maffeis C, Schutz Y, Grezani A, et al: Meal-induced thermogenesis and obesity: Is a fat meal a risk factor for fat gain in children? *J Clin End* 2001;86:214–219.

McKelvey W, Greenland S, Sandler R: A second look at the relation between colorectal adenomas and consumption of foods containing partially hydrogenated oils. *Epidemiolog* 2000;11:469–473.

Murphy S: How consideration of population variance and individuality affects our understanding of nutritional requirements in human health and disease. *J Nutr* 2001; 131:S361–S365.

Saris W, Astrup A, Prentice A, et al: Randomized controlled trial of changes in dietary carbohydrates/fat and simple vs complex carbohydrates on body weight and blood lipids: the CARMEN study. *Int J Obes* 2000;24:1310–1318.

Schrauwen P, Westerterp K: The role of high-fat diets and physical activity in the regulation of body weight. *Br J Nutr* 2000;84:417–427.

Simopoulos A: Essential fatty acids in health and chronic disease. *Food Rev In* 1997; 13:623–631.

Stoll B: Essential fatty acids, insulin resistance, and breast cancer risk. *Nutr Cancer* 1998;31:72–77.

## CHAPTER 2: THE HEALTHY WOMAN'S DIET

Block G, Abrams B: Vitamin and mineral status of women of childbearing potential, *Ann NY Acad* 1993;678:244–254.

Brody S, Preut R, Schommer K, et al: Ascorbic acid treatment decreases reactivity to stress: A randomized trial. *Psychophysl* 2001;38:S29 (meeting abstract).

Brug J, Debie S, van Assema P, et al: Psychosocial determinants of fruit and vegetable consumption among adults: Results of focus group interviews. *Food Qual P* 1996; 6:99–107.

Chapman K, Chan M, Clark C: Factors influencing dairy calcium intake in women. *J Am Col N* 1995;14:336–340.

Dittus K, Hillers V, Beerman K: Benefits and barriers to fruit and vegetable intake: Relationship between attitudes and consumption. *J Nutr Educ* 1995;27:120–126.

Ford E, Mokdad A: Fruit and vegetable consumption and diabetes mellitus incidence among U.S. adults. *Prev Med* 2001;32:33–39.

Fortes C, Forastiere F, Farchi S, et al: Diet and overall survival in a cohort of very elderly people. *Epidemiolog* 2000;11:440–445.

French S, Harnack L, Jeffery R: Fast food restaurant use among women in the Pound of Prevention study. *Int J Obes* 2000;24:1353–1359.

Fruits and vegetables: Nature's best protection. *Consumer Reports on Health* June 1998:1–5.

Fung T, Willett W, Stampfer M, et al: Dietary patterns and the risk of coronary heart disease in women. *Arch In Med* 2001;161:1857–1862.

Harman D: Role of antioxidant nutrients in aging: Overview. *Age* 1995;18:51–62.

Johnson R, Frary C: Choose beverages and foods to moderate your intake of sugars: The 2000 Dietary Guidelines for Americans—What's all the fuss about? *J Nutr* 2001; 131:2766–2771.

Joshipura K, Ascherio A, Manson J, et al: Fruit and vegetable intake in relation to risk of ischemic stroke. *J Am Med A* 1999;282:1233–1239.

Kant A: Consumption of energy-dense, nutrient-poor foods by adult Americans. *Am J Clin N* 2000;72:929–936.

Krebs-Smith S, Cook A, Subar A, et al: U.S. adults' fruit and vegetable intakes, 1989 to 1991: A revised baseline for the Healthy People 2000 Objective. *Am J Pub He* 1995;85:1623–1629.

Krebs-Smith S, Kantor L: Choose a variety of fruits and vegetables daily: Understanding the complexities. *J Nutr* 2001;131:487S–501S.

Lechner L, Brug J, de Vries H: Misconceptions of fruit and vegetable consumption: Differences between objective and subjective estimation of intake. *J Nutr Educ* 1997; 29:313–320.

Liu S, Manson J, Lee I, et al: Fruit and vegetable intake and risk of cardiovascular disease: The Women's Health Study. *Am J Clin N* 2000;72:922–928.

Markus R, Panhyysen G, Tuiten A, et al: Effects of food on cortisol and mood in vulnerable subjects under controllable and uncontrollable stress. *Physl Behav* 2000; 70:333–342.

Neumark-Sztainer D, Story M, Resnick M, et al: Correlates of inadequate fruit and vegetable consumption among adolescents. *Prev Med* 1996;25:497–505.

Nolan C, Gray-Donald K, Shatensteine B, et al: Dietary patterns leading to high-fat intake. *Can J Publ* 1995;86:389–391.

Paolisso G, Tagliamonte M, Rizzo M, et al: Oxidative stress and advancing age: Results in healthy centenarians. *J Am Ger So* 1998;46:833–838.

Patterson B, Harlan L, Block G, et al: Food choices of whites, blacks, and hispanics: Data from the 1987 National Health Interview Survey. *Nutr Cancer* 1995:23:105–119.

Preziosi P, Galan P, Deheeger M, et al: Breakfast type, daily nutrient intakes, and vitamin and mineral status of French children, adolescents, and adults. *J Am Col N* 1999; 18:171–178.

Singh R, Niaz M, Ghosh S: Effect on central obesity and associated disturbances of low-energy, fruit- and vegetable-enriched prudent diet in North Indians. *Postg Med J* 1994;70:895–900.

Subar A, Heimendinger J, Patterson B, et al: Fruit and vegetable intake in the United States: The baseline survey of the Five a Day for Better Health program. *Am J H Pro* 1995;9:352–360.

Tucker K, Hannan M, Chen H, et al: Potassium, magnesium, and fruit and vegetable intakes are associated with greater bone mineral density in elderly men and women. *Am J Clin N* 1999;69:727–736.

Ulus I, Ozyurt G, Korfali E: Decreased serum choline concentrations in humans after surgery, childbirth, and traumatic head injury. *Neurochemical Research* 1998;23:727–732.

Zhang S, Hunter D, Rosner B, et al: Intakes of fruits, vegetables, and related nutrients and the risk of non-Hodgkin's lymphoma among women. *Canc Epid B* 2000;9:477–485.

## CHAPTER 3: SUPERMARKET SAVVY

Bengmark S: Ecoimmunonutrition: A challenge for the third millennium. *Nutrition* 1998;14:563–572.

Hasler C: A new look at an ancient concept. *Chem Ind L* 1998;3:84–89.

Hasler C: Functional foods: Their role in disease prevention and health promotion. *Food Tech B* 1998;52:63–69.

Hennekens C, Buring J, Manson J, et al: Lack of effect of long-term supplementation with beta carotene on the incidence of malignant neoplasms and cardiovascular disease. *N Eng J Med* 1996;334:1145–1149.

Milner J: Do "functional foods" offer opportunities to optimize nutrition and health. *Food Tech B* 1998;52:63–70.

Position of the American Dietetic Association: Phytochemicals and functional foods. *J Am Diet A* 1995;95:493–496.

Reilly C: Functional foods: A challenge for consumers. *Trends Food* 1994;5:121–123.

Silverglade B, Heller I: Are functional foods the solution to dysfunctional diets? A review of U.S. regulatory requirements and lessons from abroad. *Food Drug L* 1997;52:313–321.

Van Poppel G, Goldbolm R: Epidemiologic evidence for beta carotene and cancer prevention. *Am J Clin N* 1995;62(suppl):1393S–1402S.

CHAPTER 4: HEALTHY, QUICK-FIX COOKING

Clark H, Harrison C, Reid C, et al: Effect of supplements of fruit and vegetables on food intake, body weight, and appetite among Scottish consumers. *P Nutr Soc* 2000; Spring:55A.

Dietary guidelines 2000: Fruits and vegetables first. www.5aday.com/meal_comparison.html

Frazao E (editor): U.S.D.A.'s *America's Eating Habits: Changes and Consequences,* Economic Research Report, Agriculture Information Bulletin Number 750. Washington, D.C., 1999.

Gorsky R, Pamuk E, Williamson D, et al: The twenty-five-year health-care costs of women who remain overweight after forty years of age. *Am J Prev M* 1996;12:388–394.

Huang K: Price and income affect nutrients consumed from meats. *Food Review.* U.S.D.A. Economic Research Service, Jan–Apr 1996, pp 37–40.

Lin B, Frazao E: Nutritional quality of foods at and away from home. *Food Review.* U.S.D.A. Economic Research Service, May–Aug 1997, pp 33–40.

Porrini M, Crovetti R, Riso P, et al: Effects of physical and chemical characteristics of food on specific and general satiety. *Physl Behav* 1995;57:461–468.

Putnam J, Allshouse J: U.S. per capita food supply trends. *Food Review.* U.S.D.A. Economic Research Service, Sept–Oct 1998, pp 2–11.

Warman P, Havard K: Yield, vitamin and mineral contents of organically and conventionally grown potatoes and sweet corn. *Agr, Eco, Env* 1998;68:207–216.

Warwick Z, Hall W, Pappas T, et al: Taste and smell sensations enhance the satiating effect of both a high-carbohydrate and a high-fat meal in humans. *Physl Behav* 1993;53:553–563.

Woese K, Lange D, Boess C, et al: A comparison of organically and conventionally grown foods: Results of a review of the relevant literature. *J Sci Food* 1997;74:281–293.

Worthington V: Effect of agricultural methods on nutritional quality: A comparison of organic with conventional crops. *Altern Th H* 1998;4:58–69.


CHAPTER 5: EATING OUT

Przybys J: Airport dining takes off. *LV Rev J,* Wednesday, September 3, 1997.


CHAPTER 6: EVERYTHING YOU NEED TO KNOW ABOUT SUPPLEMENTS

Albertson A, Tobelmann R: Consumption of grain and whole-grain foods by an American population during the years 1990 to 1992. *J Am Diet A* 1995;95:703–704.

Block G, Dresser C, Hartman A, et al: Nutrient sources in the American diet: Quantitative data from the NHANES II survey: Macronutrients and fats. *Am J Epidem* 1985; 122:27–40.

Cuskelly G, McNulty H, Scott J: Effect of increasing dietary folate on red cell folate implications for prevention of neural tube defects. *Lancet* 1996;367:657–659.

Dollahite J, Franklin D, McNew R: Problems encountered in meeting the Recommended Dietary Allowances for menus designed according to the Dietary Guidelines for Americans. *J Am Diet A* 1995;95:341–344.

Ford E: Vitamin supplement use and diabetes mellitus incidence among adults in the United States. *Am J Epidem* 2001;153:892–897.

Hunt J: Position of the American Dietetic Association: Vitamin and mineral supplementation. *J Am Diet A* 1996;96:73–77.

Junyao L, Bing L, Blot W, et al: Preliminary report on the results of nutrition prevention trials of cancer and other common diseases among residents in Linxian, China. *Chin Med J* 1995;108:780.

Karkkainen M, Lamberg-Allardt C, Ahonen S, et al: Does it make a difference how and when you take your calcium? *Am J Clin N* 2001;74:335–342.

Kennedy E, Ohls J, Carlson S, et al: The Healthy Eating Index: Design and Applications. *J Am Diet A* 1995;95:1103–1108.

Krebs-Smith S, Cleveland L, Ballard-Barbash R, et al: Characterizing food intake patterns of American adults. *Am J Clin N* 1997;65(suppl):1264S–1268S.

Kumar A, Aitas A, Hunter A, et al: Sweeteners, dyes, and other excipients in vitamin and mineral preparations. *Clin Pediat* 1996;35:443–450.

Lampe J, Martini M, et al: Urinary lignan and isoflavonoid excretion in premenopausal women consuming flaxseed powder. *Am J Clin N* 1994;60:122–128.

Looker A, Dallman P, Carroll M, et al: Prevalence of iron deficiency in the United States. *J Am Med A* 1997;277:973–976.

Manore M, Besenfelder P, Wells C, et al: Nutrient intakes and iron status in female long-distance runners during training. *J Am Diet A* 1989;89:257–259.

Mark S, Wang W, Fraumeni J, et al: Lowered risks of hypertension and cerebrovascular disease after vitamin mineral supplementation: The Linxian Nutrition Intervention Trial. *Am J Epidem* 1996;143:658–664.

Mayne S: Antioxidant nutrients and cancer incidence and mortality: An epidemiologic perspective. *Adv Pharmacol* 1997;38:657–675.

Meydani S, Meydani M, Blumberg J, et al: Vitamin E supplementation and in vivo immune response in healthy elderly subjects. *J Am Med A* 1997;277:1380–1386.

Mossad S, Machnin M, Medendorp S, et al: Zinc gluconate lozenges for treating the common cold. *Ann Int Med* 1996;125:81–88.

National Center for Nutrition and Dietetics: Straight answers about vitamin and mineral supplements. *J Am Diet A* 1997.

Nesbitt P, Thompson L: Lignans in homemade and commercial products containing flaxseed. *Nutr Cancer* 1997;29:222–227.

Patterson A, Brown W, Roberts D: Dietary and supplement treatment of iron deficiency results in improvements in general health and fatigue in Australian women of childbearing age. *J Am Col N* 2001;20:337–342.

Peet M, Murphy B, et al: Depletion of omega-3 fatty acid levels in red blood cell membranes of depressed patients. *Biol Psychi* 1998;43:315–319.

Subar A, Block G: Use of vitamin and mineral supplements: Demographics and amounts of nutrients consumed. *Am J Epidem* 1990;132:1091–1101.

Thompson L, Rickard S, et al: Variability in anticancer lignan levels in flaxseed. *Nutr Cancer* 1997;27:26–30.

Tice J, Ross E, Coxson P, et al: Cost-effectiveness of vitamin therapy to lower plasma homocysteine levels for the prevention of coronary heart disease. *J Am Med A* 2001; 286:936–943.

Watkins M, Erickson J, Thun M: Multivitamin use and mortality in a large prospective study. *Am J Epidem* 2000;151:149–162.

Weber C, Jakobsen T, Mortensen S, et al: Antioxidative effect of dietary coenzyme Q10 in human blood plasma. *Int J Vit N* 1994;64:311–315.

## CHAPTER 7: STAYING SLIM: LOSING WEIGHT FOR GOOD

Anderson R, Wadden T, Barlett S, et al: Effects of lifestyle activity vs structured aerobic exercise in obese women. *J Am Med A* 1999;281:335–340.

Atkinson R, Dietz W, Hill J, et al: Weight cycling. *J Am Med A* 1994;272:1196–1202.

Bray G, DeLany J: Opinions of obesity experts on the causes and treatment of obesity: A new survey. *Obes Res* 1995;3:S419–S423.

Drapkin R, Wing R, Shiffman S: Responses to hypothetical high-risk situations: Do they predict weight loss in a behavioral treatment program or the context of dietary lapses? *Health Psyc* 1995;14:427–434.

Dunn A, Andersen R, Jakicic J: Lifestyle physical activity interventions. History, short- and long-term effects, and recommendations. *Am J Prev M* 1998;15:398–412.

Dunn A, Marcus H, Kampert B, et al: Comparison of lifestyle and structured interventions to increase physical activity and cardiovascular fitness. *J Am Med A* 1999; 281:327–334.

Foreyt J, Goodrick G: Attributes of successful approaches to weight loss and control. *Appl Prev P* 1994;3:209–215.

Foreyt J, Goodrick G: Factors common to successful therapy for the obese patient. *Med Sci Spt* 1991;23:292–297.

French S, Jeffery R: Consequences of dieting to lose weight: Effects on physical and mental health. *Health Psyc* 1994;13:195–212.

Head S, Brookhart A: Lifestyle modification and relapse-prevention training during treatment for weight loss. *Behav Ther* 1997;28:307–321.

Hensrud D, Weinsier R, Darnell B, et al: A prospective study of weight maintenance in obese subjects reduced to normal body weight without weight-loss training. *Am J Clin N* 1994;60:688–694.

Iribbarren C, Sharp D, Burchfiel C, et al: Association of weight loss and weight fluctuation with mortality among Japanese-American men. *N Eng J Med* 1995;333:686–692.

Jeffery R, Epstein L, Wilson G, et al: Long-term maintenance of weight loss: Current status. *Health Psyc* 2000;19:5–16.

Kahn H, Tatham L, Rodriguez C, et al: Stable behaviors associated with adults' ten-year change in body mass index and likelihood of gain at the waist. *Am J Pub He* 1997;87:747–754.

Kirk S, Hill A: Exploring the food beliefs and eating behaviors of successful and unsuccessful dieters. *J Hum Nu Di* 1997;10:331–341.

Klem M, Wing R, McGuire M, et al: A descriptive study of individuals successful at long-term maintenance of substantial weight loss. *Am J Clin N* 1997;66:239–246.

Lavery M, Loewy J: Identifying predictive variables for long-term weight change after participation in a weight-loss program. *J Am Diet A* 1993;93:1017–1024.

Lee I, Manson J, Hennekens C, et al: Body weight and mortality. *J Am Med A* 1993;270:2823–2828.

Losonczy K, Harris T, Cornoni-Huntley J, et al: Does weight loss from middle age to old age explain the inverse weight mortality relation in old age? *Am J Epidem* 1995;141:312–321.

Manson J, Willett W, Stampfer M, et al: Body weight and mortality among women. *N Eng J Med* 1995;333:677–685.

McGuire M, Wing R, Klem M, et al: Long-term maintenance of weight loss: Do people who lose weight through various weight-loss methods use different behaviors to maintain their weight? *Int J Obes* 1998;22:572–577.

Miller W: How effective are traditional dietary and exercise interventions for weight loss? *Med Sci Spt* 1999;31:1129–1134.

Mokdad A, Bowman B, Ford E, et al: The continuing epidemics of obesity and diabetes in the United States. *J Am Med A* 2001;286:1195–1200.

Parham E: Enhancing social support in weight-loss management groups. *J Am Diet A* 1993;93:1152–1156.

Pasman W, Westerterp-Plantenga M, Saris W: The effectiveness of long-term supplementation of carbohydrate, chromium, fiber, and caffeine on weight maintenance. *Int J Obes* 1997;21:1143–1151.

Pratt M: Benefits of lifestyle activity vs structured exercise. *J Am Med A* 1999;281:375–376.

Raben A, Jensen N, Marckmann P, et al: Spontaneous weight loss during eleven weeks' ad libitum intake of a low fat/high fiber diet in young, normal weight subjects. *Int J Obes* 1995;19:916–923.

Rebuffe-Serive M, Hendler R, Bracero N, et al: Behavioral effects of weight cycling. *Int J Obes* 1994;18:651–658.

Rippe J, Hess S: The role of physical activity in the prevention and management of obesity. *J Am Diet A* 1998;98(suppl):S31–S38.

Rippe J, Price J, Hess S, et al: Improved psychological well-being, quality of life, and health practices in moderately overweight women participating in a twelve-week structured weight-loss program. *Obes Res* 1998;6:208–218.

Shick S, Wing R, Klem M, et al: Persons successful at long-term weight loss and maintenance continue to consume a low-energy, low-fat diet. *J Am Diet A* 1998;98:408–413.

Skender M, Goodrick K, Del Junco D, et al: Comparison of two-year weight-loss trends in behavioral treatments of obesity: Diet, exercise, and combination interventions. *J Am Diet A* 1996;96:342–346.

Willett W, Manson J, Stampfer M, et al: Weight, weight change, and coronary heart disease in women. *J Am Med A* 1995;273:461–465.

Williams G, Grow V, Freedman Z, et al: Motivational predictors of weight loss and weight-loss maintenance. *J Pers Soc* 1996;70:115–126.

Williamson D: Dietary intake and physical activity as "predictors" of weight gain in observational, prospective studies on adults. *Nutr Rev* 1996;54:S101–S109.

Williamson D, Pamuk E, Thun M, et al: Prospective study of intentional weight loss and mortality in never-smoking overweight U.S. white women aged forty to sixty-four years. *Am J Epidem* 1995;141:1128–1141.

Wing R, Hill J: Successful weight-loss maintenance. *Ann R Nutr* 2001;21:323–341.

Wing R, Jeffery R, Burton L, et al: Food provision vs structured meal plans in the behavioral treatment of obesity. *Int J Obes* 1996;20:56–62.

## CHAPTER 8: CHANGING HABITS

Boyd N, Martin L, Beaton M, et al: Long-term effects of participation in a randomized trial of a low-fat high-carbohydrate diet. *Canc Epid B* 1996;5:217–222.

Greene G, Rossi S: Stages of change for reducing dietary fat intake over nineteen months. *J Am Diet A* 1998;98:529–534.

Greene G, Rossi S, Reed G, et al: Stages of change for reducing dietary fat to 30 percent of energy or less. *J Am Diet A* 1994;94:1105–1110.

Harnack L, Block G, Lane S: Influence of selected environmental and personal factors on dietary behavior for chronic disease prevention: A review of the literature. *J Nutr Educ* 1997;29:306–312.

Heitmann B, Lissner L, Osler M: Do we eat less fat, or just report so? *Int J Obes* 2000; 24:435–442.

Keenan D, Achterberg C, Kris-Etherton P, et al: Use of qualitative and quantitative methods to define behavioral fat-reduction strategies and their relationship to dietary fat reduction in the Patterns of Dietary Change study. *J Am Diet A* 1996;96: 1245–1250.

Kelsey K, Earp J, Kirkley B: Is social support beneficial for dietary change? A review of the literature. *Fam Comm H* 1997;20:70–82.

Kristal A, Patterson R, Glanz K, et al: Psychosocial correlates of healthful diets: Baseline results from the working well study. *Prev Med* 1995;24:221–228.

Lamb R, Joshi M: The stage model and processes of change in dietary fat reduction. *J Hum Nu Di* 1996;9:43–53.

Lappalainen R, Saba A, Holm L, et al: Difficulties in trying to eat healthier: Descriptive analysis of perceived barriers for healthy eating. *Eur J Cl N* 1997;51:S36–S40.

Mhurchu C, Margetts B, Speller V: Applying the stages-of-change model to dietary change. *Nutr Rev* 1997;55:10–16.

Patterson R, Kristal A, White E: Do beliefs, knowledge, and perceived norms about diet and cancer predict dietary change? *Am J Pub He* 1996;86:1394–1400.

Sporny L, Contento I: Stages of change in dietary fat reduction: Social psychological correlates. *J Nutr Educ* 1995;27:191–199.

## CHAPTER 9: NUTRITION, EXERCISE, AND SPORTS

Alessio H, Goldfarb A, Cao G: Exercise-induced oxidative stress before and after vitamin C supplementation. *Int J Sp Nu* 1997;7:1–9.

Allen J, McLung J, Nelson A, et al: Ginseng supplementation does not enhance healthy young adults' peak aerobic exercise performance. *J Am Col N* 1998;17:462–466.

Andrews R, Greenhaff P, Curtis S, et al: The effect of dietary creatine supplementation on skeletal muscle metabolism in congestive heart failure. *Eur Heart J* 1998;19: 617–622.

Beals K, Manore M: Behavioral, psychological, and physical characteristics of female athletes with subclinical eating disorders. *Int J Sp Nu* 2000;10:128–143.

Beard J, Tobin B: Iron status and exercise. *Am J Clin N* 2000;72:S594–S597.

Blair S, Kohl H, Barlow C: Physical activity, physical fitness, and all-cause mortality in women: Do women need to be active? *J Am Col N* 1993;12:368–371.

Blomstrand E, Hassmen P, Ekblom E, et al: Influence of ingesting a solution of branched-chain amino acids on perceived exertion during exercise. *Act Physl S* 1997;159:41–49.

Borgen J: Risk and trigger factors for the development of eating disorders in female elite athletes. *Med Sci Spt* 1994;26:414–419.

Clark J: Creatine: A review of its nutritional applications in sport. *Nutrition* 1998; 14:322–324.

Cordain L: Does creatine supplementation enhance athletic performance? *J Am Col N* 1998;17:205–206.

Davis J, Welsh R, De Volve K, et al: Effects of branch-chain amino acids and carbohydrate on fatigue during intermittent, high-intensity running. *Int J Sp M* 1999; 20:309–314

Dekkers J, van Doornen L, Kemper H: The role of antioxidant vitamins and enzymes in the prevention of exercise-induced muscle damage. *Sport Med* 1996;21:213–238.

Douchi T, Yamamoto S, Oki T, et al: The effects of physical exercise on body fat distribution and bone-mineral density in postmenopausal women. *Maturitas* 2000; 35:25–30.

Dutz R, Bernardot D, Martin D, et al: Relationship between energy deficits and body composition in elite female gymnasts and runners. *Med Sci Spt* 2000;32:659–668.

Estok P, Rudy E: The relationship between eating disorders and running women. *Res Nurs H* 1996;19:377–387.

Evans W: Vitamin E, vitamin C, and exercise. *Am J Clin N* 2000;72:S647–S652.

Hetland M, Haarbo J, Christiansen C, et al: Running induces menstrual disturbances but bone mass is unaffected, except in amenorrheic women. *Am J Med* 1993;95:53+.

Johnston C, Swam P, Corte C: Substrate utilization and work efficiency during submaximal exercise in vitamin C depleted-repleted adults. *Int J Vit N* 1999;69:41–44.

Lemon P: Beyond the Zone: Protein needs of active individuals. *J Am Col N* 2000; 19:513S–521S.

Lopez-Varela S, Montero A, Chandra R, et al: Nutritional status of young female elite gymnasts. *Int J Vit N* 2000;70:185–190.

Manore M: Effect of physical activity on thiamine, riboflavin, and vitamin $B_6$ requirements. *Am J Clin N* 2000;72:S598–S606.

Micklesfield L, Lambert E, Fataar A, et al: Bone-mineral density in mature, premenopausal ultramarathon runners. *Med Sci Spt* 1995;27:688–696.

Miller K, Klibanski A: Amenorrheic bone loss. *J Clin End* 1999;84:1775–1783.

Mittleman K, Ricci M, Bailey S: Branched-chain amino acids prolong exercise during heat stress in men and women. *Med Sci Spt* 1998;30:83–91.

Myburgh K, Bachrach L, Lewis B, et al: Low bone-mineral density at axial and appendicular sites in amenorrheic athletes. *Med Sci Spt* 1993;25:1197–1202.

Nishiyama S, Inomoto T, Nakamura T, et al: Zinc status relates to hematological deficits in women endurance runners. *J Am Col N* 1996;15:359–363.

Nuviala R, Lapieza M, Bernal E: Magnesium, zinc, and copper status in women involved in different sports. *Int J Sp Nu* 1999;9:295–309.

Ousley-Pahnke L, Black D, Gretebeck R: Dietary intake and energy expenditure of female collegiate swimmers during decreased training prior to competition. *J Am Diet A* 2001;101:351–354.

Sherman S, D'Agostino R, Cobb J, et al: Physical activity and mortality in women in the Framingham Heart Study. *Am Heart J* 1994;128:879–884.

Smolak L, Murnen S, Ruble A: Female athletes and eating problems. *Int J Eat D* 2000; 27:371–380.

Sundgot-Borgen J: Eating disorders in female athletes. *Sport Med* 1994;17:176–188.

Takanami Y, Iwane H, Kawai Y, et al: Vitamin E supplementation and endurance exercise. *Sport Med* 2000;29:73–83.

Thein L, Thein J: The female athlete. *J Orthop Sp* 1996;23:134–148.

Treuth M, Hunter G, Kekes T, et al: Reduction in intra-abdominal adipose tissue after strength training in older women. *J Appl Phys* 1995;78:1425–1431.

Wiggins D, Wiggins M: The female athlete. *Clin Sp Med* 1997;16:593–612.

Williams M, Branch J: Creatine supplementation and exercise performance: An update. *J Am Col N* 1998;17:216–234.

Zhu Y, Haas J: Iron depletion without anemia and physical performance in young women. *Am J Clin N* 1997;66:334–341.

## CHAPTER 10: PREGNANCY AND BREAST-FEEDING

American College of Obstetricians and Gynecologists. Technical Bulletin 1994:189.

Biano A, Smilen S, Davis Y, et al: Pregnancy outcome and weight-gain recommendations for the morbidly obese woman. *Obstet Gyn* 1998;91:97–102.

Brown J, Kahn E: Maternal nutrition and the outcome of pregnancy. *Clin Perin* 1997; 24:433–449.

Bucher H, Guyatt G, Cook R, et al: Effect of calcium supplementation on pregnancy-induced hypertension and preeclampsia. *J Am Med A* 1996;275:1113–1117.

Carmichael S, Abrams B, Selvin S: The pattern of maternal weight gain in women with good pregnancy outcomes. *Am J Pub He* 1997;87:1984–1988.

Chappell L, Seed P, Briley A, et al: Effect of antioxidants on the occurrence of preeclampsia in women at increased risk: A randomized trial. *Lancet* 1999;354:810–816.

Choi W, Little J, Arslan A: Prenatal vitamin supplementation and pediatric brain tumors: Huge international variation in use and possible reduction in risk. *Child Nerv* 1998; 14:551–557.

Czeizel A: Periconceptional folic acid containing multivitamin supplementation. *Eur J Ob Gy* 1998;78:151–161.

Glenn F, Glenn W, Burdi A: Prenatal flouride for growth and development. *J Dent Chil* 1997;Sept–Oct:319–321.

Goldenberg R, Tamura T: Prepregnancy weight and pregnancy outcome. *J Am Med A* 1996;275:1127–1128.

Goldenberg R, Tamura T, Neggers Y, et al: The effect of zinc supplementaton on pregnancy outcome. *J Am Med A* 1995;274:463–468.

Handwerker S, Altura B, Altura B: Serum ionized magnesium and other electrolytes in the antenatal period of human pregnancy. *J Am Col N* 1996;15:36–43.

Hubel C: Oxidative stress in the pathogenesis of preeclampsia. *P Soc Exp M* 1999; 222:222–235.

Kadir R, Sabin C, Whitlow B, et al: Neural tube defects and periconceptional folic acid in England and Wales: Retrospective study. *Br Med J* 1999;319:92–93.

Kelly A, Kevany J, de Onis M, et al: A WHO collaborative study of maternal anthropometry and pregnancy outcomes. *Int J Gyn O* 1996;53:219–233.

Kovacs C, Kronenberg H: Maternal fetal calcium and bone metabolism during pregnancy, puerperium, and lactation. *Endocr Rev* 1997;18:832–872.

Leger J, Jaquet D, Marchal C, et al: Syndrome X: A consequence of intra-uterine malnutrition? *J Ped End M* 2000;13:1257–1259.

Locksmith G, Duff P: Preventing neural tube defects: The importance of periconceptional folic acid supplements. *Obstet Gyn* 1998;91:1027–1034.

Merialdi M, Caulfield L, Zavaleta N, et al: Adding zinc to prenatal iron and folate tablets improves fetal neurobehavioral development. *Am J Obst G* 1999;180:483–490.

Moutquin J, Garner P, Burrows R, et al: Report of the Canadian Hypertension Society Consensus Conference. 2. Nonpharmacologic management and prevention of hypertensive disorders in pregnancy. *Can Med A J* 1997;157:907–919.

Muscati S, Gray-Donald K, Koski K: Timing of weight gain during pregnancy: Promoting fetal growth and minimizing maternal weight retention. *Int J Obes* 1996; 20:526–532.

Nelen W, Blom H, Thomas C, et al: Methylenetetrahydrofolate reductase polymorphism affects the change in homocysteine and folate concentrations resulting from low-dose folic acid supplementation in women with unexplained recurrent miscarriages. *J Nutr* 1998;128:1336–1341.

Ortega R, Martinez R, Lopez-Sobaler A, et al: Influence of calcium intake on gestational diabetes. *Ann Nutr M* 1999;43:37–46.

Park E, Wagenbichler P, Elmadfa I: Effects of multivitamin/mineral supplementation, at nutritional doses, on plasma antioxidant status and DNA damage estimated by sister chromatid exchanges in lymphocytes in pregnant women. *Int J Vit N* 1999; 69:396–402.

Poranen A, Ekblad U, Uotila P, et al: The effect of vitamin C and E on placental lipid peroxidation and antioxidative enzymes in perfused placenta. *Act Obst Sc* 1998; 77:372–376.

Preston-Martin S, Pogoda J, Mueller B, et al: Prenatal vitamin supplementation and risk of childhood brain tumors. *Int J Canc* 1998;S11:17–22.

Ritchie L, Fung E, Halloran B, et al: A longitudinal study of calcium homeostasis during human pregnancy and lactation and after resumption of menses. *Am J Clin N* 1998; 67:693–701.

Scholl T, Hediger M, Bendich A, et al: Use of multivitamin/mineral prenatal supplements: Influence on the outcome of pregnancy. *Am J Epidem* 1997;146:134–141.

Siman C, Eriksson U: Vitamin E decreases in occurrence of malformations in the offspring of diabetic rats. *Diabetes* 1997;46:1054–1061.

Skarb S: Vitamin E and C in preeclampsia. *Eur J Ob Gy* 2000;93:37–39.

Williams M, King I, Sorensen T, et al: Risk of preeclampsia in relation to elaidic acid (trans fatty acids) in maternal erythrocytes. *Gynecol Obs* 1998;46:84–87.

## CHAPTER 11: THE MATURE WOMAN

Albertazzi P, Pansini F, Bonaccorsi G, et al: The effect of dietary soy supplementation on hot flushes. *Obstet Gyn* 1998;91:6–11.

Anderson J, Johnstone B, Cook-Newell M: Metaanalysis of the effects of soy protein intake on serum lipids. *N Eng J Med* 1995;333:276–282.

Chmouliovsky L, Habicht F, James R, et al: Beneficial effect of hormone replacement therapy on weight loss in obese menopausal women. *Maturitas* 1999;32:147–153.

Fukutake M, Takashahi M, Ishida K, et al: Quantification of genistein and genistein in soybeans and soybean products. *Food Chem T* 1996;34:457–461.

Guicheney P, Leger D, Barrat J, et al: Platelet serotonin content and plasma tryptophan in peri- and postmenopausal women: Variations with plasma estrogen levels and depressive symptoms. *Eur J Cl In* 1988;18:297–304.

Haggans C, Hutchins A, Olson B, et al: Effect of flaxseed consumption on urinary estrogen metabolites in postmenopausal women. *Nutr Cancer* 1999;33:188–195.

Heaney R, Dawson-Hughes B, Gallagher J, et al: The role of calcium in peri- and postmenopausal women: Consensus opinion of the North American Menopause Society. *Menopause* 2001;8:84–95.

Jain S, McVie R, Jaramillo J, et al: The effect of modest vitamin E supplementation on lipid peroxidation products and other cardiovascular risk factors in diabetic patients. *Lipids* 1996;31:S87–S90.

Knight D, Eden J: Phytoestrogens: A short review. *Maturitas* 1995;22:167–175.

Kuller L, Simkin-Silverman L, Wing R, et al: Women's healthy lifestyle project. *Circulation* 2001;103:32–37.

LeBoff M, Kohlmeier L, Hurwitz S, et al: Occult vitamin D deficiency in postmenopausal U.S. women with acute hip fracture. *J Am Med A* 1999;281:1505–1511.

Lu L, Tice J, Bellino F: Photoestrogens and healthy aging: Gaps in knowledge. *Menopause* 2001;8:157–170.

Murkies A, Lombard C, Strauss B, et al: Dietary flour supplementation decreases postmenopausal hot flushes: Effect of soy and wheat. *Maturitas* 1995;21:189–195.

Murkies A, Lombard C, Strauss B, et al: Postmenopausal hot flushes decreased by dietary flour supplementation: Effects of soy and wheat. *Am J Clin N* 1998;68:1532S–1533S.

Murphy S, Khaw K, May H, et al: Milk consumption and bone-mineral density in middle-aged and elderly women. *Br J Med PS* 1994;308:939–941.

Nagata C, Kabuto M, Kurisu Y, et al: Decreased serum estradiol concentration associated with high dietary intake of soy products in premenopausal Japanese women. *Nutr Cancer* 1997;29:228–233.

Nagata C, Takatsuka N, Kawakami N, et al: Soy product intake and hot flashes in Japanese women. *Am J Epidem* 2001;153:790–793.

Scheiber M, Rebar R: Isoflavones and postmenopausal bone health: A viable alternative to estrogen therapy? *Menopause* 1999;6:233–241.

Seidl M, Stewart D: Alternative treatments for menopausal symptoms. *Can Fam Phy* 1998;44:1299–1308.

Stampfer M, Hu F, Manson J, et al: Primary prevention of coronary heart disease in women through diet and lifestyle. *N Eng J Med* 2000;343:16–22.

Svendsen O, Hassager C, Christiansen C: Effect of an energy restrictive diet, with or without exercise, on lean tissue mass, resting metabolic rate, cardiovascular risk factors, and bone in overweight postmenopausal women. *Am J Med* 1993;95:131–140.

Symanski E, Hertz-Picciotto I: Blood lead levels in relation to menopause, smoking, and pregnancy history. *Am J Epidem* 1995;141:1047–1058.

Taaffe D, Pruitt L, Reim J, et al: Effect of sustained resistance training on basal metabolic rate in older women. *J Am Ger So* 1995;43:465–471.

Thune I, Brenn T, Lund E, et al: Physical activity and the risk of breast cancer. *N Eng J Med* 1997;336:1269–1275.

Woods M, Barnett J, Spiegelman D, et al: Horomone levels during dietary changes in premenopausal African-American women. *J Nat Canc* 1996;88:1369–1374.

Zheng W, Anderson K, Kushi L, et al: A prospective cohort study of intake of calcium, vitamin D, and other micronutrients in relation to incidence of rectal cancer among postmenopausal women. *Canc Epid B* 1998;7:221–225.

## CHAPTER 12: NUTRITION AFTER SIXTY-FIVE: THE ANTIAGING LIFESTYLE

Barnett Y, King C: An investigation of antioxidant status, DNA repair capacity, and mutation as a function of age in humans. *Mut Res* 1995;338:115–128.

Battisti C, Dotti M, Manneschi L, et al: Increase of serum levels of vitamin E during human aging: Is it a protective factor against death? *Arch Ger G* 1994;4(suppl):13–18.

Carmetl R, Gott P, Waters C, et al: The frequently low cobalamin levels in dementia usually signify treatable metabolic, neurologic, and electrophysiologic abnormalities. *Eur J Haema* 1995;54:245–253.

DeStefani E, Brennan P, Boffetta P, et al: Vegetables, fruits, related dietary antioxidants and risk of squamous cell carcinoma of the esophagus. *Nutr Cancer* 2000;38:23–29.

Evans W: Reversing sarcopenia: How weight training can build strength and vitality. *Geriatrics* 1996;51:46–53.

Evans W, Cyr-Campbell D: Nutrition, exercise, and healthy aging. *J Am Diet A* 1997; 97:632–638.

Fiatarone M, O'Neill E, Doyle N, et al: Exercise training and nutritional supplementation for physical frailty in very elderly people. *N Eng J Med* 1994;330:1769–1775.

Fielding R: The role of progressive resistance training and nutrition in the preservation of lean body mass in the elderly. *J Am Col N* 1995;14:587–594.

Goswami S, Dhara P: Effects of vitamin $B_1$ supplementation on reaction time in adult males. *Med Sci Res* 1994;22:279–280.

Harman D: Role of antioxidant nutrients in aging: Overview. *Age* 1995;18:51–62.

Hurley B, Roth S: Strength training in the elderly. *Sport Med* 2000;30:249–268.

Hursting S, Kari F: The anticarcinogenic effects of dietary restriction. *Mut Res* 1999; 443:235–249.

Jama J, Launer L, Witteman J, et al: Dietary antioxidants and cognitive function in a population-based sample of older persons. *Am J Epidem* 1996;144:275–280.

Kakkar R, Bains J, Sharma S: Effect of vitamin E on life span, malondialdehyde content, and antioxidant enzymes in aging Zaprionus paravittiger. *Gerontology* 1996; 42:312–321.

Kline K, Yu W, Sanders B: Vitamin E: Mechanisms of action as tumor cell growth inhibitors. *J Nutr* 2001;13:S161–S163.

Manzella D, Barbieri M, Ragno E, et al: Chronic administration of pharmacologic doses of vitamin E improves the cardiac autonomic nervous system in patients with type 2 diabetes. *Am J Clin N* 2001;73:1052–1057.

Mares-Perlman J, Lyle B, Klein R, et al: Vitamin supplement use and incident cataracts in a population-based study. *Arch Ophth* 2000;118:1556–1563.

Mattson M, Duan W, Lee J, et al: Suppression of brain aging and neurodegenerative disorders by dietary restriction and environmental enrichment. *Mech Age D* 2001; 122:757–778.

Means L, Higgins J, Fernandez T: Midlife onset of dietary restriction extends life and prolongs cognitive functioning. *Physl Behav* 1993;54:503–508.

Mezzetti A, Lapenna D, Romano F, et al: Systemic oxidative stress and its relationship with age and illness. *J Am Ger So* 1996;44:823–827.

Michels K, Giovannucci E, Joshipura K, et al: Prospective study of fruit and vegetable consumption and incidence of colon and rectal cancers. *J Nat Canc* 2000;92:1740–1752.

Olivieri O, Stanzial A, Girelli D, et al: Selenium status, fatty acids, vitamins A and E, and aging: The Nove Study. *Am J Clin N* 1994;60:510–517.

Owens J, Matthews K, Wing R, et al: Can physical activity mitigate the effects of aging in middle-aged women? *Circulation* 1992;85:1265–1270.

Reiter R: Oxidative processes and antioxidative defense mechanisms in the aging brain. *FASEB J* 1995;9:526–533.

Riggs K, Spiro A, Tucker K, et al: Relations of vitamin $B_{12}$, vitamin $B_6$, folate, and homocysteine to cognitive performance in the Normative Aging Study. *Am J Clin N* 1996; 63:306–314.

Ronco A, DeStefani E, Boffetta P, et al: Vegetables, fruits, and related nutrients and risk of breast cancer. *Nutr Cancer* 1999;35:111–119.

Salo P, Laippala P, Frey H: Effect of advanced brain atrophy and vitamin deficiency on cognitive functions in nondemented subjects. *Act Neur Sc* 1993;87:161–166.

Schmuck A, Fuller C, Devaraj S, et al: Effect of aging on susceptibility of low-density lipoproteins to oxidation. *Clin Chem* 1995;41:1628–1632.

Socci D, Crandall B, Arendash G: Chronic antioxidant treatment improves the cognitive performance in aged rats. *Brain Res* 1995;693:88–94.

Terry P, Giovannucci E, Michels K, et al: Fruit, vegetables, dietary fiber, and risk of colorectal cancer. *J Nat Canc* 2001;93:525–533.

Traber M: Does vitamin E decrease heart-attack risk? *J Nutr* 2001;131:395S–397S.

Weindruch R: Immunogerontologic outcomes of dietary restriction started in adulthood. *Nutr Rev* 1995;53:66S–71S.

Zhang S, Hunter D, Rosner B, et al: Intakes of fruits, vegetables, and related nutrients and the risk of non-Hodgkin's lymphoma among women. *Canc Epid B* 2000;9:477–485.

## CHAPTER 13: WOMEN, NUTRITION, AND MEDICATIONS

Baranowitz S, Maderson P: Acetaminophen toxicity is substantially reduced by beta carotene in mice. *Int J Vit N* 1996;65:175–180.

Feldman E: How grapefruit juice potentiates drug bioavailability. *Nutr Rev* 1997;55: 398–400.

Harper J, Levine A, Rosenthal D, et al: Erythrocyte folate levels, oral contraceptive use, and abnormal cervical cytology. *Acta Cytol* 1994;38:324–330.

Lasswell A, DeForge B, Sobal J, et al: Family medicine residents' knowledge and attitudes about drug-nutrient interactions. *J Am Col N* 1995;14:137–143.

Muggeo M, Zenti M, Travia D, et al: Serum retinol levels throughout two years of cholesterol-lowering therapy. *Metabolism* 1995;44:398–403.

Rieck J, Halkin H, Almog S, et al: Urinary loss of thiamine is increased by low doses of furosemide in healthy volunteers. *J La Cl Med* 1999;134:238–243.

Struck B: Cerebral hemorrhage associated with aspirin, ginkgo biloba and vitamin E. *J Am Ger So* 2000;48:P109 (meeting abstract).

Teresi M, Morgan D: Attitudes of health-care professionals toward patient counseling on drug-nutrient interactions. *Ann Pharmac* 1994;28:576–580.

Thomas J: Drug-nutrient interactions. *Nutr Rev* 1995;53:271–282.

Walter-Sack I, Klotz U: Influence of diet and nutritional status on drug metabolism. *Clin Pharm* 1996;31:47–64.

Wirell M, Wester P, Stegmayer B: Nutritional dose of magnesium in hypertensive patients on beta-blockers lowers systolic blood pressure. *J Intern M* 1994;236:189–195.

## CHAPTER 14: WHAT CAUSES DISEASE?

Birt D, Hendrich S, Wang W: Dietary agents in cancer prevention: Flavonoids and isoflavonoids. *Pharm Thera* 2001;90:157–177.

Buzina-Suboticanec K, Buzina R, Stavljenic A, et al: Aging, nutritional status, and immune response. *Int J Vit N* 1998;68:133–141.

Chandra R: Nutrition and the immune system: An overview. *Am J Clin N* 1997;66:460S–463S.

De la Fuente M, Fernandez M, Burgos M, et al: Immune function in aged women is improved by ingestion of vitamin C and vitamin E. *Can J Pharm* 1998;76:373–380.

Fortes C, Forastiere F, Agabiti N, et al: The effect of zinc and vitamin A supplementation on immune response in an older population. *J Am Ger So* 1998;46:19–26.

Gill H, Rutherfurd K, Prasad J, et al: Enhancement of natural and acquired immunity by lacto-bacillus rhammosus, lacto-bacillus acidophilus, and bifidobacterium lactis. *Br J Nutr* 2000;83:167–176.

Girodon F, Lombard M, Galan P, et al: Effect of micronutrient supplementation on infection in institutionalized elderly subjects: A controlled trial. *Ann Nutr M* 1997; 41:98–107.

Kubena K, McMurray D: Nutrition and the immune system. *J Am Diet A* 1996;96:1156–1164.

Lee C, Wan J: Vitamin E supplementation improves cell-mediated immunity and oxidative stress of Asian men and women. *J Nutr* 2000;130:2932–2937.

Lesourd B: Nutrition and immunity in the elderly: Modification of immune responses with nutritional treatments. *Am J Clin N* 1997;66:478S–484S.

Percival S, Cousins R: Immunomodulating effects of a dietary supplement containing zinc and echinacea. *FASEB J* 1999;13:A872 (meeting abstract).

Scrimshaw N, SanGiovanni J: Synergism of nutrition, infection, and immunity: An overview. *Am J Clin N* 1997;66:464S–477S.

Thurnham D: Micronutrients and immune function: Some recent developments. *J Clin Path* 1997;50:887–891.

## CHAPTER 15: WOMEN'S MAIN HEALTH CONCERNS

Abernathy R, Black D: Healthy body weights. *Am J Clin N* 1996;63(suppl):409S–411S/448S–451S/474S–477S.

Adish A, Esrey S, Gyorkos T, et al: Effect of consumption of food cooked in iron pots on iron status and growth of young children. *Lancet* 1999;353:712–716.

Adler A, Holub B: Effect of garlic and fish oil supplementation on serum lipid and lipoprotein concentrations in hypercholesterolemic men. *Am J Clin N* 1997;65:445–450.

Agarwal K: Iron and the brain: Neurotransmitter receptors and magnetic resonance spectroscopy. *Br J Nutr* 2001;85:S139–S145/S147–S150.

Alleva R, Tomasetti M, Battino M, et al: The roles of coenzyme Q10 and vitamin E on the peroxidation of human low-density lipoprotein subfractions. *P Nas Us* 1995; 92:9388–9391.

Anderson J, Garner S: The effects of phytoestrogens on bone. *Nutr Res* 1997;17:1617–1632.

Anderson J, Gilliland S: Effect of fermented milk (yogurt) containing lacto-bacillus aci-dophilus L1 on serum cholesterol in hypercholesterolemic humans. *J Am Col N* 1999;18:43–50.

Anderson J, Hanna T, Peng X, et al: Whole-grain foods and heart-disease risk. *J Am Col N* 2000;19:S291–S299.

Anderson J, Rondano P: Peak bone mass development of females: Can young adult women improve their peak bone mass? *J Am Col N* 1996;15:570–574.

Ascherio A, Katan M, Zock P, et al: Trans fatty acids and coronary heart disease. *N Eng J Med* 1999;340:1994–1998.

Ascherio A, Willett W: Health effects of *trans* fatty acids. *Am J Clin N* 1997;66:1006–1010.

Baik H, Russell R: Vitamin $B_{12}$ deficiency in the elderly. *Ann R Nutr* 1999;19:357–377.

Behall K, Scholfield D, Hallfrisch J: Effect of beta glucan level in oat fiber extracts on blood lipids in men and women. *J Am Col N* 1997;16:46–51.

Berger T, Polidor M, Dabbahg A, et al: Antioxidant activity of vitamin C in iron-overloaded human plasma. *J Biol Chem* 1997;272:5656–5660.

Bergstrom A, Pisani P, Tenet V, et al: Overweight as an avoidable cause of cancer in Europe. *Int J Canc* 2001;91:421–430.

Bodnar L, Scanlon K, Freedman D, et al: High prevalence of postpartum anemia among low-income women in the United States. *Am J Obst G* 2001;185:438–443.

Booth S: Skeletal functions of vitamin K–dependent proteins: Not just for clotting any-more. *Nutr Rev* 1997;55:282–284.

Booth S: Warfarin and fracture risk. *Nutr Rev* 2000;58:20–22.

Boue C, Combe N, Billeaud C, et al: Trans fatty acids in adipose tissue of French women in relation to their dietary sources. *Lipids* 2000;35:561–566.

Bouker K, Hilakivi-Clarke L: Genistein: Does it prevent or promote breast cancer? *Envir H Per* 2000;108:701–708.

Brech D: Vitamin and mineral diet adequacy and supplement use by full-time employed women with preschool children. *J Am Diet A* 1999;99:1267–1269.

Breuer-Katschinski B, Nemes K, Marr A, et al: Relation of serum antioxidant vitamins to the risk of colorectal adenoma. *Digestion* 2001;63:43–48.

Bruce W, Giacca A, Medline A: Possible mechanisms relating diet and risk of colon can-cer. *Canc Epid B* 2000;9:1271–1279.

Bruner A, Joffe A, Duggan A, et al: Randomized study of cognitive effects of iron supple-mentation on nonanemic iron-deficient adolescent girls. *Lancet* 1996;348:992–996.

Buring J, Hennekens: Antioxidant vitamins and cardiovascular disease. *Nutr Rev* 1997; 55:53S–58S.

Bushman J: Green tea and cancer in humans. A review of the literature. *Nutr Cancer* 1998;31:151–159.

Calvo M, Park Y: Changing phosphorus content of the U.S. diet: Potential for adverse effects on bone. *J Nutr* 1996;126:1168S–1180S.

Chapuy M, Preziosi P, Maamer M, et al: Prevalence of vitamin D insufficiency in an adult normal population. *Osteopor Int* 1997;7:439–443.

Chel V, Ooms M, Popp-Snijders C, et al: Ultraviolet irradiation corrects vitamin D deficiency and suppresses secondary hyperthyroidism in the elderly. *J Bone Min* 1998; 13:1238–1242.

Conlisk A, Galuska D: Is caffeine associated with bone-mineral density in young adult women? *Prev Med* 2000;31:562–568.

Connor W: Importance of n-3 fatty acids in health and disease. *Am J Clin N* 2000; (suppl)71:171S–175S.

Cramer D, Kuper H, Harlow B, et al: Carotenoids, antioxidants, and ovarian cancer risk in premenopausal and postmenopausal women. *Int J Canc* 2001;94:128–134.

Daviglus M, Stamler J, Orencia A, et al: Fish consumption and the thirty-year risk of fatal myocardial infarction. *N Eng J Med* 1997;336:1046–1053.

Dawson-Hughes B: Calcium and vitamin D nutritional needs of elderly women. *J Nutr* 1996;126:1165–1167.

Dawson-Hughes B, Harris S, Dallal G: Plasma calcidiol, season, and serum parathryoid hormone concentrations in healthy elderly men and women. *Am J Clin N* 1997; 65:67–71.

Dawson-Hughes B, Harris S, Krall E, et al: Effect of calcium and vitamin D supplementation on bone density in men and women sixty-five years of age or older. *N Eng J Med* 1997;337:670–676.

Dawson-Hughes B, Harris S, Krall E, et al: Effect of withdrawal of calcium and vitamin D supplements on bone mass in elderly men and women. *Am J Clin N* 2000; 72:745–750.

De Bruin L, Pawliszyn J, Joseph P: Detection of monocyclic aromatic amines, possible mammary carcinogens, in human milk. *Chem Res T* 1999;12:78–82.

De Stefani E, Correa P, Ronco A, et al: Dietary fiber and risk of breast cancer: A case-control study in Uruguay. *Nutr Cancer* 1997;28:14–19.

De Stefani E, Mendilaharsu M, Deneo-Pellegrini H: Sucrose as a risk factor for cancer of the colon and rectum: A case-control study in Uruguay. *Int J Canc* 1998;75:40–44.

Diaz G, Paraskeva C, Thomas M, et al: Apoptosis is induced by the active metabolite of vitamin $D_3$ and its analog EB1089 in colorectal adenoma and carcinoma cells. *Cancer Res* 2000;60:2304–2312.

Diaz M, Frei B, Vita J, et al: Antioxidants and atherosclerotic heart disease. *N Eng J Med* 1997;337:408–416.

Dimai H, Porta S, Wirnsberger G, et al: Daily oral magnesium supplementation suppresses bone turnover in young adult males. *J Clin End* 1998;83:2742–2748.

Donovan U, Gibson R: Iron status in women aged fourteen to nineteen years consuming vegetarian and omnivorous diets. *J Am Col N* 1995;14:463–472.

Dreher M, Maher C: The traditional and emerging role of nuts in healthful diets. *Nutr Rev* 1996;54:241–245.

Eaton-Evans J, McIlrath E, Jackson W, et al: Copper supplementation and the maintenance of bone-mineral density in middle-aged women. *J Tr El Exp* 1996;9:87–94.

Eichner R: Fatigue of anemia. *Nutr Rev* 2001;59:17S–19S.

Emmert D, Kirchner J: The role of vitamin E in the prevention of heart disease. *Arch Fam M* 1999;8:537–542.

Enig M: Trans fatty acids in diets and databases. *Cereal F W* 1996;41:58–63.

Fleischchauer A, Arab L: Garlic and Cancer: A critical review of the epidemiologic literature. *J Nutr* 2001;131:1032–1040.

Fleischchauer A, Poole C, Arab L: Garlic consumption and cancer prevention: Meta-analysis of colorectal and stomach cancers. *Am J Clin N* 2000;72:1047–1052.

Ford E, Giles W: Serum vitamins, carotenoids, and angina pectoris. *Ann Epidemi* 2000;10:106–116.

Fowke J, Longcope C, Hebert J: Macronutrient intake and estrogen metabolism in healthy postmenopausal women. *Breast Canc* 2001;65:1–10.

Frei B: On the role of vitamin C and other antioxidants in atherogenesis and vascular dysfunction. *P Soc Exp M* 1999;222:196–204.

Gamboa-Pinto A, Rock C, Ferruzzi M, et al: Cervical tissue and plasma concentrations of alpha-carotene and beta carotene in women are correlated. *J Nutr* 1998;128:1933–1936.

Gatto L, Hallen G, Brown A, et al: Ascorbic acid induces a favorable lipoprotein profile in women. *J Am Col N* 1996;15:154–158.

Gesensway D: Vitamin D and sunshine. *Ann Int Med* 2000;133:319–320.

Giovannucci E: Tomatoes: Tomato-based products, lycopene, and cancer: Review of the epidemiological literature. *J Nat Canc* 1999;91:317–331.

Giuliano A, Gapstur S: Can cervical dysplasia and cancer be prevented with nutrients? *Nutr Rev* 1998;56:9–16.

Glerup H, Mikkelsen K, Poulsen L, et al: Commonly recommended dietary intake of vitamin D is not sufficient if sunlight exposure is limited. *J Int Med* 2000;247:260–268.

Gogos C, Ginopoulos P, Zoumbos N, et al: The effect of omega-3 polyunsaturated fatty acids on T-lymphocytes subsets of patients with solid tumors. *Cancer Det* 1995;19:415–417.

Goodfellow J, Bellamy M, Ramsey M, et al: Dietary supplementation with marine omega-3 fatty acids improves systemic large artery endothelial function in subjects with hypercholesterolemia. *J Am Col N* 2000;35:265–270.

Gotay C, Dumitriu D: Health-food store recommendations for breast-cancer patients. *Arch Fam M* 2000;9:692–698.

Graham I, Daly L, Refsum H, et al: Plasma homocysteine as a risk factor for vascular disease. *J Am Med A* 1997;277:1775–1781.

Gueguen L, Pointillart A: The bioavailability of dietary calcium. *J Am Col N* 2000;19:S119–S136.

Gueux E, Azais-Braesco V, Bussiere L, et al: Effect of magnesium deficiency on triacylglycerol-rich lipoprotein and tissue sensitivity to peroxidation in relation to vitamin E content. *Br J Nutr* 1995;74:849–856.

Haas J, Brownlie T: Iron deficiency and reduced work capacity. *J Nutr* 2001;131:676S–690S.

Haggans C, Travelli E, Thomas W, et al: The effect of flaxseed and wheat bran consumption on urinary estrogen metabolites in premenopausal women. *Canc Epid B* 2000; 9:719–725.

Heaney R: Age considerations in nutrient needs of bone health. *J Am Col N* 1996; 15:575–578.

Heaney R: There should be a dietary guideline for calcium. *Am J Clin N* 2000;71:658–661.

Heaney R, Dawson-Hughes B, Gallagher J, et al: The role of calcium in peri- and post-menopausal women. *Menopause* 2001;8:84–95.

Heisler T, Towfigh S, Simon N, et al: Peptide YY and vitamin E inhibit hormone-sensitive and insensitive breast-cancer cells. *J Surg Res* 2000;91:9–14.

Henderson N, Price R, Cole J, et al: Bone density in young women is associated with body weight and muscle strength but not dietary intakes. *J Int Med* 1994;236:385–390.

Hertog M, Kromhout D, Aravanis C, et al: Flavonoid intake and long-term risk of coronary heart disease and cancer in the Seven Countries Study. *Arch In Med* 1995;155:381–386.

Horn-Ross P: Phytoestrogens, body composition, and breast cancer. *Canc Cause* 1995; 6:567–573.

Hu F, Stampfer M, Manson J, et al: Frequent nut consumption and risk of coronary heart disease in women: Prospective cohort study. *Br Med J* 1998;317:1341–1345.

Hu F, Stampfer M, Rimm E, et al: A prospective study of egg consumption and risk of cardiovascular disease in men and women. *J Am Med A* 1999;281:1387–1394.

Hurrell R, Reddy M, Cook J: Inhibition of non-haem iron absorption in man by polyphenolic-containing beverages. *Br J Nutr* 1999;81:289–295.

Ilich J, Kerstetter J: Nutrition in bone health revisited: A story beyond calcium. *J Am Col N* 2000;19:715–737.

Iwamoto M, Sato M, Kono M, et al: Walnuts lower serum cholesterol in Japanese men and women. *J Nutr* 2000;130:171–176.

Jacobs D, Meyer K, Kushi L, et al: Whole-grain intake may reduce the risk of ischemic heart-disease death in postmenopausal women: The Iowa Women's Health Study. *Am J Clin N* 1998;68:248–257.

Jee S, He J, Appel L, et al: Coffee consumption and serum lipids. *Am J Epidem* 2001; 153:353–362.

Jenkins D, Kendall C, Vidgen E, et al: The effect on serum lipids and oxidized low density lipoprotein of supplementing self-selected low-fat diets with soluble-fiber, soy, and vegetable protein foods. *Metabolism* 2000;49:67–72.

Jensen C, Haskell W, Whittam J: Long-term effects of water-soluble dietary fiber in the management of hypercholesterolemia in healthy men and women. *Am J Card* 1997;79:34–37.

Johanning G: Eicosapentaenoic acid and epidermal growth factor modulation of human breast-cancer cell adhesion. *Cancer Lett* 1997;118:95–100.

Jumaan A, Holmberg L, Zack M, et al: Beta-carotene intake and risk of postmenopausal breast cancer. *Epidemiolog* 1999;10:49–53.

Kaltwasser J, Werner E, Schalk K, et al: Clinical trial on the effect of regular tea drinking on iron accumulation in genetic haemochromatosis. *Gut* 1998;43:699–704.

Kameda M, Miyazawa K, Mori Y, et al: Vitamin $K_2$ inhibits osteoclastic resorption by inducing osteoclast apoptosis. *Bioc Biop R* 1996;220:515–519.

Kanai T, Takagi T, Masuhiro K, et al: Serum vitamin K level and bone-mineral density in postmenopausal women. *Int J Gyn O* 1997;56:25–30.

Kanetsky P, Gammon M, Mandelblatt J, et al: Dietary intake and blood levels of lycopene: Association with cervical cancer among non-Hispanic, black women. *Nutr Cancer* 1998;31:31–41.

Kannar D, Wattanapenpaiboon N, Savige G, et al: Hypocholesterolemic effect of an enteric-coated garlic supplement. *J Am Col N* 2001;20:225–231.

Kato I, Dnistrian A, Schwartz M, et al: Risk of iron overload among middle-aged women. *Int j Vit N* 2000;70:119–125.

Kato I, Dnistrian A, Schwartz M, et al: Serum folate, homocysteine and colorectal cancer risk in women. A nested case-control study. *Br J Canc* 1999;79:1917–1922.

Katz D, Nawaz H, Boukhalil J, et al: Acute effects of oats and vitamin E on endothelial responses to ingested fat. *Am J Prev M* 2001;20:124–129.

Khaw K, Welch A, Luben R, et al: Relation between plasma ascorbic acid and mortality in men and women in EPIC-Norfolk prospective study. *Lancet* 2001;257:657–663.

Kiechl S, Willeit J, Egger G, et al: Body iron stores and the risk of carotid atherosclerosis. *Circulation* 1997;96:3300–3307.

Kiel D, Powell J, Oiao N, et al: Dietary silicon and bone-mineral density. *J Bone Min* 2001;16:S510 (meeting abstract).

Klevay L: Cardiovascular disease from copper deficiency. *J Nutr* 2000;130:S489–S492.

Klipstein-Grobusch K, Gelejnse J, den Breeijen J, et al: Dietary antioxidants and risk of myocardial infarction in the elderly: The Rotterdam study. *Am J Clin N* 1999;69:261–266.

Klipstein-Grobusch K, Grobbee D, den Breeijen J, et al: Dietary iron and risk of myocardial infarction in the Rotterdam study. *Am J Epidem* 1999;149:421–428.

Kretchevsky S: Beta carotene, carotenoids, and the prevention of coronary heart disease. *J Nutr* 1999;129:5–8.

Kretsch M, Fong A, Green M, et al: Cognitive function, iron status, and hemoglobin concentration in obese dieting women. *Eur J Clin N* 1998;52:512–518.

Kris-Etherton P, Taylor D, Zhao G: Is there an optimal diet for the hypertriglyceridemic patient? *J Card Risk* 2000;7:333–337.

Kruger M, Coetzer H, de Winter R, et al: Calcium, gamma-linoleic acid and eicosapentaenoic acid supplementation in senile osteoporosis. *Aging-Clin* 1998;10:385–394.

Kugiyama K, Motoyama T, Hirashima O, et al: Vitamin C attenuates abnormal vasomotor reactivity in spasm coronary arteries in patients with coronary spastic angina. *J Am Col N* 1998;32:103–109.

Kuper H, Titus-Ernstoff L, Harlow B, et al: Population based study of coffee, alcohol, and tobacco use and risk of ovarian cancer. *Int J Canc* 2000;88:313–318.

Kwasniewska A, Charzewska J, Tukendorf A, et al: Dietary factors in women with dysplasia colli uteri associated with human papillomavirus infection. *Nutr Cancer* 1998;30:39–45.

Kwasniewska A, Tukendorf A, Semczuk M: Folate deficiency and cervical intraepithelial neoplasia. *Eur J Gyn On* 1997;18:526–530.

Lasztity R, Hidvegi M, Bata A: Saponins in food. *Food Rev In* 1998;14:371–390.

Leveille S, LaCroix A, Koepsell T, et al: Dietary vitamin C and bone-mineral density in postmenopausal women in Washington state, U.S.A. *J Epidem C* 1997;51:479–485.

Levi F, Pasche C, Lucchini F, et al: Dietary intake of selected micronutrients and breast-cancer risk. *Int J Canc* 2001;91:260–263.

Levine A, Harper J, Ervin C, et al: Serum 25-hydroxyvitamin D, dietary calcim intake, and distal colorectal adenoma risk. *Nutr Cancer* 2001;39:35–41.

Levine G, Frei B, Koulouris S, et al: Ascorbic acid reverses endothelial vasomotor dysfunction in patients with coronary artery disease. *Circulation* 1996;93:1107–1113.

Lichtenstein A: Trans fatty acids, plasma lipid levels, and risk of developing cardiovascular disease. *Circulation* 1997;95:2588–2590.

Lipkin M, Newmark H: Vitamin D, calcium, and prevention of breast cancer. *J Am Col N* 1999;18:S392–S397.

Lipworth L, Martinez M, Angell J, et al: Olive oil and human cancer: An assessment of the evidence. *Prev Med* 1997;26:181–190.

Lloyd T, Rollings N, Eggli D, et al: Bone status among postmenopausal women with different habitual caffeine intakes. *J Am Col N* 2000;19:256–261.

Looker A, Dallman P, Carrol M, et al: Prevalence of iron deficiency in the United States. *J Am Med A* 1997;277:973–976.

Lu L, Anderson K, Grady J, et al: Decreased ovarian hormones during a soy diet: Implications for breast cancer. *Cancer Res* 2000;60:4112–4121.

Lu L, Tice J, Bellino F: Phytoestrogens and healthy aging: Gaps in knowledge. *Menopause* 2001;8:157–170.

Malafa M, Neitzel L: Vitamin E succinate promotes breast-cancer tumor dormancy. *J Surg Res* 2000;93:163–170.

Marcus P, Newcomb P: The association of calcium and vitamin D, and colon and rectal cancer in Wisconsin women. *Int J Epid* 1998;27:788–793.

Massey L, Whiting S: Dietary salt, urinary calcium, and bone loss. *J Bone Min* 1996; 11:731–736.

McCann S, Moysich K, Mettlin C: Intakes of selected nutrients and food groups and risk of ovarian cancer. *Nutr Cancer* 2001;39:19–28.

McClain C, Morris P, Hennig B: Zinc and endothelial function. *Nutrition* 1995;11:117–120.

McClean J, Barr S, Prior J: Calcium, exercise, and bone density in young women: Are they related? *Med Sci Spt* 2001;33:1292–1296.

McGill H, McMahan A, Herderick E, et al: Origin of atherosclerosis in childhood and adolescence. *Am J Clin N* 2000;72:1307–1315.

Merz-Demlow B, Duncan A, Wangen K, et al: Soy isoflavones improve plasma lipids in normocholesterolemic, premenopausal women. *Am J Clin N* 2000;71:1462–1469.

Meydani M: Vitamin E and atherosclerosis: Beyond prevention of LDL oxidation. *J Nutr* 2001;131:S366–S368.

Mezquita-Raya P, Torres M, Luna J, et al: Relation between vitamin D insufficiency, bone density, and bone metabolism in healthy postmenopausal women. *J Bone Min* 2001; 16:1408–1415.

Miller W, Sharpe R: Environmental estrogens and human reproductive cancers. *Endocr-R Ca* 1998;5:69–96.

Morton D, Barrett-Connor E, Schneider D: Vitamin C supplement use and bone-mineral density in older women: The Rancho Bernardo Study. *J Bone Min* (meeting abstract).

Munday J, James K, Fray L, et al: Daily supplementation with aged garlic extract, but not raw garlic, protects low density lipoproteins against in vitro oxidation. *Atheroscler* 1999;143:399–404.

Ness A, Powles J: Fruit and vegetables, and cardiovascular disease: A review. *Int J Epidem* 1997;26:1–13.

Neven L: Isoflavones: An overview of benefits for health and market. *Agr Food In* 1998; 9:39–41.

Nguyen T, Center J, Eisman J: Osteoporosis in elderly men and women: Effects of dietary calcium, physical activity, and body-mass index. *J Bone Min* 2000;15:322–331.

Nishiyama S, Irisa K, Matsubasa T, et al: Zinc status relates to hematological deficits in middle-age women. *J Am Col N* 1998;17:291–295.

Nygard O, Refsum H, Ueland P, et al: Coffee consumption and plasma total homocysteine: The Hordaland Homocysteine Study. *Am J Clin N* 1997;65:136–143.

Oakley G, Erickson J, Adams M: Urgent need to increase folic acid consumption. *J Am Med A* 1995;274:1717–1718.

Packer L, Weber S, Rimbach G: Molecular aspects of alpha tocotrienol antioxidant action and cell signalling. *J Nutr* 2001;131:S369–S373.

Pak C, Sakhaee K, Adams B, et al: Treatment of postmenopausal osteoporosis with slow-release sodium fluoride. *Ann Int Med* 1995;123:401–408.

Patterson A, Brown W, Roberts D: Dietary and supplement treatment of iron deficiency results in improvements in general health and fatigue in Australian women of childbearing age. *J Am Col N* 2001;20:337–342.

Peng Y, Peng Y, Childers J, et al: Concentrations of carotenoids, tocopherols, and retinol in paired plasma and cervical tissue of patients with cervical cancer, precancer, and noncancerous diseases. *Canc Epid B* 1998;7:347–350.

Pennington J: Intakes of minerals from diets and foods: Is there a need for concern? *J Nutr* 1996;126:2304–2308.

Prasad K, Mantha S, Muir A, et al: Reduction of hypercholesterolemic atherosclerosis by CDC-flaxseed with very low alpha-linoleic acid. *Atheroscler* 1998;136:367–375.

Princen H, van Duyvenvoorde W, Buytenhek R, et al: Supplementation with low doses of vitamin E protects LDL from lipid peroxidation in men and women. *Art Throm V* 1995;15:325–333.

Recker R, Hinders S, Davies K, et al: Correcting calcium nutritional deficiency prevents spine fractures in elderly women. *J Bone Min* 1996;11:1961–1966.

Report of the National Cholesterol Education Program Expert Panel on detection, evaluation, and treatment of high blood cholesterol in adults. *Arch In Med* 1988;148:36–69.

Rimm E, Stampfer M: Antioxidants for vascular disease. *Med Clin Na* 2000;84:239+.

Rimm E, Willett W, Hu F, et al: Folate and vitamin $B_6$ from diet and supplements in relation to risk of coronary heart disease among women. *J Am Med A* 1998;279:359–364.

Robinson K, Arheart K, Refsum H, et al: Low circulating folate and vitamin $B_6$ concentrations. *Circulation* 1998;97:437–443.

Ronco A, De Stefani E, Boffetta P, et al: Vegetables, fruits, and related nutrients and risk of breast cancer. *Nutr Cancer* 2000;35:111–119.

Rubenowitz E, Axelsson G, Rylander R: Magnesium and calcium in drinking water and death from acute myocardial infarction in women. *Epidemiolog* 1999;10:31–36.

Rubenowitz E, Molin I, Axelsson G, et al: Magnesium in drinking water in relation to morbidity and mortality from acute myocardial infarction. *Epidemiolog* 2000;11:416–421.

Safe S: Interactions between hormones and chemicals in breast cancer. *Ann R Pharm* 1998; 38:121–158.

Samman S, Sandstrom B, Toft M, et al: Green tea or rosemary extract added to foods reduces nonheme-iron absorption. *Am J Clin N* 2001;73:607–612.

Sasazuki S, Kodama H, Yoshimasu K, et al: Relation between green tea consumption and the severity of coronary atherosclerosis among Japanese men and women. *Ann Epidemi* 2000;10:401–408.

Sato Y, Asoh T, Kondo I, et al: Vitamin D deficiency and risk of hip fractures among disabled elderly stroke patients. *Stroke* 2001;32:1673–1677.

Scheiber M, Rebar R: Isoflavones and postmenopausal bone health. *Menopause* 1999;6:233–241.

Sellers T, Kushi L, Cerhan J, et al: Vitamin B intake, alcohol, and risk of breast cancer in a prospective study of postmenopausal women. *Epidemiolog* 2001;12:420–428.

Serafini M, Maiani G, Ferro-Luzzi A: Alcohol-free red wine enhances plasma antioxidant capacity in humans. *J Nutr* 1998;128:1003–1007.

Seshadri N, Robinson K: Homocysteine, B vitamins, and coronary artery disease. *Med Clin Na* 2000;84:215+.

Shapira D, Clark R, Wolff P, et al: Visceral obesity and breast-cancer risk. *Cancer* 1994; 74:632–639.

Singh P, Fraser G: Dietary risk factors for colon cancer in a low-risk population. *Am J Epidem* 1998;148:761–774.

Sinha R, Kulldorgf M, Chow W, et al: Dietary intake of heterocyclic amines, meat-derived mutagenic activity, and risk of colorectal adenomas. *Canc Epid B* 2001;10:439–446/ 559–562.

Slattery M, Boucher K, Caan B, et al: Eating patterns and risk of colon cancer. *Am J Epidem* 1998;148:4–16.

Slattery M, Edwards S, Boucher K, et al: Lifestyle and colon cancer. *Am J Epidem* 1999; 159:869–877.

Slavin J, Martini M, Jacobs D, et al: Plausible mechanisms for the protectiveness of whole grains. *Am J Clin N* 1999;70:412–419, S459–S463.

Song K, Milner J: The influence of heating on the anticancer properties of garlic. *J Nutr* 2001;131:1054–1057.

Specker B: Evidence for an interaction between calcium intake and physical activity on changes in bone-mineral density. *J Bone Min* 1996;11:1539–1544.

Stampfer M, Hu F, Manson J, et al: Primary prevention of coronary heart disease in women through diet and lifestyle. *N Eng J Med* 2000;343:16–22.

St. Clair R: Estrogens and atherosclerosis: Phytoestrogens and selective estrogen receptor modulators. *Curr Op Lip* 1998;9:457–463.

Stefanick M, Mackey S, Sheehan M, et al: Effects of diet and exercise in men and post-menopausal women with low levels of HDL cholesterol and high levels of LDL cholesterol. *N Eng J Med* 1998;339:12–20.

Stone K, Duong T, Sellmeyer D, et al: Broccoli may be good for bones. *J Bone Min* 1999;14:F272 (meeting abstract).

Storm D, Eslin R, Porter E, et al: Calcium supplementation prevents seasonal bone loss and changes in biochemical markers of bone turnover in elderly New England women. *J Clin End* 1998;83:3817–3825.

Tavani A, Negri E, LaVecchia C: Coffee intake and risk of hip fracture in women in Northern Italy. *Prev Med* 1995;24:396–400.

Terry P, Giovannucci E, Michels K, et al: Fruit, vegetables, dietary fiber, and risk of colorectal cancer. *J Nat Canc* 2001;93:525–533.

Thomson S, Heimburger D, Cornwell P, et al: Effect of total plasma homocysteine on cervical dysplasia risk. *Nutr Cancer* 2000;37:128–133.

Title L, Cummings P, Giddens K, et al: Effect of folic acid and antioxidant vitamins on endothelial dysfunction in patients with coronary artery disease. *J Am Col C* 2000; 36:758–765.

Todd S, Woodward M, Tunstall-Pedoe H, et al: Dietary antioxidant vitamins and fiber in the etiology of cardiovascular disease and all causes mortality. *Am J Epidem* 1999; 150:1073–1080.

Trevisanato S, Kim Y: Tea and health. *Nutr Rev* 2000;58:1–10.

Tribble D: Antioxidant consumption and risk of coronary heart disease; Emphasis on vitamin C, vitamin E, and beta carotene: A statement of health-care professionals from the American Heart Association. *Circulation* 1999;99:591–595.

Tsai M: Moderate hyperhomocysteinemia and cardiovascular disease. *J La Cl Med* 2000; 135:16–25.

Tucker K, Hannan M, Chen H, et al: Potassium, magnesium, and fruit and vegetable intakes are associated with greater bone-mineral density in elderly men and women. *Am J Clin N* 1999;69:727–736.

Turley J, Fu T, Ruscetti F, et al: Vitamin E succinate induces fas-mediated apoptosis in estrogen receptor negative human breast cancer cells. *Cancer Res* 1997;57:881–890.

Ubbink J, Delport R, Vermaak W, et al: Bio-availability of calcium and magnesium from magnesium citrate/calcium malate. *So Afr Med J* 1997;87:1271–1276.

Van Asselt D, Merkus F, Russel F, et al: Nasal absorption of hydroxycobalamin in healthy elderly adults. *Br J Cl Ph* 1998;45:83–86.

Van den Berg M, Franken D, Boers G, et al: Combined vitamin $B_6$, plus folic acid therapy in young patients with arteriosclerosis and hyperhomocysteinemia. *J Vasc Surg* 1994; 20:933–940.

Van Loo J, Cummings J, Delzenne N, et al: Functional food properties of nondigestible oligosaccharides: A consensus report from the ENDO project (DGXII AIRII-CT94-1095). *Br J Nutr* 1999;81:121–132.

Vesper H, Schmelz E, Nikolova-Karakashian M, et al: Sphingolipids in food and the emerging importance of sphingolipids to nutrition. *J Nutr* 1999;129:1239–1250.

Visioli F, Galli C: The effect of minor constituents of olive oil on cardiovascular disease: New findings. *Nutr Rev* 1998;56:142–147.

Viteri F: Iron supplementation for the control of iron deficiency in populations at risk. *Nutr Rev* 1997;55:195–209.

Viteri F, Ali F, Tuijague J: Long-term weekly iron supplementation improves and sustains nonpregnant women's iron status as well or better than currently recommended short-term daily supplementation. *J Nutr* 1999;129:2013–2020.

Wang J, Schramm D, Holt R, et al: A dose-response effect from chocolate consumption on plasma epicatechin and oxidative damage. *J Nutr* 2000;130:2115–2119.

Watkins B, Li Y, Lipman H, et al: Omega-3 polyunsaturated fatty acids and skeletal health. *Exp Bio Med* 2001;226:485–497.

Watkins B, Li Y, Siefert M: Dietary omega-3 fatty acids and bone health. *Curr Org Ch* 2000; 4:1125–1144.

Weggemans R, Zock P, Katan M: Dietary cholesterol from eggs increases the ratio of total cholesterol to high-density lipoprotein cholesterol in humans. *Am J Clin N* 2001; 73:885–891.

Weisburger J: Eat to live, not live to eat. *Nutrition* 2000;16:767–773.

White E, Kristal A, Shikany J, et al: Correlates of serum alpha and gamma tocopherol in the Women's Health Initiative. *Ann Epidemi* 2001;11:136–144.

Whiting S: The inhibitory effect of dietary calcium on iron bioavailabity. *Nutr Rev* 1995; 53:77–80.

Willett W, Stampfer M, Manson J, et al: Coffee consumption and coronary heart disease in women. *J Am Med A* 1996;275:458–462.

Wollowski I, Rechkemmer G, Pool-Zobel B: Protective role of probiotics and prebiotics in colon cancer. *Am J Clin N* 2001;73:S451–S455.

Wu A, Ziegler R, Horn-Ross P, et al: Tofu and risk of breast cancer in Asian-Americans. *Canc Epid B* 1996;5:901–906.

Xu X, Duncan A, Merz B, et al: Effects of soy isoflavones on estrogen and phytoestrogen metabolism in premenopausal women. *Canc Epid B* 1998;7:1101–1108.

Zhang S, Tang G, Russell R, et al: Measurement of retinoids and carotenoids in breast adipose tissue and comparison of concentrations in breast-cancer cases and control subjects. *Am J Clin N* 1997;66:626–632.

Zhu Y, Haas J: Iron depletion without anemia and physical performance in young women. *Am J Clin N* 1997;66:334–341.

Zhu Y, Haas J: Response of serum transferrin receptor to iron supplementation in iron-depleted, nonanemic women. *Am J Clin N* 1998;67:271–275.

## CHAPTER 16: OTHER HEALTH CONDITIONS

Abraham G, Flechas J: Management of fibromyalgia: Rationale for the use of magnesium and malic acid. *J Nutr* 1992;3:49–59.

Agelli M: Vitamin C and vitamin B supplements helped prevent recurrence of urinary and vaginal tract infections. *Clin Res* 1994;42:A346 (meeting abstract).

Age-Related Eye Disease Study Research Group: A randomized, placebo-controlled, clinical trial of high-dose supplementation with vitamins C and E, beta carotene, and zinc for age-related cataracts and vision loss. *Arch Ophth* 2001;119:1439–1452.

Allison D, Kreibich K, Heshka S, et al: A randomized placebo-controlled clinical trial of an acupressure device for weight loss. *Int J Obes* 1995;19:653–658.

Alpert J, Fava M: Nutrition and depression: The role of folate. *Nutr Rev* 1997;55:145–149.

Anderson J: Chromium in the prevention and control of diabetes. *Diabete Met* 2000; 26:22–27.

Anderson R: Chromium, glucose intolerance, and diabetes. *J Am Col N* 1998;17:548–555.

Anderson R, Cheng N, Bryden N, et al: Elevated intakes of supplemental chromium improve glucose and insulin variables in individuals with type 2 diabetes. *Diabetes* 1997;46:1786–1791.

Appel L, Moore T, Obarzanek E, et al: A clinical trial of the effects of dietary patterns on blood pressure. *N Eng J Med* 1997;336:1117–1124.

Archer S, Green D, Chamberlain M, et al: Association of dietary fish and n-3 fatty acid intake with hemostatic factors in the Coronary Artery Risk Development in Young Adults (CARDIA) study. *Art Throm V* 1998;18:1119–1123.

Baldewicz T, Goodkin K, Feaster D, et al: Plasma pyridoxine deficiency is related to increased psychological distress in recently bereaved homosexual men. *Psychosom Med* 1998;60:297–308.

Bar-Natan R, Lomnitski L, Sofer Y, et al: Interaction between beta carotene and lipoxygenase in human skin. *Int J Bio C* 1996;28:935–941.

Beatty S, Koh H, Henson D, et al: The role of oxidative stress in the pathogenesis of age-related macular degeneration. *Surv Ophtha* 2000;45:115–134.

Beebe D: Nuclear cataracts and nutrition: Hope for intervention early and late in life. *Inv Ophth V* 1998;39:1531–1534.

Belch J, Hill A: Evening primrose oil and borage oil in rheumatologic conditions. *Am J Clin N* 2000;71:S352–S356.

Belda J, Roma J, Vilela C, et al: Serum vitamin E levels negatively correlate with severity of age-related macular degeneration. *Mech Age D* 1999;107:159–164.

Bendich A: The potential for dietary supplements to reduce premenstrual syndrome (PMS) symptoms. *J Am Col N* 2001;19:3–12.

Benton D, Fordy J, Haller J: The impact of long-term vitamin supplementation on cognitive functioning. *Psychophar* 1995;117:298–305.

Benton D, Parker P: Breakfast, blood glucose, and cognition. *Am J Clin N* 1998;67(suppl):S772–S778.

Biachi L, Melli R, Pizzala R, et al: Effects of beta carotene and alpha tocopherol on photogenotoxicity induced by 8-methoxypsoralen: The role of oxygen. *Mut Res* 1996;369:183–194.

Bone R, Landrum J, Kilburn M, et al: Effect of dietary supplementation with lutein on macular pigment density. *Inv Ophth V* 1996;37:532-B444 (meeting abstract).

Bottiglieri T: Folate, vitamin $B_{12}$, and neuropsychiatric disorders. *Nutr Rev* 1996;54:382–390.

Bou-Holaigah I, Rowe P, Kan J, et al: The relationship between neurally medicated hypotension and the chronic fatigue syndrome. *J Am Med A* 1995;274:961–967.

Bowen D, Kestin M, McTiernan, et al: Effects of dietary fat intervention on mental health in women. *Canc Epid B* 1995;4:555–559.

Bro R, Shank L, McLaughlin T, et al: Effects of a breakfast program on on-task behaviors of vocational high school students. *J Educ Res* 1996;90:111–115.

Brown N, Bron A, Harding J, et al: Nutrition, supplements and the eye. *Eye* 1998;12:127–133.

Brubaker R, Bourne W, Bachman L, et al: Ascorbic acid content of human corneal epithelium. *Inv Ophth V* 2000;41:1681–1683.

Bruner A, Joffee A, Duggan A, et al: Randomized study of cognitive effects of iron supplementation in nonanemic iron-deficient adolescent girls. *Lancet* 1996;348:992–996.

Bucher H, Cook R, Guyatt G, et al: Effects of dietary calcium supplementation on blood pressure. *J Am Med A* 1996;275:1113–1117.

Burke K, Combs O, Gross E, et al: The effects of topical and oral L-selenomethione on pigmentation and skin cancer induced by ultraviolet irradiation. *Nutr Cancer* 1992; 17:123–137.

Carmel R: Current concepts in cobalamin deficiency. *Ann R Med* 2000;51:357–375.

Chan P, Huang T, Chen Y, et al: Randomized, double-blind, placebo-controlled study of the safety and efficacy of vitamin B complex in the treatment of nocturnal leg cramps in elderly patients with hypertension. *J Clin Phar* 1998;38:1151–1154.

Chapuy M, Preziosi P, Maamer M, et al: Prevalence of vitamin D insufficiency in an adult normal population. *Osteopor Int* 1997;7:439–443.

Chausmer A: Zinc, insulin, and diabetes. *J Am Col N* 1988;17:109–115.

Cho E, Hung S, Willett W, et al: Prospective study of dietary fat and the risk of age-related macular degeneration. *Am J Clin N* 2001;73:209–218.

Christen W, Ajani U, Glynn R, et al: Prospective cohort study of antioxidant vitamin supplement use and the risk of age-related maculopathy. *Am J Epidem* 1999; 149:476–484.

Christensen L, Pettijohn L: Mood and carbohydrate craving. *Appetite* 2001;36:137–145.

Clement-LaCroix P, Michel L, Moysan A, et al: UVA-induced immune suppression in human skin: Protective effect of vitamin E in human epidermal cells in vitro. *Br J Derm* 1996;134:77–84.

Coffee linked to rheumatoid arthritis. *Sci News* 2000;158:155.

Cohen B, Babb S, Yurgelun-Todd D, et al: Brain choline uptake and cognitive function in middle age. *Biol Psychi* 1997;41:307.

Cope G, Thorpe G, Holder R, et al: Serum and tissue antioxidant capacity in cervical intraepithelial neoplasia. *Ann Clin Bi* 1999;36:86–93.

Copeland D, Stouikides C: Pyridoxine in carpal tunnel syndrome. *Ann Pharmac* 1994; 28:1042–1044.

Cross G, Marley J, Miles H, et al: Changes in nutrient intake during the menstrual cycle of overweight women with premenstrual syndrome. *Br J Nutr* 2001;85:475–482.

Cumming R, Mitchell P, Smith W: Diet and cataract. *Ophthalmol* 2000;107:450–456.

Cunningham J: Micronutrients as nutriceutical interventions in diabetes mellitus. *J Am Col N* 1998;17:7–10.

Darlington L, Stone T: Antioxidants and fatty acids in the amelioration of rheumatoid arthritis and related disorders. *Br J Nutr* 2001;85:251–269.

Davis C, Vincent J: Chromium in carbohydrate and lipid metabolism. *J Biol Chem* 1997; 2:675–679.

Deutch B, Jorgensen E, Hansen J, et al: Menstrual discomfort in Danish women reduced by dietary supplements of omega-3 pufa and $B_{12}$. *Nutr Res* 2000;20:621–631.

Do zinc lozenges shorten common colds? *Sci News* 2000;158:155.

Dreher F, Gabard S, Schwindt D, et al: Topical melatonin in combination with vitamins E and C protects skin from ulraviolet-induced erythema: A human study in vivo. *Br J Derm* 1998;139:332–339.

Driver H, Taylor S: Sleep disturbances and exercise. *Sport Med* 1996;21:1–6.

Edmonds S, Winyard P, Guo R, et al: Putative analgesic activity of repeated oral doses of vitamin E in the treatment of rheumatoid arthritis. Results of a prospective placebo controlled double-blind trial. *Ann Rheum D* 1997;56:649–655.

Edwards R, Peet M, Shay J, et al: Omega-3 polyunsaturated fatty acid levels in the diet and in red blood cell membranes of depressed patients. *J Affect D* 1998;48:149–155.

Eichner R: Fatigue of anemia. *Nutr Rev* 2001;59:S17–S19.

Fava M, Borus J, Alpert J, et al: Folate, vitamin $B_{12}$, and homocysteine in major depressive disorder. *Am J Psychi* 1997;154:426–428.

Fischer K, Colombani P, Langhans W, et al: Cognitive performance and its relationship with postprandial metabolic changes after ingestion of different macronutrients in the morning. *Br J Nutr* 2001;85:393–405.

Ford E: Vitamin supplement use and diabetes mellitus incidence among adults in the United States. *Am J Epidem* 2001;153:892–897.

Ford E, Mokdad A: Fruit and vegetable consumption and diabetes mellitus incidence among U.S. adults. *Prev Med* 2001;32:33–39.

Ford E, Will J, Bowman B, et al: Diabetes mellitus and serum carotenoids: Findings from the Third National Health and Nutrition Examination Survey. *Am J Epidem* 1999;149:168–176.

Ford E, Williamson D, Liu S: Weight change and diabetes incidence: Findings from a national cohort of U.S. adults. *Am J Epidem* 1997;146:214–222.

Frye C, Demolar G: Menstrual cycle and sex differences influence salt preference. *Physl Behav* 1994;55:193–197.

Fugh-Berman A, Cott J: Dietary supplements and natural products as psychotherapeutic agents. *Psychos Med* 1999;61:712–728.

Furushiro M, Suzuki S, Shishido Y, et al: Effects of oral administration of soybean lecithin transphosphotidylated phosphatidylserine on impaired learning of passive avoidance in mice. *Jpn J Pharm* 1997;75:447–450.

Galbraith H: Nutritional and hormonal regulation of hair follicle growth and development. *P Nutr Soc* 1998;57:195–205.

Gallai V, Sarchielli P, Morucci P, et al: Magnesium content of mononuclear blood cells in migraine patients. *Headache* 1994;34:160–165.

Garcia M, Ward G, Ma Y, et al: Effect of docosahexaenoic acid on the synthesis of phosphatidylserine in rat brain in microsomes and C6 glioma cells. *J Neurochem* 1998;70:24–30.

Garfinkel D, Laudon M, Nof D, et al: Improvement of sleep quality in elderly people by controlled-release melatonin. *Lancet* 1995;346:541–544.

Garfinkel M, Singhal A, Katz W, et al: Yoga-based intervention for carpal tunnel syndrome. *J Am Med A* 1998;280:1601–1603.

Gerber J: Nutrition and migraine: Review and recommended strategies. *JNMS-J Neur* 1997;5:87–94.

Giuliano A, Gapstur S: Can cervical dysplasia and cancer be prevented with nutrients? *Nutr Rev* 1998;56:9–16.

Goebels N, Soynka M: Dementia associated with vitamin $B_{12}$ deficiency. *J Neurop Clin* 2000;12:389–394.

Grahn B, Paterson P, Pass K, et al: Zinc and the eye. *J Am Col N* 2001;20:106–118.

Grant K, Chandler R, Castle A, et al: Chromium and exercise training: Effect on obese women. *Med Sci Spt* 1997;29:992–998.

Grant W: The role of meat in the expression of rheumatoid arthritis. *Br J Nutr* 2000; 84:589–595.

Greco R: Topical vitamin C. *Plas R Surg* 2000;105:464–465.

Green M, Rogers P: Impairments in working memory associated with spontaneous dieting behavior. *Psychol Med* 1998;28:1063–1070.

Hajjar I, Grim C, George V, et al: Impact of diet on blood pressure and age-related changes in blood pressure in the U.S. population. *Arch In Med* 2001;161:589–593.

Hashimoto S, Kohsaka M, Morita N, et al: Vitamin $B_{12}$ enhances the phase-response of circadian melatonin rhythm to a single bright light exposure in humans. *Neurosci L* 1996:220:129–132.

Heap L, Peters T, Wessely S: Vitamin B status in patients with chronic fatigue syndrome. *J Roy S Med* 1999;92:183–185.

Hemila H: Vitamin C intake and susceptibility to the common cold. *Br J Nutr* 1997; 77:59–72.

Heumberger R, Mares-Perlman J, Klein R, et al: Relationship of dietary fat to age-related maculopathy in the third National Health and Nutrition Examination Survey. *Arch Ophth* 2001;119:1833–1838.

Hibbeln J, Linnoila M, Umhau J, et al: Essential fatty acids predict metabolites of serotonin and dopamine in cerebrospinal fluid among healthy control subjects and early- and late-onset alcoholics. *Biol Psychi* 1998;44:235–242.

Hibbeln J, Umhau J, Linnoila M, et al: A replication study of violent and nonviolent subjects: Cerebrospinal fluid metabolites of serotonin and dopamine are predicted by plasma essential fatty acids. *Biol Psychi* 1998;44:243–249.

Hu F, Hankinson S, Stampfer M, et al: Prospective study of cataract extraction and risk of coronary heart disease in women. *Am J Epidem* 2001;153:875–881.

Huisman A, White K, Algra A, et al: Vitamin D levels in women with system lupus erythematosus and fibromyalgia. *J Rheumatol* 2001;28:2535–2539.

Hypponen E, Laara E, Reuanen A, et al: Intake of vitamin D and risk of type 1 diabetes. *Lancet* 2001;358:1500–1503.

Itoh K, Kawasaki T, Nakamura M: The effects of high oral magnesium supplementation on blood pressure, serum lipids, and related variables in apparently healthy Japanese subjects. *Br J Nutr* 1997;78:737–750.

Jaax S, Scott L, Wolf J, et al: General guidelines for a low-fat diet effective in the management and prevention of nonmelanoma skin cancer. *Nutr Cancer* 1997;27:150–156.

Jacques P: The potential preventive effects of vitamins for cataract and age-related macular degeneration. *Int J Vit N* 1999;69:198–205.

Jacques P, Chylack L, Hankinson S, et al: Vitamin C, stroke, and early age-related nuclear opacities. *Arch Ophth* 2001;119:1009–1019/1191–1199.

Jacques P, Taylor A, Hankinson S, et al: Long-term vitamin C supplement use and prevalence of early age-related lens opacities. *Am J Clin N* 1997;66:911–916.

Jain S, McVie R, Jaramillo J, et al: Effect of modest vitamin E supplementation on blood glycated hemoglobin and triglyceride levels and red cell indices in type 1 diabetic patients. *J Am Col N* 1996;15:458–461.

Jama J, Launer L, Witteman J, et al: Dietary antioxidants and cognitive function in a population-based sample of older persons: The Rotterdam Study. *Am J Epidem* 1996;144:275–280.

Jarisch R, Wantke F: Wine and headache. *Int A Al Im* 1996;110:7–12.

Joseph J, Denisova N, Fisher D, et al: Age-related neurodegeneration and oxidative stress. *Neurobiol A* 1998;16:747–755.

Joseph J, Shukitt-Hale B, Denisova N, et al: Long-term dietary strawberry, spinach, or vitamin E supplementation retards the onset of age-related neuronal signal-transduction and cognitive behavioral deficits. *J Neurosc* 1998;18:8047–8055.

Kalmjin S, Feskens E, Launer L, et al: Polyunsaturated fatty acids, antioxidants, and cognitive function in very old men. *Am J Epidem* 1997;145:33–41.

Kanarek R: Psychological effects of snacks and altered meal frequency. *Br J Nutr* 1997;77(suppl):S105–S118.

Kaplan B, Simpson J, Ferre R, et al: Effective mood stabilization with a broad-based nutritional supplement. *Biol Psychi* 2001;49:388 (meeting abstract).

Katayama I, Miyazaki Y, Nishioka K: Topical vitamin $D_3$ (tacalcitol) for steroid-resistant prurigo. *Br J Derm* 1996;135:237–240.

Katiyar S, Ahmad N, Mukhtar H: Green tea and skin. *Arch Dermat* 2000;136:989–994.

Kaye W, Gendall K, Fernstrom M, et al: Effects of acute tryptophan depletion on mood in bulimia nervosa. *Biol Psychi* 2000;47:151–157.

Keniston R, Leklem J, Nathan P: Vitamin $B_6$, vitamin C, and carpal tunnel syndrome. *J Occ Envir M* 998;40:305–309.

Keniston R, Nathan P, Leklem J, et al: Vitamin $B_6$, vitamin C, and carpal tunnel syndrome. *J Occup Env* 1997;39:949–959.

Kiuchi T, Sei H, Seno H, et al: Effect of vitamin $B_{12}$ on the sleep-wake rhythm following an eight-hour advance of the light-dark cycle in the rat. *Physl Behav* 1997;61:551–554.

Korol D, Gold P: Glucose, memory, and aging. *Am J Clin N* 1998;67(suppl):S764–S771.

Kremer J: N-3 fatty acid supplements in rheumatoid arthritis. *Am J Clin N* 2000;71 (suppl):349S–351S.

Kretsch M, Green M, Fong A, et al: Cognitive effects of a long-term weight-reducing diet. *Int J Obes* 1997;21:14–21.

Kwasniewski A, Tukendorf A, Semczuk M: Content of alpha tocopherol in blood serum of human papillomavirus-infected women with cervical dysplasia. *Nutr Cancer* 1997; 28:248–251.

Kwasniewski A, Tukendorf A, Semczuk M: Folate deficiency and cervical intraepithelial neoplasia. *Eur J Gyn O* 1997;18:526–530.

La Rue A, Koehler K, Wayne S, et al: Nutritional status and cognitive functioning in a normal aging sample: A six-year reassessment. *Am J Clin N* 1997;65:20–29.

Lauritzen C, Reuter H, Repges R, et al: Treatment of premenstrual tension syndrome with vitex agnus castus: Controlled, double-blind study versus pyridoxine. *Phytomed* 1997; 4:183–189.

Lee J, Jiang S, Levine N, et al: Carotenoid supplementation reduces erythema in human skin after stimulated solar radiation exposure. *P Soc Exp M* 2000;223:170–174.

Leiberman H: The effects of ginseng, ephedrine, and caffeine on cognitive performance, mood and energy. *Nutr Rev* 2001;59:91–102.

Lin A, Uhde T, Slate S, et al: Effects of intravenous caffeine administered to healthy males during sleep. *Depress Anxiety* 1997;5:21–28.

Linos A, Kaklamani V, Kaklamani E, et al: Dietary factors in relation to rheumatoid arthritis. *Am J Clin N* 2000;70:1077–1082.

Liu S, Manson J, Stampfer M, et al: A prospective study of whole-grain intake and risk of type 2 diabetes mellitus in U.S. women. *Am J Pub He* 2000;90:1409–1415.

Longas M, Bhuyan D, Bhuyan K, et al: Dietary vitamin E reverses the effects of ultraviolet light irradiation on rat skin glycosaminoglycans. *Bioc Biop A* 1993;115:239–244.

Lou W, Quintana A, Geronemus R, et al: Effects of topical vitamin K and retinol on laser-induced purpura on nonlesional skin. *Derm Surg* 1999;25:942–944.

Lucero K, Hicks R: Relationship between habitual sleep duration and diet. *Perc Mot Sk* 1990;71(3 pt 2):1377–1378.

Lyle B, Mares-Perlman J, Klein B, et al: Serum carotenoids and tocopherols and incidence of age-related nuclear cataracts. *Am J Clin N* 1999;69:272–277.

Maes M, deVos N, Pioli R, et al: Lower serum vitamin E concentrations in major depression. *J Affect D* 2000;58:241–246.

Maes M, Vandoolaeghe E, Neels H, et al: Lower serum zinc in major depression is a sensitive marker of treatment resistance and of the immune/inflammatory response in that illness. *Biol Psychi* 1997;42:349–358.

Marean M, Cumming C, Fox E, et al: Fluid intake in women with premenstrual syndrome. *Women Heal* 1995;23:75.

Mares-Perlman J, Brady W, Klein B, et al: Diet and nuclear lens opacities. *Am J Epidem* 1995;141:322–334.

Mares-Perlman J, Fisher A, Klein R, et al: Lutein and zeaxanthin in the diet and serum and their relation to age-related maculopathy in the third National Health and Examination Survey. *Am J Epidem* 2001;153:424–432.

Mares-Perlman J, Klein R, Klein B, et al: Association of zinc and antioxidant nutrients with age-related, macular degeneration. *Arch Ophth* 1996:114:991–997.

Markus C, Panhuysen G, Tuiten A, et al: Does carbohydrate-rich, protein-poor food prevent a deterioration of mood and cognitive performance of stress-prone subjects when subjected to a stressful task? *Appetite* 1998;31:49–65.

Martin L, Kaplan B, Crawford S, et al: A randomized controlled trial of a nutritional supplement in the management of fibromyalgia. *J Rheumatol* 2001;28:35 (meeting abstract).

Masaki K, Losonczy K, Izmirlian G, et al: The association of vitamin E and C supplement use with cognitive function and dementia. *J Am Ger Soc* 1998;46:P18 (meeting abstract).

Masse P, Ziv I, Cole D, et al: A cartilage matrix deficiency experimentally induced by vitamin $B_6$ deficiency. *P Soc Exp M* 1998;217:97–103.

McCully K, Sisto S, Natelson B: Use of exercise for treatment of chronic fatigue syndrome. *Sport Med* 1996;21:35–48.

McGahon B, Martin D, Horrobin D, et al: Age-related changes in synaptic function: Analysis of the effect of dietary supplementation with omega-3 fatty acids. *Neuroscienc* 1999;94:305–314.

McMurray D, Jolly C, Chapkin R: Effects of dietary n-3 fatty acids on T-cell receptor-mediated signaling a murine model. *J Infec Dis* 2000;182(suppl):S103–S107.

Meck W, Williams C: Perinatal choline supplementation increases the threshold for thinking in spatial memory. *Neuroreport* 1997;8:3053–3059.

Mele A, Szklo M, Visani G, et al: Hair dye use and other risk factors for leukemia and preleukemia. *Am J Epidem* 1994;139:609–619.

Merchant R, Carmack C, Wise C: Dietary supplementation with *Chlorella pyrenoidosa* for patients with fibromyalgia syndrome. *FASEB J* 1998;12:253.

Merchant R, Carmack C, Wise C: Nutritional supplementation with *Chlorella pyrenoidosa* for patients with fibromyalgia syndrome. *Sc J Rheum* 2000;29:308–313.

Mikhail M, Palan P, Basu J, et al: Decreased beta carotene levels in exfoliated vaginal epithelial cells in women with vaginal candidiasis. *Am J Reprod* 1994;32:221–225.

Miller G, DiRienzo D, Reusser M, et al: Benefits of dairy product consumption on blood pressure in humans. *J Am Col N* 2000;19:S147–S164.

Miller J: Vitamin E and memory: Is it vascular protection? *Nutr Rev* 2000;58:109–111.

Monroe B: Alcohol, thiamin, and fibromyalgia. *J Am Col N* 1998;17:300.

Motluk A: Flabby minds. *New Sci* 2001;169:10.

Mulherin D, Thurnham D, Situnayake R: Glutathione reductase activity, riboflavin status, and disease activity in rheumatoid arthritis. *Ann Rheum D* 1996;55:837–914.

Muller H, de Toledo F, Resch K: Fasting followed by vegetarian diet in patients with rheumatoid arthritis. *Sc J Rheum* 2001;30:1–10.

Nachbar F, Korting H: The role of vitamin E in normal and damaged skin. *J Mol Med-J* 1995;73:7–17.

Nalini G, Hariprasad C, Nagarajan A, et al: The antioxidant status in rheumatoid arthritis. *J Clin Bio* 1997;23:69–75.

Naveh Y, Schapira D, Ravel Y, et al: Zinc metabolism in rheumatoid arthritis: Plasma and urinary zinc and relationship to disease activity. *J Rheumatol* 1997;24:643–646.

Ness A, Chee D, Elliott P: Vitamin C and blood pressure: An overview. *J Hum Hyper* 1997; 11:343–350.

Ohta Y, Okada H, Majima Y, et al:Anticataract action of vitamin E. *Ophthal Res* 1996; 28(suppl):16–25.

Ortiz A, Shea B, Suarez-Almazor M, et al: The efficacy of folic acid and folinic acid in reducing methotrexate gastrointestinal toxicity in rheumatoid arthritis: A meta-analysis of randomized controlled trials. *J Rheumatol* 1998;25:36–43.

Packer L, Tritschler H, Wessel K: Neuroprotection by the metabolic antioxidant alpha-lipoic acid. *Free Rad B* 1997;22:359–378.

Paleologos M, Cumming R, Lazarus R: Cohort study of vitamin C intake and cognitive impairment. *Am J Epidem* 1998;148:45–50.

Paolisso G, Balbi V, Volpe C, et al: Metabolic benefits deriving from chronic vitamin C supplementation in aged non-insulin dependent diabetics. *J Am Col N* 1995;14:387–392.

Paolisso G, Barbagallo M: Hypertension, diabetes mellitus, and insulin resistance: The role of intracellular magnesium. *Am J Hypert* 1997;10:346–355.

Paolisso G, Giugliano D: Oxidative stress and insulin action. *Diabetolog* 1996;39:357–363.

Paolisso G, Tagliamonte M, Barbieri M, et al: Chronic vitamin E administration improves brachial reactivity and increases intracellular magnesium concentration in type II diabetic patients. *J Clin End* 2000;85:109–115.

Paolisso G, Tagliamonte M, Rizzo M, et al: Oxidative stress and advancing age: Results in healthy centenarians. *J Am Ger Soc* 1998;46:833–838.

Patterson A, Brown W, Powers J, et al: Iron deficiency, general health and fatigue. *Qual Life R* 2000;9:491–497.

Peet M, Murphy B, Shay J, et al: Depletion of omega-3 fatty acid levels in red blood cell membranes of depressive patients. *Biol Psychi* 1998;43:315–319.

Pence B, Delver E, Dunn D: Effects of dietary selenium on UVB-induced skin carcinogenesis and epidermal antioxidant status. *J Invest Derm* 1994;102:759–761.

Peng Y, Peng Y, Childers J, et al: Concentrations of carotenoids, tocopherols, and retinol in paired plasma and cervical tissue of patients with cervical cancer, precancer, and noncancerous diseases. *Canc Epid B* 1998;7:347–350.

Penninx B, Guralnik J, Ferrucci L, et al: Vitamin $B_{12}$ deficiency and depression in physically disabled older women. *Am J Psychi* 2000;157:660–661/715–721.

Pere A, Lindgren L, Tuomainen P, et al: Dietary potassium and magnesium supplementation in cyclosporine-induced hypertension and nephrotoxicity. *Kidney Int* 2000; 58:2462–2472.

Perig W, Perrig P, Stahelin H: The relation between antioxidants and memory performance in the old and very old. *J Am Ger So* 1997;45:718–724.

Pinto A, Rock C, Ferruzzi M, et al: Cervical tissue and plasma concentrations of alpha carotene and beta carotene in women are correlated. *J Nutr* 1998;128:1933–1936.

Pollitt E: Iron deficiency and educational deficiency. *Nutr Rev* 1997;55:133–140.

Pollitt E, Mathews R: Breakfast and cognition: An integrative summary. *Am J Clin N* 1998;67(suppl):S804–S813.

Potischman N, Brinton L: Nutrition and cervical neoplasia. *Cancer Cause* 1996;7:113–126.

Ramesh G, Das U: Effect of evening primrose and fish oils on two stage skin carcinogenesis in mice. *Pros Leuk E* 1998;59:155–161.

Rangarajan M, Zatz J: Skin delivery of vitamin E. *J Cosmet Sci* 1999;50:249–279.

Reinhard P, Schweinsberg F, Wernet D, et al: Selenium status in fibromyalgia. *Tox Lett* 1998;96,97:177–180.

Ricciarelli R, Maroni P, Ozer N, et al: Age-dependent increase of collagenase expression can be reduced by alpha tocopherol via protein kinase C inhibition. *Free Rad B* 1999; 27:729–737.

Rock C, Michael C, Reynolds R, et al: Prevention of cervical cancer. *Cr R Onc H* 2000;33:169–185.

Rogers P: A healthy body, a healthy mind. *P Nutr Soc* 2001;60:135–143.

Rose F: Food and headache. *Headache Q* 1997;8:319–329.

Rouhiainen P, Rouhiainen H, Salonen J: Association between low plasma vitamin E concentration and progression of early cortical lens opacities. *Am J Epidem* 1996;144: 496–500.

Sakurauchi Y, Matsumoto Y, Shinzato T, et al: Effects of L-carnitine supplementation on muscular symptoms in hemodialyzed patients. *Am J Kidney* 1998;32:258–264.

Salonen J, Nyyssonen K, Tuomainen T, et al: Increased risk of non-insulin dependent diabetes mellitus at low plasma vitamin E concentrations. *Br Med J* 1995;311:1124–1127.

Sandow P, Afra J, Ambrosini A, et al: Prophylactic treatment of migraine with beta-blockers and riboflavin. *Headache* 2000;40:30–35.

Sano M, Ernesto C, Thomas R, et al: A controlled trial of selegiline, alpha-tocopherol, or both as treatment for Alzheimer's disease. *N Eng J Med* 1997;336:1216–1222.

Sargeant L, Wareham N, Bingham S, et al: Vitamin C and hyperglycemia in the prospective investigation into cancer: Norfolk (EPIC-Norfolk) Study. *Diabet Care* 2000; 23:726–732.

Sarzi-Puttini P, Comi D, Boccassini L, et al: Diet therapy for rheumatoid arthritis. *Sc J Rheum* 2000;29:302–307.

Sawynok J: Pharmacological rationale for the clinical use of caffeine. *Drugs* 1995;49:37–50.

Schoenen J, Jacquy J, Lenaerts M: Effectiveness of high-dose riboflavin in migraine prophylaxis. *Neurology* 1998;50:466–470.

Sharma A, Sharb S, Chugh S, et al: Evaluation of oxidative stress before and after control of glycemia and after vitamin E supplementation in diabetic patients. *Metabolism* 2000;49:160–162.

Shephard R: Chronic fatigue syndrome: An update. *Sport Med* 2001;31:167–194.

Shukitt-Hale B, Askew E, Lieberman H: Effects of thirty days of undernutrition on reaction time, moods, and symptoms. *Physl Behav* 1997;62:783–789.

Sicard B, Perault M, Enslen M, et al: The effects of 600 mg of slow-release caffeine on mood and alertness. *Aviat Sp En* 1996;67:859–862.

Singh J, Hustler B, Waring J, et al: Dietary and physiological studies to investigate the relationship between calcium and magnesium signaling in the mammalian myocardium. *Mol C Bioch* 1997;176:127–134.

Smith A: Breakfast cereal, caffeinated coffee, mood, and cognition. *Nutrition* 2000; 16:228–229.

Smith A: Breakfast consumption and intelligence in elderly persons. *Psychol Rep* 1998; 82:424–426.

Smith J, Terpening C, Schmidt S, et al: Relief of fibromyalgia symptoms following discontinuation of dietary excitotoxins. *Ann Pharmac* 2001;35:702–706.

Snowden W: Evidence from an analysis of 2000 errors and omissions made in IQ tests by a small sample of schoolchildren, undergoing vitamin and mineral supplementation, that speed of processing is an important factor in IQ performance. *Pers Indiv* 1997; 22:131–134.

Solzbach U, Hornig B, Jeserich M, et al: Vitamin C improves endothelial dysfunction of epicardial coronary arteries in hypertensive patients. *Circulation* 1997;96:1513–1519.

Spring B, Lieberman H, Swope G, et al: Effects of carbohydrates on mood and behavior. *Nutr Rev* 1986;May (suppl):51–60.

Stahl W, Heinrich U, Jungmann H, et al: Carotenoids and carotenoids plus vitamin E protect against ultraviolet light–induced erythma in humans. *Am J Clin N* 2000;71:795–798.

Stahl W, Heinrich U, Jungmann H, et al: Increased dermal carotenoid levels assesed by noninvasive reflection spectrophotometry correlate with serum levels in women ingesting Betatene. *J Nutr* 1998;128:903–907.

Steenvoorden D, Beijersbergen van Henegouwen G: The use of endogenous antioxidants to improve photoprotection. *J Photoch B* 1997;41:1.

Stone J, Doube A, Dudson D, et al: Inadequate calcium, folic acid, vitamin E, zinc, and selenium intake in rheumatoid arthritis patients: Results of a dietary survey. *Sem Arth Rh* 1997;27:180–185.

Strickland F, Pelley R, Kripke M: Prevention of ultraviolet-induced suppression of contact and delayed hypersensitivity by aloe barbadensis gel extract. *J Inves Der* 1994; 102:197–204.

Striffler J, Polansky M, Anderson R: Dietary chromium decreases insulin resistance in rats fed a high-fat, mineral-imbalanced diet. *Metabolism* 1998;47:396–400.

Tanabe K, Yamamoto A, Suzuki N, et al: Efficacy of oral magnesium administration on decreased exercise tolerance in a state of chronic sleep deprivation. *Jpn Circ J* 1998; 62:341–346.

Tanskanen A, Hibbeln J, Tuomilehto J, et al: Fish consumption and depressive symptoms in the general population in Finland. *Psych Serv* 2001;52:529–531.

Tessier F, Moreaux V, Aragon I, et al: Decrease in vitamin C concentration in human lens during cataract progression. *Int J Vit N* 1998;68:309–315.

Thiele J, Podda M, Packer L: Tropospheric ozone: An emerging environmental stress to skin. *Biol Chem* 1997;378:1299–1305.

Thiele J, Traber M, Tsang K, et al: In vivo exposure to ozone depletes vitamins C and E and induces lipid peroxidation in epidermal layers of murine skin. *Free Rad B* 1997; 23:385–391.

Thomson S, Heimburger D, Cornwell P, et al: Effect of total plasma homocysteine on cervical dysplasia risk. *Nutr Cancer* 2000;37:128–133.

Thun M, Mohan A, Eugenia N, et al: Hair dye use and risk of fatal cancers in U.S. women. *J Nat Canc* 1994;86:210–215.

Thys-Jacobs S: Alleviation of migraines with therapeutic vitamin D and calcium. *Headache* 1994;34:590–592.

Thys-Jacobs S: Micronutrients and the premenstrual syndrome: The case for calcium. *J Am Col N* 2000;19:220–227.

Van Goor L, Woiski M, Lagaay A, et al: Review: Cobalamin deficiency and mental impairment in elderly people. *Age Ageing* 1995;24:536–542.

Van Leer E, Seidell J, Kromhout D: Sodium, potassium, magnesium, and blood pressure in the Netherlands. *Int J Epid* 1995;24:1117–1123.

Vatassery G: Vitamin E and other endogenous antioxidants in the central nervous system. *Geriatrics* 1998;53:S25–S27.

Voderholzer U, Hornyak M, Thiel B, et al: Impact of experimentally induced serotonin deficiency by tryptophan depletion on sleep EEG in healthy subjects. *Neuropsych* 1998;18:112–124.

Vuksan V, Sievenpiper J, Wong J, et al: American ginseng attenuates postprandial glycemia in a time-dependent but not dose-dependent manner in healthy individuals. *Am J Clin N* 2001;73:753–758.

Vuksan V, Stavro M, Sievenpiper J, et al: American ginseng improves glycemia in individuals with normal glucose tolerance. *J Am Col N* 2000;19:738–744.

Walker A, de Souza M, Vickers M, et al: Magnesium supplementation alleviates premenstrual symptoms of fluid retention. *J Women Hg* 1998;7:1157–1165.

Warburton D: Effects of caffeine on cognition and mood without caffeine abstinence. *Psychophar* 1995;119:66–70.

Weber S, Thiele J, Cross C, et al: Vitamin C, uric acid, and glutathione gradients in murine stratum corneum and their susceptibility to ozone exposure. *J Inves Der* 1999;113:1128–1132.

Wei H: Photoprotective action of isoflavone genistein: Models, mechanisms, and relevance to clinical dermatology. *J Am Acad D* 1998;39:271–272.

Weig M, Werner E, Frosch M, et al: Limited effect of refined carbohydrate dietary supplementation on colonization of the gastrointestinal tract of healthy subjects by Candida albicans. *Am J Clin N* 1999;69:1170–1173.

Wells A, Read N: Influences of fat, energy, and time of day on mood and performance. *Physl Behav* 1996;59:1069–1076.

Wells A, Read N, Idzikowski C, et al: Effects of meals on objective and subjective measures of daytime sleepiness. *J Appl Phys* 1998;84:507–515.

Wells A, Read N, Macdonald I: Effects of carbohydrate and lipid on resting energy expenditure, heart rate, sleepiness and mood. *Physl Behav* 1998;63:621–628.

Wyatt K, Dimmock P, Jones P, et al: Efficacy of vitamin B$_6$ in the treatment of premenstrual syndrome: Systematic review. *Br Med J* 1999;318:1375–1381.

Wyon D, Abrahamsson L, Jartelius M, et al: An experimental study of the effects of energy intake at breakfast on the test performance of ten-year-old children in school. *Int J F S M* 1997;48:5–12.

Yamori Y, Mizushima S: A review of the link between dietary magnesium and cardiovascular risk. *J Card Risk* 2000;7:31–35.

Yang W, Drouin M, Herbert M, et al: The monosodium glutamate symptom complex: Assessment in a double-blind, placebo-controlled, randomized study. *J Allerg Cl* 1997;99:757–762.

Zeisel S: Choline: Needed for normal development of memory. *J Am Col N* 2000;19:S528–S531.

Zhao J, Jin X, Yaping E, et al: Photoprotective effect of black tea extracts against UVB-induced phototoxicity in skin. *Phytochem P* 1999;70:637–644.

Ziambaras K, Dagogo-Jack S: Reversible muscle weakness in patients with vitamin D deficiency. *West J Med* 1997;167:435–439.

# Index

# About the Author

Elizabeth Somer, M.A., R.D., is a nationally recognized nutrition expert and award-winning writer. She appears regularly on *The Today Show* and is a former consultant to *Good Morning America,* is a contributing editor to *Shape* magazine, and is the author of six books. She lives with her family in Salem, Oregon. Her Web site can be found at www.elizabethsomer.com.